国家级特色专业建设项目
国家级实验教学示范中心建设成果
高等院校临床医学专业实践类教材系列

英汉对照妇产科实践指南

Bilingual Clerk Book of Obstetrics and Gynecology

主　编　凌　奕　金　松

副主编　王华民　陈彩霞

主　审　黄元华

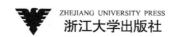

ZHEJIANG UNIVERSITY PRESS
浙江大学出版社

高等院校临床医学专业实践类教材系列
编写说明

    海南医学院组织编写的这套临床医学专业五年制本科实践类教材是一套以岗位胜任力为导向，以实践能力培养为核心，以技能操作训练为要素、统一规范并符合现代医学发展需要的系列教材。这套教材包括《临床技能学》、《临床见习指南》（分为外科学、内科学、妇产科学、儿科学四个分册）、《系统解剖学实验教程》、《形态学实验教程》、《生物化学与分子生物学实验教程》、《病原生物学与免疫学实验教程》、《预防医学实验教程》、《英汉对照妇产科实践指南》，共 11部。本套教材的编写力求体现实用、可操作性等特点。在编写中结合临床医学专业教育特色，体现了早临床、多临床、反复临床的教改思想，在尽可能不增加学生负担的前提下，注重实践操作技能的培养。我们希望通过本套教材的编写及使用，不断探索临床医学实践教学的新思路，为进一步推进医药卫生人才培养模式变革作出新的贡献。

    本套教材适用于五年制临床医学专业的医学生，同时也是低年资住院医师作为提高工作能力的参考书。

    限于编写人员的知识水平和教学经验，本套教材一定存在许多错误，敬请各位教师、学生在使用过程中，将发现的问题及时反馈给我们，以便再版时更正和完善。

高等院校临床医学专业实践类教材建设委员会主任

陈志斌

2013 年 3 月

本套教材目录

前　　言

随着改革开放及医学全球化的迅速发展,广大师生对于专业英语的提高与应用的要求日益增长,编写合适的双语教材显得十分必要。编者所在的海南医学院妇产科教研室双语教学团队积极探索双语教学方法,近年来在专业国际合作与交流,妇产科本科生双语教学,留学生、研究生教学,以及国外到我校实习生的带教,卫生系统骨干医师英语培训等教学实践中,积累了丰富的教学资料和教学经验,是我院双语教学建设示范课程。我们特编写《英汉对照妇产科实践指南》,供上述广大需要中英双语妇产科临床实践的中外师生使用。

本书分基础、生理产科、病理产科及胎儿医学、妇科及计划生育等共 5 章 41节,其中,第 2 章中的 2.1～2.3、2.5,第 3 章中的 3.3、3.5、3.7～3.17 及第 4 章中的 4.6、4.14 由凌奕编写,第 3 章中的 3.1、3.2、3.4、3.6,第 4 章中的 4.1～4.5、4.11、4.13、4.15、4.16 及第 5 章由周知编写,第 1 章、第 4 章中的 4.12 及参考文献由张宇编写,第 2 章中的 2.4 由张宏玉编写,第 4 章中的 4.7～4.10 由张峻霄编写。编写组全部成员均参与了本书的构思、编写、审稿及校稿工作。每一节包含关键词汇、知识要点、实践应用案例、思考题、答案及案例分析,部分章节添加循证医学思维知识拓展部分。全书力求突出重点,理论联系实际,以案例为导向,加深读者对概念的理解,锻炼妇产科临床思维,增强学习的兴趣和效果。中英文采取对称排列的方式,方便实用。该书既是妇产科双语学习教材,也是学习临床医学英语的良好参考书,可以参考本书指导临床实习和见习,有助于专业英语学习。

本书在编写过程中得到了海南医学院领导的高度重视与支持,美国犹他大学医学院国际医学教育专家 Devon Hale 教授给予通讯指导;教务处及教材编写委员会给予了鼎力支持与帮助。限于编者水平,书中难免存在错误和不足之处,敬请读者谅解并指正,以便日后完善改进。

编　者
2013 年 8 月

本书编写组成员

主　编　凌　奕　金　松

副主编　王华民　陈彩霞

主　审　黄元华

编　者　马燕琳　包　珊　张峻霄　张　宇

　　　　张宏玉　李月萍　周　知　陈曼玲

　　　　陈雪银　陈泽俊　陈　蔚　胡春霞

　　　　钟业超

秘　书　王　丽　叶海鸥　曾蓉蓉

CONTENTS
目　录

Chapter 1　Foundation

1.1　Applied Anatomy

Key words

1. bony pelvis
2. coccyx
3. pelvic inlet
4. pelvic outlet
5. uterus
6. vagina
7. fornix
8. fallopian tube
9. ovary
10. perineum

1.1.1　Main content

The bony pelvis is composed of the 2 pelvic bones with the sacrum and coccyx posteriorly. The pelvic brim divides the "false pelvis" above (part of the abdominal cavity) and the "true pelvis" below.

(1) Pelvic inlet：It is also known as the pelvic brim. Formed by the sacral promontory posteriorly, iliopectinea lines laterally and the symphysis pubis anteriorly.

(2) Pelvic outlet：It is formed by the coccyx posteriorly, the ischial tuberosities laterally and the pubic arch anteriorly. The pelvic outlet has 3 wide notches. The sciatic notches are divided into the greater and lesser sciatic foramina by the sacrotuberous and sacrospinous ligaments which can be considered as part of the perimeter of the outlet clinically.

第 1 章　基　　础

1.1　应用解剖

关键词

1. 骨性骨盆
2. 尾骨
3. 骨盆入口
4. 骨盆出口
5. 子宫
6. 阴道
7. 穹窿
8. 输卵管
9. 卵巢
10. 会阴

1.1.1　主要内容

骨盆是由骶骨、尾骨及两块髋骨组成。尾骨后方盆腔边缘分"假骨盆"（位于骨盆分界线以上，属于腹腔的一部分）和位于骨盆分界线以下的"真骨盆"。

（1）骨盆入口：也称为骨盆边缘形成的口径，后方为骶骨，两侧为髂耻线，前方为耻骨联合。

（2）骨盆出口：后方为尾骨，两侧为坐骨结节，前方为耻骨弓。骨盆出口有 3 个宽的结节，2 个坐骨结节，被骶结节和骶棘韧带分成大孔和小孔，临床上可作为出口周径的参数。

(3) The pelvic cavity: It lies between the inlet and the outlet. It has a deep posterior wall and a shallow anterior wall giving a curved shape. The contents of the pelvic cavity: the pelvic cavity contains the rectum, sigmoid colon, coils of the ileum, ureter, bladder, female reproductive organs, fascia, and peritoneum.

1.1.2　Female internal genital organs

(1) Vagina: The vagina is a thin-walled distensible fibromuscular tube that extends upwards and backwards from the vestibule of the vulva to the cervix. It is about 8 cm long and lies posterior to the bladder and anterior to the rectum. The vagina serves as an eliminatory passage for menstrual flow, forms part of the birth canal, and receives the penis during sexual intercourse.

(2) The fornix: This is the vaginal recess around the cervix and is divided into anterior, posterior and lateral regions which, clinically, provide access points for examining the pelvic organ.

(3) Uterus: The uterus is a thick-walled, hollow, pear-shaped muscular organ consisting of the cervix, body and fundus. In the nulliparous female, it is about 8 cm long, about 5 cm wide, and about 2.5 cm thick. The uterus is covered with peritoneum that forms an anterior uterovesical fold, a fold between the uterus and rectum termed the pouch of Douglas, and the broad ligaments laterally. The uterus receives, retains, and nourishes the fertilized ovum.

(4) Uterine orientation: In most females, the uterus lies in an anteverted and anteflexed position.

(5) Anteversion: The long axis of the uterus is angled forward.

(6) Retroversion: The fundus and body are angled backwards and therefore lie in the pouch of Douglas. It occurs in about 15% of the female population. A full bladder may mimic retroversion

（3）盆腔：位于骨盆入口和出口之间。骨盆腔形成前浅后深的弯曲的形态。盆腔的内容：盆腔包含直肠、乙状结肠、回肠、输尿管、膀胱、女性生殖器官、筋膜和腹膜。

1.1.2　女性内生殖器官

（1）阴道：阴道是一个有弹性的壁薄的肌纤维管，它向上和向后延伸，从阴唇的前庭延伸到宫颈，长约 8 cm，它位于膀胱的后方、直肠的前方。阴道是月经血排出及分娩的通道，也是性交器官。

（2）穹窿：它是环绕宫颈的阴道隐窝，按其位置分为前后及两侧几部分，在临床上，可经此穿刺或引流以检查盆腔情况。

（3）子宫：子宫是有腔壁厚的梨形的肌性器官，包括子宫颈、子宫体和子宫底。未孕妇女子宫长约 8 cm，宽约 5 cm，厚约 2.5 cm。子宫前腹膜向前反折覆盖膀胱，形成膀胱子宫陷凹。子宫和直肠之间的皱褶称为道格拉斯陷凹，其侧方为阔韧带。子宫主要作用是接收、保留和滋养受精卵。

（4）子宫位置：大多数女性子宫为前倾前屈的位置。

（5）子宫前倾：子宫的长轴倾角向前。

（6）子宫后倾：子宫底和子宫体的角度是向后的，因此靠着道格拉斯陷凹。临床上膀胱充盈可显示后倾位发生在约 15% 的

clinically.

（7）Anteflexion：The long axis of the body of the uterus is angled forward on the long axis of the cervix.

（8）Retroflexion：The body of the uterus is angled backward on the cervix.

（9）Fallopian tubes：The fallopian or "uterine" tubes are paired tubular structures，about 10 cm long. The fallopian tubes extend laterally from the cornua of the uterine body，in the upper border of the broad ligament and open into the peritoneal cavity near the ovaries. The fallopian tube is divided into 4 parts：

①Infundibulum：Distal，funnel-shaped portion with finger-like "fimbriae".

②Ampulla：The widest and longest part of tube outside the uterus.

③Isthmus：Thick-walled with a narrow lumen and therefore，least distensible part. It enters the horns of the uterine body.

④Intramural：It is the part which pierces the uterine wall. The main functions of the oviduct tube are to receive the ovum from the ovary，provide a site where fertilization can take place （usually in the ampulla）and transport the ovum from the ampulla to the uterus. The tube also provides nourishment for the fertilized ovum.

（10）Ovaries：The ovaries are whitish-grey，almond-shaped organs measuring about 4 cm×2 cm which are responsible for the production of the female germ cells，i. e. ova，and the female sex hormones，oestrogen and progesterone. They are suspended on the posterior layer of the broad ligament by a peritoneal extension （mesovarium）and supported by the suspensory ligament of the ovary （a lateral extension of the broad ligament and mesovarium）and the round ligament which stretches from the lateral wall of the uterus to the media aspect of the ovary.

妇女当中。

（7）前屈：宫体的长轴与宫颈的长轴成向前的夹角。

（8）后屈：宫体的长轴与宫颈的长轴成向后的夹角。

（9）输卵管：输卵管约 10 cm 长，是成对的肌性管道，由宫角向两侧延伸，位于阔韧带边缘的上方，靠近卵巢的部位开向腹腔，根据输卵管形态分为 4 个部分：

①漏斗部：在输卵管的远端，成漏斗状，伞端像手指一样。

②壶腹部：是最大和最长的部分，子宫峡部外侧。

③峡部：厚壁，管腔狭窄。

④间质部：该部分穿过子宫壁。输卵管的主要功能是接受卵巢排出的卵子，能进行受精（通常在壶腹部）和运输卵子，将来自壶腹部的卵子输送到子宫，并为受精卵提供营养。

（10）卵巢：卵巢白灰色，呈杏仁形，约 4 cm×2 cm，是产生女性配子（卵子）、女性雌激素和孕激素的器官。其后方为腹膜皱褶形成的阔韧带，它由外侧的骨盆漏斗韧带和内侧的卵巢固有韧带悬于盆壁与子宫之间，借韧带系膜与子宫两侧的阔韧带相连。

(11) Perineum: The perineum lies inferior to the pelvic inlet and is separated from the pelvic cavity by the pelvic diaphragm. Seen from below with the thighs abducted, it is a diamond-shaped area bounded anteriorly by the pubic symphysis, posteriorly by the tip of the coccyx and laterally by the ischiai tuberosities. The perineum is artificially divided into the anterior urogenital triangle containing the external genitalia in females and an anal triangle containing the anus and ischiolorectal fossae.

1.1.3　Female external genital organs

These are sometimes collectively known as the "vulva". It consists of:

(1) Labia majora: A pair of fat-filled folds of skin extending on either side of the vaginal vestibule from the mons towards the anus.

(2) Labia minora: A pair of flat folds containing a core of spongy connective tissue with a rich vascular supply. Lie medial to the labia majora.

(3) Vestibule of the vagina: Lies between the labia minora, contains the urethral meatus and vaginal orifice. Receives mucous secretions from the greater and lesser vestibular glands.

(4) Clitoris: It is a short, erectile organ; the female homologue of the male penis. Like the penis, a crus arises from each ischiopubic ramus and join in the midline forming the "body" capped by the sensitive "glands".

(5) Bulbs of vestibule: Masses of elongated erectile tissue, 3 cm long, lying along the sides of the vaginal orifice.

（11）会阴：会阴位于骨盆入口的下方，由盆膈将其与盆腔分开。从下面看是一个菱形区域，前方为耻骨联合下缘，后方为尾骨尖，两侧为坐骨结节。人为地划分为尿道生殖前三角（女性外生殖器）和坐骨肛门窝。

1.1.3　女性外生殖器官

这些有时被统称为"外阴"，包括：

（1）大阴唇：两股内侧一对纵行隆起的皮肤皱襞，起自阴阜，止于会阴。

（2）小阴唇：为位于大阴唇内侧的一对扁平皱襞，富含神经和丰富的血管。

（3）阴道前庭：位于大小阴唇之间，包含尿道口和阴道口，大小前庭腺有黏液分泌。

（4）阴蒂：短，勃起的器官，与男性阴茎同源。如同阴茎一样，两侧阴蒂脚附着于两侧耻骨支上，在中间形成头部敏感腺体的体部。

（5）前庭球：又称球海绵体，位于前唇两侧由具有勃起性的静脉丛组成。由一对细长的勃起组织组成，长约 3 cm，沿阴道口的两侧分布。

1. 2　Applied Physiology

Key words

1. menstruation
2. endometrium
3. fertilization
4. menstrual cycle
5. gonadotrophin-releasing-hormone，GnRH
6. follicle stimulating hormone，FSH
7. luteinising hormone，LH
8. ovulation
9. human chorionic gonadotrophin

1. 2. 1　Main content

The menstrual cycle

Menstruation is the shedding of the functional superficial 2/3 of the endometrium after sex hormone withdrawal. This process which consists of 3 phases, is typically repeated 300-400 times during a woman's life. Coordination of the menstrual cycle depends on a complex interplay between the hypothalamus, the pituitary gland, the ovaries, and the uterine endometrium. Cyclical changes in the endometrium prepare it for implantation in the event of fertilization and menstruation in the absence of fertilization.

It should be noted that several other tissues are sensitive to these hormones and undergo cyclical change (*e. g.* the breasts and the lower part of the urinary tract).

The endometrial cycle can be divided into 3 phases.

Phases of the menstrual cycle：The first day of the menses is considered to be day 1 of the menstrual cycle.

The proliferative or follicular phase. This begins at the end of the menstrual phase (usually day 4) and ends at ovulation (days 13-14). During this phase,

1. 2　应用生理

关键词

1. 月经
2. 子宫内膜
3. 受精
4. 月经周期
5. 促性腺激素释放激素
6. 卵泡刺激素
7. 促黄体生成激素
8. 排卵
9. 人绒毛膜促性腺激素

1. 2. 1　主要内容

月经周期

月经是由于性激素撤退后子宫内膜功能层表面的 2/3 部分脱落形成。这过程包括 3 个阶段：增生期、排卵期和分泌期，在女性的一生中规律性地重复 300～400 次。月经周期的协调依赖于下丘脑、垂体、卵巢、子宫内膜和子宫之间复杂的相互作用。子宫内膜的周期性变化在受精时为着床做准备，未受精时即形成月经。

应该注意那些对性激素敏感并且也经历此种周期性变化的组织（如乳房和下部的尿路）。

子宫内膜周期可分为 3 个阶段。

月经周期阶段：经期第一天被认为是月经周期的第一天。

增生期或卵泡期开始于月经末（通常是 4 天）至排卵结束（13～14 天）。在这一阶段，子宫

the endometrium thickens and ovarian follicles mature.

The hypothalamus is the initiator of the follicular phase. Gonadotrophin-releasing hormone （GnRH） is released from the hypothalamus in a pulsatile fashion to the pituitary portal system surrounding the anterior pituitary gland. GnRH causes release of follicle stimulating hormone （FSH）. FSH is secreted into the general circulation and interacts with the granulosa cells surrounding the dividing oocytes.

FSH enhances the development of 15-20 follicles each month and interacts with granulosa cells to enhance aromatization of androgens into oestrogen and oestradiol.

Only one follicle with the largest reservoir of oestrogen can withstand the declining FSH environment whilst the remaining follicles undergo atresia at the end of this phase.

Follicular oestrogen synthesis is essential for uterine priming, but it is also part of the positive feedback that induces a dramatic preovulatory leuteinising hormone （LH） surge and subsequent ovulation.

The luteal or secretory phase. The luteal phase starts at ovulation and lasts through to 28th day of the menstrual cycle. The major effects of the LH surge are the conversion of granulose cells from predominantly androgen-converting cells to predominantly progesterone-synthesizing cells. High progesterone levels exert negative feedback on GnRH which, in turn, FSH/LH secretion.

At the beginning of the luteal phase, progesterone induces the endometrial glands to secrete glycogens, mucus, and other substances. These glands become tortuous and have large lumina due to secretory activity. Spiral arterioles extend into the superficial layer of the endometrium.

内膜增厚和卵泡成熟。

下丘脑是卵泡期的启动者。促性腺激素释放激素（GnRH）以脉冲的方式从下丘脑释放到垂体前叶周围的垂体门脉系统，GnRH 导致卵泡刺激素（FSH）释放。FSH 分泌进入外周体循环并与分离的卵母细胞周围的颗粒细胞相互作用。

每个月 FSH 促进 15～20 卵泡发育并且激活颗粒细胞芳香化酶，促进雌激素及雌二醇的合成。

在这个阶段只有具备最大雌激素储备力的卵泡，能承受 FSH 下降环境，而其余的卵泡在这个阶段结束时渐渐闭锁。

卵泡雌激素的合成是子宫增生的基础，也是正反馈的一部分。正反馈导致促黄体生成激素高峰以及随后的排卵这一排卵期前的动态变化。

黄体期或分泌期：黄体期开始于排卵期，从排卵期开始持续到下次月经周期前的第 14 天。LH 峰的主要作用是将以雄激素转化细胞为主转换成以孕酮合成细胞为主。高水平的孕酮对 GnRH 产生负反馈调节，抑制 FSH/LH 分泌。

在黄体期开始，孕酮诱导子宫内膜腺体分泌糖原、黏液等其他物质。这些腺体由于分泌活动增强使之变得更屈曲、更长，螺旋动脉延伸到子宫内膜表层。

In the absence of fertilization by day 23 of the menstrual cycle, the superticial endometrium begins to degenerate and consequently decrease ovarian hormone levels. As oestrogen and progesterone levels fall, the endometrium undergoes involution.

If the corpus luteum is not rescued by human chorionic gonadotrophin (hCG) hormone from the developing placenta, menstruation occurs 14 days after ovulation. If conception occurs, placental HCG maintains luteal function until placental production of progesterone is well established.

The menstrual phase. This phase sees the gradual withdrawal of ovarian sex steroids which causes slight shrinking of the endometrium, and therefore the blood flow of spiral vessels is reduced. This, together with spiral arteriolar spasms, leads to distal endometrial ischaemia and stasis.

Extravasation of blood and endometrial tissue breakdown lead to onset of menstruation.

The menstrual phase begins as the spiral arteries rupture, releasing blood into the uterus and the apoptosing endometrium is sloughed off.

During this period, the functional layer of the endometrium is completely shed. Arteriolar and venous blood, remnants of endometrial stroma and glands, leucocytes and red blood cells are all present in the menstrual flow. Shedding usually lasts about 3-4 days.

在未受精的情况下,月经第23天其表层子宫内膜开始退化,因此卵巢激素水平下降。由于雌激素和孕激素水平下降,子宫内膜经历退化。

如果黄体不能被生长中胎盘释放的人绒毛膜促性腺激素所保留,排卵后14天月经发生。如果怀孕,胎盘的人绒毛膜促性腺激素维持黄体功能直到胎盘正常生成孕酮。

月经期:这一阶段卵巢性类固醇逐步减少,导致子宫内膜轻微萎缩,并因此螺旋血管血流减少。可能伴有螺旋小动脉痉挛,导致子宫内膜远端局部缺血和淤血。

血液外渗和子宫内膜组织剥落引起月经来临。

月经期以螺旋动脉破裂,释放血液进入子宫以及子宫内膜脱落开始。

在这期间,子宫内膜功能层完全脱落。小动脉和静脉血液,残存的子宫内膜基质和腺体,白细胞和红细胞都是在月经期出现,脱落通常持续3~4天。

Chapter 2　Normal Pregnancy

第 2 章　生理产科

2. 1　Physiology of Pregnancy

2. 1　妊娠生理

Key words

1. fertilization
2. implantation
3. zygote
4. placenta
5. placental barrier
6. human chorionic gonodotrophin，hCG
7. ductus venosus
8. embryonic period
9. the umbilical cord
10. supine hypotension

关键词

1. 受精
2. 植入
3. 受精卵
4. 胎盘
5. 胎盘屏障
6. 人绒毛膜促性腺激素
7. 静脉导管
8. 胚胎期
9. 脐带
10. 仰卧位低血压

The earliest sign of pregnancy is missing a menstrual period. For women who are of reproductive age and have regular periods and normal sex activity，missing a period for $\geqslant 1$ wk is presumptive evidence of pregnancy (conception).

妊娠最早期的表现通常是停经。具有正常月经周期和正常性行为的生育期妇女，停经大于一周以上应怀疑妊娠(怀孕)。

2. 1. 1　Fertilization & implantation

2. 1. 1　受精与植入

Fertilization is the union of the ovum and a spermtozoon (zygote). It is the beginning of pregnancy. Fertilization usually occurs in the ampullar portion of the fallopian tube.

受精是卵子与精子的结合(受精卵)。受精是妊娠的开始。受精通常在输卵管的壶腹部发生。

Once fertilization is complete，the zygote migrates toward the body of the uterus aided by the muscular contractions of the fallopian tubes. It takes 3 to 4 days for the zygote to reach the body of the uterus.

受精完成后，受精卵借助输卵管的收缩作用移动到宫腔内，这个过程大约需要 3～4 天。

During this time，cleavage begins，once it reaches the uterine endometrium，it is formed a structure termed a blastocyst. Then，implantation occurs，the

在向子宫移动的同时，受精卵开始分裂。当到达子宫内膜时，受精卵已经分裂增殖形成囊

outside cell of the blastocyst（trophoblast cell）produce proteolytic enzymes that dissolve the endometrium they touch. This action burrow the blastocyst into the endometrim. This process is the implantation. It may occur about 10-14 days after fertilization. It is common to have a light bleeding at this moment and some women may believe they are starting a menstruation period，but generally this bleeding is extremely light and lasts only a day or so.

The normal implantation point is ususlly high in the body of the uterus. If it is low in the uterus, the growing placenta may occlude the cervix and make birth of the fetus difficult，this condition is termed placenta previa.

2.1.2 Fetal life-support system

To support the fertilized ovum（zygote）and the future fetus，a fetal life-support system is formed by the plancenta, fetal membrane, amniotic fluid, and umbilical cord.

2.1.3 Placental architecture

Maternal and fetal blood do not mix placental barrier（Figure 2-1-1）.

胚。这时,受精卵开始植入。囊胚的外层细胞(滋养细胞)产生蛋白消化酶分解接触到的子宫内膜,把囊胚埋进子宫内膜内,这个过程称为植入。在妊娠10～14天完成。

这个时期常常会出现少量的阴道流血,有些妇女会误认为月经来潮,但通常这种出血非常少,只有一二天的时间。

植入的正常部位通常位于子宫体腔较高的位置(近宫底)。如果植入的部位偏低(接近宫颈),胎盘生长可能会盖住宫颈口,妨碍胎儿娩出,这称为前置胎盘。

2.1.2 胎儿生命支持系统

胎儿的生命支持系统由胎盘、胎膜、羊水和脐带组成,支持受精卵及未来胎儿的发育。

2.1.3 胎盘构成

母体血液与胎儿血液互不相通:相隔胎盘屏障,如图2-1-1所示。

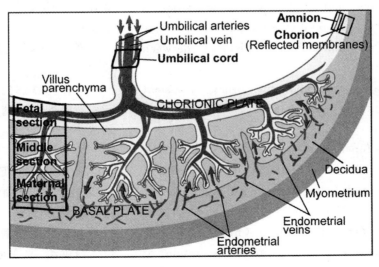

Figure 2-1-1　Placental architecture

图 2-1-1　胎盘结构

Fetal blood flows through capillary networks within highly branched terminal chorionic villi.

Maternal blood flows outside of the intervillous spaces：
- Uterine arteriols bring blood in
- Uterine venules drain blood back

In the intervillous spaces，maternal blood jets from the endometrial arteries（spiral arteries），the blood surrounds the villi and nutrients osmose from maternal blood into the villi，then it enters endomentrium veins and returned to the maternal circulation.

Uterine perfusion and the placenta circulation，are most efficient when mother lies on her left side or up-right position other than supine. This position lifts the uterus from the inferior vena cava and prevents blood being trapped in the low part of the body. If the mother lies on her back and the weight of the uterus compresses the vena cava，placental circulation can be so sharply reduced that supine hypotension occurs.

2.1.4 Placental functions

Placenta is responsible for exchange of nutrients，gases and metabolic waste products between maternal and fetal circulation.

Maintains immunological distance between mother and fetus.

Serves as special endocrine organ：transient hypothalamo-pituitary-gonada axis.

Endocrine functions：
—Human chorionic gonodotrophin （hCG）：Secreted early and helps to maintain synthesis of progesterone.
—Human placental lactogen （hPL）：Increase supply of glucose，altering maternal secretion of insulin.
—Insulin-like growth factors （IGF）：IGF

胎儿的血液循环在复杂分支的绒毛内血管网内进行。

母体血液自绒毛外面流经绒毛间隙：自子宫动脉进入，经子宫静脉返回。

在绒毛间隙内，母体血液自子宫螺旋动脉射血，血液流经绒毛周围，营养物质自母血渗透至绒毛内血管，随后血液经子宫内膜静脉返回母体循环。

母亲处于侧卧位和直立体位时子宫的血液灌注和胎盘循环要好于处在平卧位。这种体位使子宫的重量离开下腔静脉，从而避免血液淤积于身体的下部。如果母亲仰卧，子宫的重量将压迫下腔静脉，胎盘的循环会迅速下降，导致仰卧位低血压。

2.1.4 胎盘功能

胎盘的功能是承担母亲与胎儿间营养物质、气体和代谢产物的交换。

保持母亲与胎儿间的免疫隔离。

并作为特殊的内分泌器官：承担暂时性下丘脑-垂体-性腺轴功能。

内分泌功能：
人绒毛膜促性腺激素（hCG）：孕早期开始分泌，协助维持孕激素的合成。

人胎盘生乳素（hPL）：增加母体糖供给，改变母体胰岛素分泌水平。

胰岛素样生长因子（IGF）：

signaling system is a major regulator of growth in fetus and infant.

2.1.5　Umbilical cord

The umbilical cord provides a circulatory from the fetus to the chorionic villi.

It contains one vein (carring oxygenated, nutrient-rich blood from the placental villi to the fetus) and two arteries (carrying deoxygenated, nutrient depleted blood away from the fetus back to the placental villi), the rest of the cord body is formed of Wharton's jelly, which gives the cord body and prevents pressure on the vein and arteries.

2.1.6　Amniotic fluid

Amniotic fluid is constantly being formed and reabsorbed. It is an important protective mechanism for the fetus. It shields pressure (blow) from mother's abdomen, provide stable temperature, and allow the fetus free of movement, moreover, it protects the umbilical cord from pressure, thus protecting fetal oxygenation. Even if the membrane ruptureed before birth, some amniotic fluid is lost, and some will left because new fluid is constantly being formed.

2.1.7　Fetal development

The following list describes specific changes of fetal development that occur in the womb:

Embryonic period: from the fertilization to 9 weeks period.

• Week 1 to 4: It will develop into the nervous system (brain, spinal cord), hair, and skin; heart and primitive circulatory system rapidly form, this is the very life support system that will carry the fetus throughout his or her life.

• Week 5 to 10 of pregnancy (gestational age):

IGF 信号系统是调节胎儿生长的主要因子。

2.1.5　脐带

脐带是胎儿到绒毛膜之间的循环通道。

脐带由一根脐静脉（携带富含氧、营养物质的血液自胎盘绒毛到胎儿）和两条动脉（将低氧和贫营养物质的血液自胎儿带回到胎盘绒毛）组成。脐带的其他部分由 Wharton 胶组成，形成脐带的主体并保护脐动、静脉防止受压。

2.1.6　羊水

羊水持续不断地产生和吸收。它是保护胎儿的一种重要机制。它阻挡来自母亲腹部的压力（打击）。

羊水给胎儿提供稳定的温度，并使胎儿有自由活动的空间，更重要的是，羊水保护脐带免受压迫，从而防止胎儿缺氧。即使胎膜破裂后部分羊水流出，仍然有部分羊水会留在宫腔内，因为羊水会不断持续地产生。

2.1.7　胎儿发育

下面的列表描述胎儿在宫内发育情况：

胚胎期：自受精到 9 周时间。

1~4 周：将发育形成神经系统（大脑、脊髓）、头发及皮肤；心脏及最初的循环系统形成并开始工作，这是最重要的生命支持系统，将支持胎儿度过整个孕期。

5~10 周：

○ The brain, spinal cord, and heart begin to develop.

○ The gastrointestinal tract begins to develop.

○ Arm and leg buds become visible.

○ The eyes and ear structures begin to form.

○ The heart continues to develop and beats at a regular rhythm.

○ The lungs begin to form.

○ All essential organs have begun to form.

○ Facial features continue to develop.

○ The intestines rotate.

The end of the 10th week of pregnancy (8th week of embryonic age) marks the end of the "embryonic period" and the beginning of the "fetal period".

大脑、脊髓、心脏开始发育。

胃肠道开始形成。

肢芽开始出现。

眼睛和耳开始形成。

心脏继续发育,开始有规律地搏动。

开始形成肺。

其他生命基本结构开始形成。

面部结构继续发育。

内肠完成旋转。

第 10 孕周末(第 8 周胎龄)是胚胎期的结束,开始进入胎儿期。

◆ Weeks 11 to 20 of pregnancy (gestational age):

○ The face is well formed.

○ Limbs are long and thin.

○ Genitals appear well differentiated.

○ The head makes up nearly half of the baby's size.

○ More muscle tissue and bones have developed.

○ The baby begins to make active movements.

○ The baby can hear.

11~20 周:

面部发育良好。

肢体细长。

能够很好地区分性别。

头部占据大约一半的身长。

更多的肌肉组织和骨形成。

胎儿开始活动。

胎儿开始出现听力。

◆ Week 21 to 26 of pregnancy (gestational age):

○ Nails appear on the fingers and toes.

○ The mother can feel the baby moving.

○ The fetal heartbeat can be heard with a stethoscope.

○ Bone marrow begins to make blood cells.

○ The lower airways of the baby's lungs develop but still do not produce surfactant (a substance that allows the alveoli to open for gas exchange).

21~26 周:

指(趾)端开始出现指甲。

母亲开始感知胎动。

能够听到胎心。

骨髓开始产生血细胞。

胎儿的下呼吸道开始发育,但仍然没有产生表面活性物质,能够让肺泡开放进行气体交换。

◆ Weeks 27 to 37 of pregnancy (gestational age):

○ Rapid brain development occurs.

○ The eyelids open and close.

27~37 周:

大脑迅速发育。

眼皮能够睁开和关闭。

○ The respiratory system has developed to the point where gas exchange is possible.

○ Rhythmic breathing movements occur，but the lungs are not fully mature.

◆ Week 38-42 of pregnancy (gestational age)：
○ The lungs are fully mature.
○ Body fat increases.
○ Lanugo is gone except for that on the upper arms and shoulders.
○ Finger nails extend beyond fingertips.
○ Small breast buds are present on both sexes.

2.1.8　Fetal circulation

Highly oxygenated blood arriving from placenta enters the fetus through the umbilical vein, the umbilical vein carries the blood to the inferior vena cava through the Ductus venosus, then to the right atrium, from there, most of blood flow to left atrium through the foramen ovale (Figure 2-1-2).

肺部发育具备一定的气体交换功能。

出现有规律的呼吸样运动，但肺仍然没有完全成熟。

38～42 周：
肺部完全发育成熟。
身体脂肪增加。
胎毛开始消失，只存在于上臂和肩部。
指甲超出指端。
两侧乳房结节出现。

2.1.8　胎儿循环

富含氧气的血液自胎盘经过脐静脉进入胎儿，经过静脉导管进入下腔静脉窦，再到右心房，大部分血液经卵圆孔进入左心房。如图 2-1-2 所示。

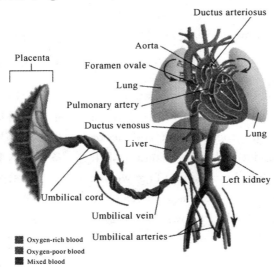

Figure 2-1-2　Fetal circulation
图 2-1-2　胎儿循环

From left atrium, it follows the course of normal circulation into the left ventricle and into the aorta.

进入左心房的血液，经正常成人的血液循环通道，经左心室到主动脉。

Deoxygenated blood from the fetus body is returned to the heart by the vena cava. The blood enters the right atrium and then to the right ventricle, then into the pulmonary artery as in adult manner. However, larger portion of blood here is shunted away from the ductus arteriosus into the aorta and then into the descending aorta.

Most of the blood flow from the descending aorta is transported by the umbilical arteries to the placental villi, where the blood is oxygenated again.

2.1.9　Maternal changes during pregnancy

Maternal physiological changes in pregnancy are the normal adaptations that a woman undergoes during pregnancy to better accommodate the embryo or fetus. The body must change its physiological and homeostatic mechanisms in pregnancy to ensure the fetus is provided for. Increases in blood sugar, breathing and cardiac output are all required. Levels of progesterone and estrogens rise continually throughout pregnancy, suppressing the hypothalamic axis and subsequently the menstrual cycle.

2.1.10　Gain in weight

One of the most noticeable alterations in pregnancy is the gain in weight. The enlarging uterus, the growing fetus, the placenta and liquor amnii, the acquisition of fat and water retention, all contribute to this increase in weight. The weight gain varies from person to person and can be anywhere from 5 pounds (2.3 kg) to over 100 pounds (45 kg).

2.1.11　Metabolic

During pregnancy, both protein metabolism and carbohydrate metabolism are affected.

An increased requirement for nutrients is given by fetal growth and fat deposition. Pregnant women require a caloric increase of 300 kcal/day and an

经过循环后的低氧血液自胎体经上、下腔静脉返回心脏,进入右心房,大部分进入右心室,然后进入肺动脉(如成人循环)。但是,在这里,大部分的血液经动脉导管至主动脉,再到腹主动脉。

流经腹主动脉的血液大部分经脐动脉到胎盘绒毛,在这里,重新被氧合。

2.1.9　妊娠期母体变化

母亲在妊娠期的变化是一个生理性的调适过程,母亲在孕期经过一系列的变化来更好地适应胚胎与胎儿的发育。机体必须改变其生理和内环境以保证胎儿的需要。血糖水平增加、呼吸与心功能的增加都是必要的。孕激素和雌激素水平在孕期持续不断地升高,从而抑制下丘脑垂体轴和月经周期。

2.1.10　体重增加

孕期一个最明显的变化就是体重增加。增大的子宫、不断生长的胎儿、胎盘及羊水、脂肪储备和水钠潴留,都有助于体重增加。体重的增加个体差异较大,从 5 磅(2.3 kg)到超过 100 磅(45 kg)。

2.1.11　代谢

妊娠期间,蛋白代谢和碳水化合物的代谢均发生改变。

胎儿的生长和脂肪的储备都需要增加营养物质供给。妊娠期妇女需要每天增加 300 kcal/d 碳

increase in protein to 70 or 75 g/day.

2.1.12 Cardiovascular

Cardiac output (CO) increases 30% to 50%, beginning by 6 wk gestation and peaking between 16 and 28 wk (usually at about 24 wk). After 30 wk, CO becomes sensitive to body position. Positions that cause the enlarging uterus to obstruct the vena cava the most (*e. g.*, the recumbent position) cause CO to decrease the most.

To increase CO, heart rate increases from the normal 70 to as high as 90 beats/min, and stroke volume increases. During the 2nd trimester, BP usually drops and systemic vascular resistance decreases.

2.1.13 Hematologic

Total blood volume increases proportionally with CO, but the increase in plasma volume is greater (close to 50%) than that in RBC mass (about 25%); thus, Hb is lowered by dilution, from about 13.3 to 12.1 g/dl. This dilutional anemia decreases blood viscosity.

Iron requirements increase by a total of about 1 g during the entire pregnancy and are higher during the 2nd half of pregnancy, about 6 to 7 mg/day. Iron supplements are needed to prevent a further decrease in Hb levels because the amount absorbed from the diet and recruited from iron stores is usually insufficient to meet the demands of pregnancy.

2.1.14 Urinary

GFR increases 30% to 50%, peaks between 16 and 24 wk gestation, and remains at that level until nearly term.

水化合物和 70 或 75 g/d 的蛋白质。

2.1.12 循环系统

心排出量增加 30%～50%，自孕 6 周开始增加，16～28 周达高峰。30 周后，心排出量对母亲体位变化很敏感，能够导致子宫重量压迫下腔静脉的体位（例如在仰卧位）可导致心排出量减少。

为了增加心排出量，心率增快自 70 次/分到 90 次/分。每搏输出量也随之增加。在孕中期，血压通常会下降，体循环阻力下降。

2.1.13 血液

全身血容量增加，但血浆的增加（约 50%）要高于红细胞的增加（约 25%），从而导致 Hb 被稀释而下降，自 13.3 下降到 12.1 g/dl。这种稀释性的贫血降低血液黏滞度。

孕期铁的需要总量增加约为 1 g，大部分需要是在孕中晚期，大约 6～7 mg/d。需要补充铁剂以防止血色素水平下降，因为自食物中很难获取足够的铁来满足妊娠的需要。

2.1.14 泌尿系统

GFR 增加 30%～50%。在孕 16～24 周达高峰，保持这一水平直到近足月。

2.1.15　Gastrointestinal

During pregnancy, woman can experience nausea and vomiting (morning sickness). Additionally, there is prolonged gastric empty time, decreased gastroesophageal sphincter tone, which can lead to acid reflux, and decreased colonic motility, which leads to increased water absorption and constipation.

2.1.16　Respiratory

Lung function changes partly because progesterone increases and partly because the enlarging uterus interferes with lung expansion. Progesterone signals the brain to lower CO_2 levels. To lower CO_2 levels, tidal and minute volume and respiratory rate increase, vital capacity and plasma PO_2 do not change.

2.1.17　Endocrine

The pituitary gland enlarges by about 135% during pregnancy. The maternal plasma prolactin level increases by 10-fold. The primary function of increased prolactin is to ensure lactation. The level returns to normal postpartum, even in women who breastfeed.

Test

1. The function of placenta are as which of the following　　　　　（　　）

A. enables the fetus to take O_2 and nutrients from the maternal body

B. serve as the excretory organ

C. secretes large amounts of hormones such as hCG estrogen

D. form a barrier against the infection to the fetus

2. The structure of the placenta includes which of the following　（　　）

2.1.15　消化系统

妊娠期间,妇女会有恶心呕吐(晨吐反应),另外,胃排空时间延长,胃食管括约肌张力下降,会导致返酸。结肠活动下降,水分吸收增多,容易发生便秘。

2.1.16　呼吸系统

肺功能的改变部分是因为孕激素水平增加,部分是因为增大的子宫妨碍肺的扩张。孕激素发出信号给大脑,降低 CO_2 水平,从而导致潮气量和每分容量及呼吸频率的增加,总呼吸容量和血氧水平没有变化。

2.1.17　内分泌系统

孕期垂体增大 135%,母血中泌乳素水平增高 10 倍,泌乳素水平增高的主要功能是保证产后泌乳。产后泌乳素水平恢复正常,在母乳喂养的妇女也是如此。

A. the amnion

B. the chorion

C. the basal decidua

D. the umbilical cord

Definition

Capacity：The process in which ejaculated sperm must undergo in order to fertilize an oocyte. Sperm become "fertilization competent" as they reside in the female reproductive tract through a series of physiological changes during this process.

Acrosome reaction：The process that occurs in the acrosome of the sperm as it approaches the egg. The reaction results in the release of numerous enzymes and facilitate the sperm to penetrate zona pellucida of the oocyte and fertilize it.

Describe placental endocrine functions.

Key points：1. hCG：The first placental hormone produced. It can be detected as early as the first missed menstrual period （shortly after implantation has occurred）. It arrive the peak at 8-10th week of pregnancy. It support the pregnancy by ensuring ovarian production of progesterone until the placenta is well formed around the tenth week.

2. Estrogen and progesterone：During early pregnancy they are produced by corpus lutein. After tenth week they are primarily produced by placenta. Estrogen can increase uterine blood flow. Progesterone inhibits the smooth muscle in the uterus from contracting and decreases prostaglandin formation thus it can support the pregnancy.

3. Other hormones：human placental lactogen （hPL）, pregnancy specific β-glycoprotein （PS β1G）, human chorionic thyrotropin （HCT）, oxytocinase, heat stable alkaline phosphatase （HSAP）, etc.

Describe the maternal changes of reproductive system during pregnancy.

Key points：

1. Uterus：size, weight, uterine cavity, isthmus uteri.

2. ovary.

3. oviduct.

4. vagina.

2.2　Antenatal Care

Key words

1. antenatal care
2. cardiotocography
3. tachycardia
4. bradycardia
5. Hb electrophoresis
6. ultrasound
7. iron
8. folate
9. fetal monitoring
10. early decelerations
11. late decelerations
12. variable decelerations

2.2　产前保健

关键词

1. 产前检查
2. 胎心监护
3. 心动过速
4. 心动过缓
5. 血红蛋白电泳
6. 超声
7. 铁
8. 叶酸
9. 胎儿监护
10. 早期减速
11. 晚期减速
12. 变异减速

2.2.1　Antenatal care

The aims of antenatal care are to: Detect any disease in the mother, ameliorate the discomforts of pregnancy, monitor and promote fetal well-being, and prepare mothers for birth. Monitor trends to prevent or detect any early complications of pregnancy, especially blood pressure which is the most important variable of eclampsia. Is thromboprophylaxis needed?

Who should give antenatal care? Midwives may manage care, calling in doctors only if a specific need arises. Book the first prenatal care appointment by 12 weeks of pregnancy: visit the general practitioner within 2 weeks if the pregnancy is already ≥ 12 weeks. The 1st antenatal visit is very comprehensive. Find a language interpreter if she needs one. Avoid using relatives (confidentiality issues).

History: Usual cycle length; LMP (a normal period?); Contraception; Drugs; Past history, e.g. Surgery to abdomen or pelvis.

Family history: Outcome and complications of past pregnancies.

Is there family history of diabetes, hypertension, fetal abnormality, or twins?

Does she have concurrent illness? If there is past or family history of DVT or embolism, screen for thrombophilia.

Is gestational diabetes (GDM) a risk? Screen (75 g glucose tolerance test) at 8±28 wks) if she has previous (GDM); at 24 wks if BMI≥30, or previous baby≥4.5 kg. Diabetes in first-degree relatives, or family origin (FO) from area of high risk of diabetes also make the test necessary.

Examination: Check heart, lungs, BP, weight (record BMI), and abdomen. Is a cervical smear needed? Varicose veins?

2.2.1　产前检查

产前检查的目的是:发现母亲疾病,改善孕期不适症状,监测和促进胎儿健康,帮助孕妇做分娩准备。通过监控变化趋势来发现或阻止怀孕的任何早期并发症,血压是最重要的变量(子痫的参数)。同时也观察是否需要抗凝治疗?

由谁做产检?助产士可以做,特殊情况下叫医生到场。自孕 12 周前开始预约产前检查。第一次产检非常重要,若已超过 12 孕周,需 2 周内就诊。第一次产检应非常仔细。需要时需找一名翻译,但避免让亲戚翻译以增加可信度。

病史询问:包括月经史、避孕史、用药史、过去史(盆腔及腹部手术史)、孕产史、家族史(糖尿病、高血压及内科病史、多胎妊娠史)、现病史。

是否有并发症,如果既往家族中有血栓形成病史,进行血栓形成倾向筛查。

是否有妊娠糖尿病风险?如既往有关病史,24 周体重指数≥30,曾经生产过≥4.5 kg 新生儿,一级亲属有糖尿病史,家族来源于糖尿病高风险地区时,孕8～28 周进行糖耐量试验。

检查:检查心、肺、血压、体重(记录 BMI)和腹部。是否需要宫颈涂片?孕妇有静脉曲张吗?

Laboratory tests：Blood：Hb，Rh blood type（antibodies if Rh-ve），syphilis & rubella serology，HBsAg HIV test（counseling，OHCM）；sickle test if the patients is black，Hb electrophoresis and 25-hydroxyvitamin D if relevant. Arrange tests to exclude Down's. Offer early ultrasound to establish dates，exclude multiple pregnancy and aid with Down's tests and arrange 18-20 week anomaly scan.

Suggestion：Parentcraf/relaxation classes；dental visit. Enquire about problems and anxieties. Consider need for iron and folate.

Advise on：Smoking，alcohol，diet，correct use of seat belts（above the bump，below the bump，but not over it）and adequate rest. Ensure knowledge of social security benefits. Usual exercise and travel are ok（avoid going to malarious areas）up to 34 weeks on most airlines. Intercourse is fine if no vaginal bleeding.

Later visits：Check urine for albumin，BP，fundal height. Check lie and presentation at 36 weeks. Do Hb and Rh antibodies at 28 & 34 weeks and give anti-D then if needed. Visits start at ＜12 weeks then at 16，25，28，31，34，36，38，40 and 41 weeks（for primips）.

The head is usually engaged by 37 weeks in Caucasian primips（if not，consider：large（or malpositioned）head，small pelvis or obstruction placenta praevia，or wrong estimation of dates）.

2.2.2　Fetal monitoring

In high-risk pregnancy，antepartum cardiotocography and biophysical profiles by ultrasound are used to monitor fetal activity and responsiveness. The aim is to detect intrauterine hypoxia prenatally.

Cardiotocography（CTG）：Doppler ultrasound detects fetal heart beats and a tocodynamometer over

实验室检查:血液检查包括 Hb、Rh 血型、梅毒和风疹血清学检查,HBsAg 和 HIV 检测;黑人中查镰状细胞贫血测试和血红蛋白电泳,必要时查血红蛋白电泳和维生素 D 的相关检查。安排唐氏综合征筛查。早孕时做 B 超以确定孕龄、胎儿数目和协助唐氏筛查,18～20 周做胎儿畸形 B 超筛查。

建议:参加孕妇学校及口腔科检查。若有焦虑应寻求帮助,根据需要,补充铁和叶酸。

提供关于烟、酒精和饮食方面的建议,告知正确使用安全带和充足的休息。增长与社会保障福利相关的知识。通常可以旅行和运动(避开疟疾区)。多数航空公司允许孕 34 周前乘坐飞机。如果没有阴道出血可以保持性生活。

孕中晚期的检查:测尿蛋白、血压、体重、宫高。第 36 周时测胎产式和胎先露。第 28 和 34 周时查血红蛋白和 Rh 抗体,必要的时候给予抗 D 治疗。进行产检的时间为 12 周前和第 16、25、28、31、34、36、38、40 和 41 周(初产妇)。

在大多数情况下白人初产妇女 37 周胎头入盆,如果没有入盆,要注意胎头大、骨盆小,或前置胎盘阻碍,或孕龄估计错误。

2.2.2　胎儿监护

胎儿检测:高危妊娠者产前胎心监护(CTG)和生物物理评分可以用来检测胎儿的活力和反应,目的是检测宫内胎儿是否缺氧。

胎儿 CTG:多普勒超声检测胎儿心跳,分娩力计可以放在宫

the uterine fundus records any contractions. A continuous trace is printed over about 30 min (*e. g.* a paper speed of 1 cm/min) with the mother lying semi-recumbent, or in the left lateral position or half-sitting position. A normal trace in an afebrile mother at term who is not having drugs has a base rate of 110-160 beats/min, with a variability of ＞5 beats/min, and at least 2 acceleration (a common response to movement or noise) of an amplitude ≥15 beats/min over a 20 min period (Fetal heart rate falls by about 1 beat/min/week from 28 weeks.) Tests need to be done every 24h antenatally to identify the changing fetal heart rate pattern associated with hypoxia (loss of baseline variability with decelerations, *etc.*).

Intrapartum monitoring：Death and disability due to complication occur in ＜ 1 ∶ 300 labours. Intrapartum fetal heart rate monitoring aims to detect patterns known to be associated with fetal distress-a diagnosis supported by fetal hypoxia (acidosis) on blood sampling.

Intermittent auscultation (JA)：At the end of contractions (to listen for decelerations). Doppler or Pinard stethoscope is used for low-risk labours, every 15 min in 1st stage, 5 min throughout 2nd stage. If abnormality noted (below) or intrapartum problems occur, start continuous fetal heart rate monitoring. But this method has poor predictive value, overdiagnosing fetal distress may happen even if used together with fetal blood sampling. Its value is uncertain even in high-risk labours, for which it is used throughout the labour, ideally with scalp electrode. Where scalp electrode is used it is also possible to monitor fetal electrocardiogram：It's reported waveform is associated with severe metabolic acidosis, fetal electrocardiogram monitoring can help to avoid fetal blood sampling test, decrease neonatal encephalopathy and fewer operative vaginal deliveries (but not caesarean

底部检测记录宫缩,持续监护 30 min(走纸速度 1cm/min)。孕妇采取半卧位或左侧卧位,正常未用药无发热的孕妇胎心基线为 110～160 次/min,变异度为 5 次/min,在 20min 内至少有两次振幅≥15 次/min 的加速(系胎动或噪声引起)。如有异常,自 28 周起胎心率下降 1 次/(min・孕周)。每 24 h 检查一次,确定是否有与缺氧相关的改变(例如基线变异消失、减速等)。

宫内监护:大约 1/300 的分娩中会出现胎死宫内和胎儿受损。胎心监护的目标是监测头皮血是否有与胎儿酸中毒和胎儿窘迫相关的类型。

间断性听诊:在宫缩过去后,用听筒听胎心音(减速),第一产程 15 min 一次,第二产程 5 min 一次,如果有异常则持续胎心监护。这种方法诊断率较低,即使与胎儿头皮血测定合用仍然有过度诊断胎儿窘迫的可能。即使在高危妊娠中它的价值也是不确定的。同时也可进行胎儿心电图检查,通过分析可发现 ST 段与部分重度代谢性酸中毒有关,它可以减少胎儿头皮血测量,减少新生儿颅内出血和阴道助产率(但不减少剖宫产率)。检查指征:高危妊娠、听诊发现异常(心律＜110 或＞160 次/min)或存在减速胎类。

sections). Indications: High-risk pregnancy; use of oxytocin; abnormality with IA (decelerations noted or heart rate <110 or >160 beats/min; fresh meconium passed. Disadvantages: Limited maternal a mobility and effort.

Management of poor trace:

1. Lie the mother on her left side and give O_2. Stop using oxytocin. If there is uterine hypercontractility give tocolysis, 0.25 mg of terbutaline (SC).

2. Take fetal blood sample. If yon do not have facility to do the test, consider rapid delivery if the trace does not improve.

Fetal blood sampling: Fetal acidosis indicates hypoxia. Scalp blood pH of 7.3-7.4 is normal. If pH is 7.25-7.29, repeat the test after 45 min. If it is 7.2-7.24 consider caesarean section. pH levels <7.2 require immediate delivery unless in second stage when a lever as low as 7.15 may be acceptable.

Fetal heart rate patterns and their clinical significance: The normal pattern is described above. Accelerations suggest intact sympathetic activity and are rarely associated with hypoxia.

Loss of baseline variability: Baseline variability of >5 beats/min shows response to vagal tone, sympathetic stimuli, and catecholamines in a well-oxygenated fetal brainstem. Loss of baseline variability may reflect a preterm fetus who is sleeping, drug effects (*e. g.* diazepam, morphine, phenothiazine), or hypoxia.

Baseline tachycardia: Heart rate >170 beats/min is associated with maternal fever, or β-sympathomimetic drug use, chorioamnionitis (loss of variation too), and acute/subacute hypoxia. Persistent rates >200 are associated with fetal cardiac arrhythmia.

Baseline bradycardia: heart rate <110 beats/min

胎心监护异常的处理：

1. 孕妇左侧位休息、吸氧、停用催产素，如果子宫高张性收缩，给予宫缩抑制剂 0.25 mg 皮下注射。

2. 采胎儿头皮血，如果没有条件可做好尽快分娩的准备。

胎儿头皮血检查：胎儿酸中毒反映胎儿低氧血症，正常值为 pH 7.3～7.4，如果 pH 7.25～7.29，45 min 后重复检测一次，若 pH 7.2～7.24，考虑剖宫产。若 pH<7.2，需立即分娩。但在第二产程 pH 低至 7.15 都是可以接受的。

胎监图形和临床表现：正常胎监图形如上所述，反映胎儿交感神经活动未受损害，而很少合并低氧血症。

基线变异消失：基线变异>5 次/min 反映胎儿正常活动，对交感神经及胆碱原物质反应。基线变异消失，反映早产胎儿在睡眠状态或用快镇静药或缺氧。

胎心基线过快：心率>170 次/min，见于孕妇发热、β-交感神经兴奋药、绒毛膜羊膜炎和急性-亚急性胎儿窘迫，持续胎心>200 次/min 与胎儿心律失常有关。

胎心基线过缓，心律<110

is rarely associated with fetal hypoxia (except in placental abruption), it may reflect fetal vagal tone, fetal heart block, or, spasmodic, cord compression.

Early decelerations coinciding with uterine contractions reflect increased vagal tone as fetal intracranial pressure rises with the contraction. Late decelerations, when the nadir of the deceleration develops some 30 sec after the peak of the uterine contraction, reflect fetal hypoxia, the degree and duration reflecting its severity. Variable decelerations both in degree and relation to uterine contractions, may represent umbilical cord compression around the limbs or presenting part.

Pathological CTG pattern: This has 2 suspicious features (baseline rate: 100-109 or 161-180 beats/minute; variability<5 beats/minute for ≥40 minutes but < 90 minutes; early, variable, or a prolonged deceleration of <3 minutes) or 1 abnormal feature (rate<100 or>180 beats/minute; sinusoidal pattern for >10 minutes; variability<5 beats/minute for ≥ 90 minutes; atypical variable decelerations or a single deceleration of>3 minutes).

次/min,与胎儿缺氧(胎盘早剥除外)有关,见于胎儿活力降低、胎心阻滞、脐带受压等。

早期减速与宫缩成正比,当宫缩增加时胎儿颅内压增高,胎儿活力增加。晚期减速,减速发生在宫缩峰值消失 30 s 之后,反映胎儿缺氧。晚期减速的程度和持续时间反映了胎儿缺氧的程度。变异减速反映脐带在胎儿肢体或先露部位受压与宫缩压力有关。

病理性 CTG 图形:有两种可疑特征:①基线为 100～109 或 161～180 次/min,大于 40 min 小于 90 min,基线变异<5 次/min,早发的、变异的或延期的减速持续小于 3 min 等。②异常基线(小于 100 次/min 或大于 180 次/min),正弦波型持续超过 10 min;细变异<5 次/min 超过 90 min;不典型变异减速或单次延长减速超过 3 min。

Turning the pyramid of prenatal care

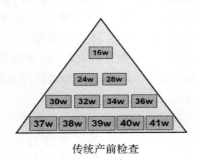

传统产前检查　　　　　　　　　新型产前检查

Figure 2-2-1　Traditional pyramid of prenatal care　　Figure 2-2-2　New pyramid of prenatal care

Early estimation of patient-specific risks for these pregnancy complications would improve pregnancy outcome by shifting antenatal care from a series of routine visits to a more individualized patient

将传统的产前检查即一系列的常规产检转向为产前检查的常规趋向于更加注意根据孕妇个体和特殊疾病来决定产前检查的时

and disease-specific approach both in terms of the schedule and content of such visits. A small proportion of women identified as being at high-risk for a variety of pregnancy complications can have close surveillance in specialist clinics.

The great majority of women would be identified as being at low-risk for pregnancy complications and in this group the number of medical visits can be substantially reduced.

Each visit would have a predefined objective and the findings will generate likelihood ratios that can be used to modify the individual patient and disease-specific estimated risk from the initial assessment at 11-13 weeks. In this respect，the 11-13 weeks assessment is likely to be the basis for a new scientific approach to antenatal care that could reduce maternal and perinatal mortality and morbidity.

This section presents the emerging evidence on the potential value of the 11-13 weeks assessment and sets the basis for a challenge to overturn the 80 years old pyramid of antenatal care.

2.3　Diagnosis of Pregnancy

Key words

1. fetal attitude
2. fetal lie
3. fetal presentation
4. fetal position
5. first trimester
6. second trimester
7. third trimester

Stage：

≤12 w	Early pregnancy
13-27 w	Mid-term pregnancy
≥28 w	Late pregnancy

间和内容。孕妇个体风险评估参数在早孕期的预测能够改善妊娠结局,少数具有不同妊娠并发症高风险的孕妇在专科门诊严密随诊。

绝大多数的孕妇筛查后为低危人群,因而产检次数可大幅度减少。

每次产检将有明确的目的,检查结果将转换成在 11～13 周检查基础上的个体化的疾病针对性的风险导致。而初次检查的特殊疾病的评估源于 11～13 周的产检评估,也就是说 11～13 周的评估是产前检查的基础,能够降低母胎的发病率和死亡率。

于是新出现了 11～13 周的评估重点,建立了新的产前检查三角,对过去延用了 80 年的旧三角模式提出了挑战。

2.3　妊娠诊断

关键词

1. 胎儿的姿势
2. 胎产式
3. 胎先露
4. 胎方位
5. 早期妊娠
6. 中期妊娠
7. 晚期妊娠

分期：

≤12 周	早期妊娠
13～27 周	中期妊娠
≥28 周	晚期妊娠

Diagnosis of Early Pregnancy　　　　　妊娠早期诊断
　　　[History and symptoms]　　　　　　病史和症状
　　　[Physical examination and signs]　检查和体征
　　　[Accessory examinations]　　　　　辅助检查
　　　[Differential diagnosis]　　　　　　鉴别诊断
[History and symptoms]　　　　　　　　病史和症状
　　　1. Amenorrhea　　　　　　　　　　1.闭经
　　　2. Morning sickness：nausea, vomiting　　2.恶心,呕吐
　　　3. Urinary frequency and urgency　3.尿频,尿急

[Examination and signs]　　　　　　　检查和体征
　　　1. Breast changes　　　　　　　　1.乳房的变化
　　　2. Genitalia　　　　　　　　　　　2.生殖器
Breast changes　　　　　　　　　　　乳房的变化
　　　enlargement，vascular engorgement, colostrum　　　增大,血管充血,初乳

Diagnosis of Early Pregnancy　　　　　妊娠早期诊断
　　　Skin changes　　　　　　　　　　皮肤变化
　　　Chloasma　　　　　　　　　　　黄褐斑

Diagnosis of Early Pregnancy　　　　　妊娠早期诊断
[Accessory examinations]　　　　　　　辅助检查
　　　1. Ultrasound：B-ultrasound　　　1.B超
　　　2. Doppler ultrasound　　　　　　2.经颅多普勒超声
　　　3. Pregnancy test　　　　　　　　3.妊娠试验
　　　4. Cervical mucus phlegm test　　4.宫颈黏液痰测试
　　　5. Basic body temperature，BBT　5.基础体温,BBT

Diagnosis of Early Pregnancy　　　　　妊娠早期诊断
[Differential diagnosis]　　　　　　　鉴别诊断
　　　1. Ovarian cyst　　　　　　　　　1.卵巢囊肿
　　　2. Uterine leiomyoma　　　　　　2.子宫肌瘤
　　　3. Urinary retention　　　　　　　3.尿潴留
　　　4. Pseudopregnancy　　　　　　　4.假孕

Diagnosis of Mid-term and Late Pregnancy　　中期和晚期妊娠诊断
[History and symptoms]　　　　　　　病史和症状
　　　Early pregnancy experience　　　妊娠早期经历
　　　Abdominal enlargement　　　　　腹部增大

Perception of fetal movement	感觉胎动
[Physical examination and signs]	检查和体征
Enlargement of the uterus	子宫增大
Fetal movement	胎动
Fetal body	胎儿肢体
Fetal heart sounds	胎心音
[Accessory examinations]	辅助检查
Ultrasound	超声
Fetal electrocardiography，FECG	胎儿心电图
Diagnosis of mid-term and late Pregnancy	中期和晚期妊娠诊断

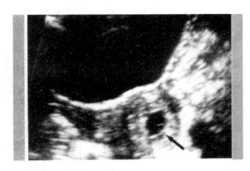

图 2-3-1　超声检查下的 5 周囊胚(箭头处)

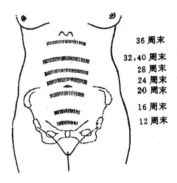

图 2-3-2　妊娠周数与宫底高度

[Symptoms]	症状
Early pregnancy experience	妊娠早期经历
Diagnosis of mid-term and late pregnancy	中期和晚期妊娠诊断
Enlargement of the uterus	子宫增大
[Examinations and signs]	检查和体征
Fetal heart sounds	胎心音
Fetal Attitude	胎儿的姿势
Fetal Lie	胎产式
Fetal Presentation	胎先露
Fetal Position	胎方位

Fetal Attitude：The posture of the fetus in the uterus.

胎儿的姿势:是指胎儿在子宫内的位置。

Fetal Lie：Relationship of the long axis of the fetus to the long axis of the uterus.

胎产式:胎儿的长轴与子宫长轴的关系。

Fetal Presentation：The fetal part that first

胎先露:指胎儿最先进入骨

enters the bony pelvic.

Fetal Position：Relationship of an arbitrary reference point on the fetus to a specific point in the maternal pelvic.

Test

Fetal position is definited 　　（　　）

A. the relationship between maternal longitudinal axis and that of the fetal

B. the relationship between maternal

产道的部分。

胎方位：胎儿先露部指示点与孕妇骨盆的关系。

pelvis and point of fetal presentation

C. the fetal portion that the first coming into pelvis inlet

D. the attitude of fetal in uterus

Answer：B

2.4　Normal Labour

2.4　正常分娩

Key words

1. normal labour
2. latent stage of first stage of labour
3. active stage of firtst stage of labour
4. active second stage of labour
5. pasive second stage of labour
6. third stage of labour
7. support care during labour
8. no supine position for delivery
9. delayed cord clamping
10. in labour assessment
11. shoulder dystocia
12. persistent occipit posterior position

关键词

1. 正常分娩
2. 第一产程潜伏期
3. 第一产程活跃期
4. 第二产程的活跃期（主动期）
5. 第二产程的潜伏期（被动期）
6. 第三产程
7. 产程中的支持性照顾
8. 非平卧位分娩
9. 晚断脐
10. 临产评估
11. 肩难产
12. 持续性枕后位

2.4.1　Prepration for delivery

2.4.1　分娩准备

2.4.1.1　Review the arrangements for delivery

- How will she get there? Will she have to pay for transport?
- How much it will cost to deliver at the facility? How will she pay?
- Who will go with her for support during labour and delivery?
- Who will help while she is away to care for her home and other children?

2.4.1.1　分娩的准备工作

- 如何到达医院,是否要自己付交通费用(是否能够负担费用)?
- 在医院分娩的费用支付方式。

- 谁在分娩过程中陪伴她?

- 在她分娩期间,谁来照顾她的家庭和其他孩子?

2.4.1.2　Advise when to go

- If the woman lives near the facility, she should go at the first signs of labour.
- If living far from the facility, she should go 2-3 weeks before baby due date and stay either at the maternity waiting home or with family or friends near the facility.
- Advise to ask for help from the community.

2.4.1.3　Advise what to bring

- Home-based maternal record.
- Clothes for mother and baby.
- Food and water for woman and support person.

2.4.1.4　Advise on labour signs

Advise to go to the facility or contact the skilled birth attendant if any of the following signs:
- a bloody sticky discharge.
- painful contractions every 20 minutes or less.

- water have broken.

2.4.1.5　Advise on danger signs

Advise to go to the hospital/health centre immediately, day or night, without waiting if any of the following signs:
- vaginal bleeding.
- convulsions.
- severe headache with blurred vision.
- fever and too weak to get out of bed.
- severe abdominal pain.

- fast or difficult breathing.

She should go to the health centre as soon as possible if any of the following signs:
- fever.
- abdominal pain.
- feels ill.

2.4.1.2　给予建议什么时候准备入院

- 如果她居住的地方离医院很近，在有临产的征兆后再准备入院。
- 如果离医院很远（交通不便），可考虑提前二三周住在医院附近的母婴之家或亲戚朋友家。

- 如果需要，可到附近的社区诊所请求帮助。

2.4.1.3　要准备的物品

- 孕期检查记录本。
- 自己和婴儿的衣服、包被。
- 孕妇和陪护人所需要的食物和水。

2.4.1.4　告之分娩的征兆

如果出现以下症状，与医院内的服务人员联系：
- 黏稠的血性分泌物（见红）。
- 每 20 min 一次或更短时间 1 次的有痛感的子宫收缩。
- 有阴道流水（破水）。

2.4.1.5　告之哪些是危险的表现

如果出现以下情况，不管是白天还是晚上，不要延误，要紧急来院就诊：
- 阴道流血。
- 抽搐。
- 剧烈的头痛伴有眼花。
- 发热并且无力，不能起床活动。
- 严重的腹疼（不是规律性的子宫收缩）。
- 呼吸增快或呼吸困难。

如果出现以下情况，要尽快上医院就诊：
- 发热。
- 腹痛。
- 感到不适。

- swelling of fingers，face，legs.

2.4.2　Examing the woman in labour

2.4.2.1　Ask，check record

History of this labour

- When did contractions begin?
- How frequent are contractions? How strong?
- Have your waters broken? If yes，when? Were they clear or green?
- Have you had any bleeding? If yes，when? How much?
- Is the baby moving?
- Do you have any concern?

Check record，or if no record

- Ask when the delivery is expected.
- Determine if preterm (less than 8 months pregnant).
- Review the birth plan.

If prior pregnancies

- Number of prior pregnancies/deliveries.
- Any prior caesarean section，forceps，or vacuum，or other complication such as postpartum haemorhage?
- Any prior third degree tear?

Current pregnancy

- RPR status.
- HB results.
- Tetanus immunization status.
- HIV status.
- Infant feeding plan.
- Receiving any medicine.

2.4.2.2　Look，listen，feel

- Observe the woman's response to contractions：
- → Is she coping well or is she distressed?
- → Is she pushing or grunting?
- Check abdomen for：
- → caesarean section scar.
- → horizontal ridge across lower abdomen (if present，

- 手指或面部、腿部水肿。

2.4.2　产妇临产评估检查

2.4.2.1　问诊与检查评估

现孕史

- 什么时间开始出现子宫收缩?
- 子宫收缩的频率、强度。
- 是否破水? 如果有破水，什么时间? 清水还是绿色的?
- 有无阴道出血? 如果有出血，出血量和开始出血的时间。
- 胎动情况。
- 还有其他什么症状?

检查孕期保健记录本(有没有以下信息)。如果没有记录本，询问：

- 预产期时间。
- 判断是否早产(小于 8 月妊娠)。

- 复习分娩计划。

如果以前有怀孕生产史：

- 孕史，分娩史。
- 有无剖宫产史、产钳、胎头吸引或其他并发症(例如产后出血)?
- 有无三度会阴裂伤?

本次妊娠情况

- RPP 检查。
- HB。
- 破伤风接种情况。
- HIV 检查。
- 婴儿的哺育计划。
- 是否用药?

2.4.2.2　视诊、听诊和触诊检查

- 观察产妇宫缩时的表现：
- →是否能够正常地应对或者很紧张?
- →是否开始屏气用力或喊叫呻吟?
- 腹部检查：
- →是否有剖宫产刀口?
- →下腹部横刀口(如果有，排空膀

empty bladder and observe again).

- Feel abdomen for:
→ contractions frequency, duration, any continuous contractions?
→ fetal lie—longitudinal or transverse?
→ fetal presentation—head, breech, other?
→ more than one fetus?
→ fetal movement.
- Listen to the fetal heart beat:
→ Count number of beats in 1 minute.
→ If less than 100 beats per minute, or more than 180 bpm, turn woman on her left side and count again.
- Measure blood pressure.
- Measure temperature.
- Look for pallor.
- Look for sunken eyes, dry mouth.
- Pinch the skin of the forearm: does it go back quickly.

2.4.2.3 Perform vaginal examination and decide stage of labour

- Explain to the woman that you will give her a vaginal examination and ask for her consent.
- Look at vulva for:
→ bulging perineum.
→ any visible fetal parts.
→ vaginal bleeding.
→ leaking amniotic fluid; if yes, is it meconium stained, foul-smelling?
→ warts, keloid tissue or scars that may interfere with delivery.
- DO NOT shave the perineal area.
- Prepare:
→ clean gloves, swabs, pads.
- Wash hands with soap before and after each examination.
- Wash vulva and perineal areas.
- Put on gloves.
- Position the woman with legs flexed and apart.

胱再次观察）。

- 腹部触诊：
→子宫收缩的频率、持续时间，是否有持续性的宫缩？
→胎产式：纵产式还是横产式？
→胎先露：头、臀或其他先露？
→单胎，还是双胎或多胎？
→胎动情况（是否感觉到胎动）。
- 胎心听诊：
→听诊一分钟内胎心搏动的次数。
→如果少于 100 次/min，让产妇侧卧，再次听诊 1 min。
- 测量血压。
- 体温。
- 产妇面色，是否苍白无力？
- 眼窝有无内陷，口唇是否干裂？
- 前臂皮肤弹性评估：捏起皮肤，看是否能够快速恢复。

2.4.2.3 阴道检查与产程分期判断

- 向产妇解释要进行一次阴道检查，征得产妇同意。
- 观察会阴部：
→ 有无会阴膨胀？
→ 是否可见先露部分？
→ 有无阴道流血？
→ 有无羊水流水；如果有，是否有胎粪污染、异常味道？
→会阴部瘢痕、硬结或伤口可能妨碍分娩。
- 不要剃除阴毛。
- 准备：
→ 清洁的手套、棉签、垫巾。
- 检查前后都要用肥皂和清水洗手。
- 用清水和肥皂清洁会阴及阴道口。
- 戴手套。
- 产妇膀胱截石位，两腿分开。

※ DO NOT perform vaginal examination if bleeding now or at any time after 7 months of pregnancy.

- Perform gentle vaginal examination (do not start during a contraction):
→ Determine cervical dilatation in centimetres.
→ Feel for presenting part. Is it hard, round and smooth (the head)? If not, identify the presenting part.
→ Feel for membranes—are they intact?
→ Feel for cord— is it felt? Is it pulsating? If so, act immediately as on.

2.4.2.4　Respond to obstetrical problems on admission

- Bulging thin perineum, vagina gaping and head visible, full cervical dilatation, Imminent delivery. See second stage of labour.
- Cervical dilatation:
→ multigravida≥5 cm.
→ primigravida ≥6 cm.

　　Late active labour
　　Record in partograph.
- Cervical dilatation ≥4 cm.
　　early active labour
　　Record in partograph.
See first stage of labour—active labour.
Start plotting partograph.
- Cervical dilatation: 0-3 cm,
contractions weak and＜2 in 10 minutes,
not yet in active labour, Record in
(treat as in latent stage).

If any of the following condition exist: obstructed labour:
- Transverse lie.
- Continuous contractions.
- Constant pain between contractions.

※如果有阴道流血,不要做阴道检查(临产时和孕7月以后的任何时间)。

- 轻柔的检查(不要在宫缩时进行)。
→ 评估宫口开大情况。
→ 胎儿先露部位,头还是其他部位。
→ 检查胎膜是否完整。
→ 检查有无脐带先露,如果能够触到,有无搏动? 如果触及脐带并且有搏动,迅速按脐带脱垂处理。

2.4.2.4　入院时产科情况处理

- 如果:会阴膨隆变薄,阴道口分开,胎头可见,宫口开全,即将分娩,见第二产程处理。
- 如果:宫口开大
→ 经产妇≥5 cm。
→ 初产妇≥6 cm。
　　第一产程活跃期的晚期,开始描记产程图,继续观察产程进展。
- 如果:宫口开大≥4 cm。
　　第一产程活跃期的早期
　　检查结果记录在产程图上,
　　开始描记产程图,
　　继续观察产程进展。
- 如果:宫口开大 0～3 cm,
　　并且宫缩较弱,小于 2 次/10 min,没有进入活跃期。
　　检查结果记录在病历上(按潜伏期管理原则处理)。
　　出现以下任何一种情况,难产的表现:
- 横位。
- 持续性的没有间隔的宫缩。
- 在两次宫缩间隔仍然感到腹痛

- Sudden and severe abdominal pain.
- Horizontal ridge across lower abdomen.
- Labour >24 hours.

If distressed, insert an IV line and give fluids.

- If in labour >24 hours, give appropriate IM/IV antibiotics.
- Refer urgently to hospital.

For all the situations below, refer urgently to hospital if in early labour, manage only in late labour.

SIGN:

- Rupture of membranes and any of:
→ Fever >38 ℃.
→ Foul-smelling vaginal discharge.

DIAGNOSIS:

- Risk of uterine and fetal infection.

MANAGE:

- Give appropriate IM/IV antibiotics.
- If late labour, deliver and refer to hospital after delivery.
- Plan to treat new born.

SIGN:

- Rupture of membranes at <8-months of pregnancy.

DIAGNOSIS:

Risk of uterine and fetal infection.

MANAGE:

- Give appropriate IM/IV antibiotics.
- If late labour, deliver.
- Discontinue antibiotic for mother after delivery if no signs of infection.
- Plan to treat new born.

SIGN:

- Diastolic blood pressure >90 mmHg.

DIAGNOSIS:

- pre-eclampsia.

严重。

- 急性发生的严重的腹痛。
- 腹部下段发现病理性缩复环。
- 产程持续大于 24 h。

处理：建立静脉通道。

- 产程超过 24 h，给予预防性应用抗生素。
- 转到上级医院。

　　若出现以下情况，如果产妇处于产程的早期，迅速转到上级医院处理。如果是接近分娩，给予紧急处理，在分娩后情况稳定迅速转院。

表现：

　　胎膜早破，并且体温大于＞38 ℃。

　　阴道分泌物有异味。

诊断：

　　有子宫和新生儿感染可能。

处理：

- 静脉或肌内注射给予抗生素。
- 如果临近分娩，分娩处理后迅速转到上级医院。
- 准备治疗新生儿。

表现：

- 妊娠小于 8 月，胎膜早破。

诊断：

- 有子宫和新生儿感染危险。

处理：

- 静脉或肌内注射应用抗生素。
- 如果临近分娩，接产处理。
- 如果产后母亲没有感染的征象，停用抗生素。
- 准备治疗新生儿。

表现：

- 舒张压>90 mmHg。

诊断：

- 子痫前期。

MANAGE：

■ Assess further and manage as on.

SIGN：

■ Severe pallor and conjunctival pallor and/or haemoglobin <7 g/dl.

DIAGNOSIS：

■ Severe anaemia.

MANAGE：

■ Manage as on.

SIGN：

■ Breech or other malpresentation.

■ Multiple pregnancy.

■ Fetal distress.

■ Prolapsed cord.

DIAGNOSIS：

■ Obstetrical complication.

MANAGE：

■ Follow specific instructions.

SIGN：

■ Warts，keloid tissue that may interfere with delivery.

■ Prior third degree tear.

DIAGNOSIS：

■ Risk of obstetrical complication.

MANAGE：

■ Do a generous episiotomy and carefully control delivery of the head.

SIGN：

■ Bleeding any time in third trimester.

■ Prior delivery by：

→ caesarean section.

→ forceps or vacuum delivery.

■ Age less than 14 years.

DIAGNOSIS：

■ Risk of obstetrical complication.

MANAGE：

■ If late labour, deliver.

■ Have help available during delivery.

处理：

■ 按相关处理原则处理。

表现：

■ 严重的面色苍白或中央性苍白或血色素低于<7 g/dl。

诊断：

■ 严重贫血。

处理：

■ 按相关处理原则处理。

表现：

■ 臀位或其他异常胎位。

■ 多胎妊娠。

■ 胎儿宫内窘迫。

■ 脐带脱垂。

诊断：

■ 有产科异常并发症。

处理：

■ 按相关处理原则处理。

表现：

■ 会阴瘢痕有可能影响胎儿娩出。

■ 前次有三度会阴裂伤。

诊断：

■ 可能有产科并发症。

处理：

■ 作一个恰当的会阴侧切并小心地控制胎头娩出。

表现：

■ 妊娠晚期出现过阴道流血。

■ 前次妊娠是：剖宫产，产钳，或胎头吸引分娩。

■ 产妇年龄小于 14 岁。

诊断：

■ 有产科并发症的危险。

处理：

■ 如果临近分娩，给予接产处理，分娩过程中有二线医生协助。

SIGN：

- Labour before 8 completed months of pregnancy (more than one month before estimated date of delivery).

DIAGNOSIS：

- Preterm labour.

MANAGE：

- Reassess fetal presentation (breech more common).
- If woman is lying，encourage her to lie on her left side.
- Call for help during delivery.
- Conduct delivery very carefully as small baby may pop out suddenly. In particular，control delivery of the head.
- Prepare equipment for resuscitation of new born.

SIGN：

- Fetal heart rate <120 or >160 beats per minute.

DIAGNOSIS：

- Posible fetal distres.

MANAGE：

- Manage as on.

SIGN：

- Rupture of membranes at term and before labour.

DIAGNOSIS：

- Rupture of membranes.

MANAGE：

- Give appropriate IM/IV antibiotics if rupture of membrane >18 hours.
- Plan to treat the new born.

SIGN：

- If two or more of the following signs：
  → thirsty.
  → sunken eyes.
  → dry mouth.
  → skin pinch goes back slowly.

DIAGNOSIS：

- Dehydration.

表现：

- 妊娠不足 8 月（比预产期提前一个月分娩）。

诊断：

- 早产。

处理：

- 评估胎儿先露部位（注意早产有更多的臀位）。
- 如果产妇愿意平卧，鼓励她侧卧位。
- 在分娩过程中要有二线医生协助。
- 接产过程要注意观察，因为胎儿较小可能突然娩出。必要时，小心地控制胎头，慢慢娩出。
- 准备新生儿复苏抢救用品。

表现：

- 胎心率低于 120 次/min 或高于 160 次/min。

诊断：

- 胎儿宫内窘迫的可能。

处理：

- 按相关措施处理。

表现：

- 足月，胎膜在临产前破裂。

诊断：

- 足月胎膜破裂。

处理：

- 如果破膜时间长于 18 h，给予预防性应用抗生素。
- 准备治疗新生儿。

表现：

- 如果出现下列情况之一：
  → 感觉渴。
  → 眼窝内隐。
  → 口唇干裂。
  → 皮肤捏起后恢复缓慢。

诊断：

- 脱水。

MANAGE：

- Give oral fluids.
- If not able to drink, give 1 litre IV fluids over 3 hours.

SIGN：

- HIV test positive.
- Taking ARV treatment or prophylaxis.

DIAGNOSIS：

- HIV-positive.

MANAGE：

- Ensure that the woman takes ARV drugs as prescribed.
- Support her choice of infant feeding.

SIGN：

- No fetal movement.
- No fetal heart beat on repeated examination.

DIAGNOSIS：

- Posible fetal death.

MANAGE：

- Explain to the parents that the baby is not doing well.

2.4.3 Give supportive care throughout labour

Use this chart to provide a supportive, encouraging atmosphere for birth, respectful of the woman's wishes.

2.4.3.1 Communication

- Explain all procedures, seek permission, and discuss findings with the woman.
- Keep her informed about the progress of labour.
- Praise her, encourage and reassure her that things are going well.
- Ensure and respect privacy during examinations and discussions.
- If known HIV positive, find out what she has told the companion. Respect her wishes.

处理：

- 经口饮水。
- 如果不能经口饮水，经静脉输入液体 1000 ml，3 h 内输完。

表现：

- HIV 阳性。
- 正在服用 ARV 治疗药物或预防性用药。

诊断：

- HIV 阳性。

处理：

- 保证产妇能够正确地服用药物。
- 帮助她选择婴儿的哺育方法。

表现：

- 无胎动。
- 没有听到胎心，再次评估仍然未能听到胎心。

诊断：

- 可能死胎。

处理：

- 告之产妇及家人胎儿的情况不好，要进一步评估。

2.4.3 产程中的支持性照顾

本节内容为产程中要为产妇提供支持性照顾，鼓励自然分娩，尊重产妇的选择和意愿。

2.4.3.1 交流沟通

- 任何检查和医疗行为都要向产妇解释，获得知情同意，并告之结果，并与产妇讨论。
- 让产妇明确自己的产程进展。
- 给予赞扬、鼓励和给予肯定，告知产程进展情况良好。
- 在检查和讨论病例时注意保护隐私。
- 如果产妇是 HIV 阳性，询问产妇是否已经告之家人。尊重产

2.4.3.2 Cleanliness

- Encourage the woman to bath or shower or wash herself and genitals at the onset of labour.
- Wash the vulva and perineal areas before each examination.
- Wash your hands with soap before and after each examination. Use clean gloves for vaginal examination.
- Ensure cleanliness of labour and birthing area(s).
- Clean up spills immediately.
- DO NOT give enema.

2.4.3.3 Mobility

- Encourage the woman to walk around freely during the first stage of labour.
- Support the woman's choice of position (left lateral, squatting, kneeling, standing supported by the companion) for each stage of labour and delivery.

2.4.3.4 Urination

- Encourage the woman to empty her bladder frequently. Remind her every 2 hours.

2.4.3.5 Eating, drinking

- Encourage the woman to eat and drink as she wishes throughout labour.
- Nutritious liquid drinks are important, even in late labour.
- If the woman has visible severe wasting or tires during labour, make sure she eats and drinks.

2.4.3.6 Breathing technique

- Teach her to notice normal breathing.

- Encourage her to breathe out more slowly, and to relax with each breath.
- If she feels dizzy, unwell, is feeling pins-and-needles (tingling) in her face, hands and feet,

妇个人的意愿。

2.4.3.2 保持产妇清洁舒适

- 鼓励产妇在产程开始时沐浴清洁身体,包括会阴部。
- 在每次阴道检查前要清洁会阴阴道口。
- 在每次检查前后,检查者要用肥皂和清水洗手,每次检查都要戴手套。
- 保持待产和分娩场所的清洁舒适。
- 在有分泌物或呕吐物时,及时清除。
- 不要给予产妇灌肠。

2.4.3.3 产程中鼓励产妇活动

- 在第一产程期间,鼓励产妇自由活动。
- 在产程中和分娩时,鼓励产妇按自己的意愿选择体位(左侧卧位,蹲位,跪,有陪伴者协助站立位)。

2.4.3.4 排尿

- 鼓励产妇自己排尿,每 2 h 提醒 1 次。

2.4.3.5 进食,进水

- 鼓励产妇根据自己的意愿进食和饮水。
- 液体食物是重要的,即使进入第二产程,仍然要进食。
- 如果产妇在产程中表现疲乏无力,注意评估产妇是否进食和饮水。

2.4.3.6 呼吸放松技术

- 教会产妇在产程中如何正常地呼吸。
- 鼓励她慢慢地呼吸,每次呼吸中间注意放松。
- 如果她感到头晕,不适,感到面部、手和脚部有针刺感,鼓励她

encourage her to breathe more slowly.

- To prevent pushing at the end of first stage of labour, teach her to pant, to breathe with an open mouth, to take in 2 short breaths followed by a long breath out.
- During delivery of the head, ask her not to push but to breathe steadily or to pant.

2.4.3.7　Pain and discomfort relief

- Suggest change of position.
- Encourage mobility, as comfortable for her.

- Encourage companion to:
→ massage the woman's back if she finds this helpful.
→ hold the woman's hand and sponge her face between contractions.
- Encourage her to use the breathing technique.

- Encourage warm bath or shower, if available.

- If woman is distressed or anxious, investigate the cause.
- If pain is constant (persisting between contractions) and very severe or sudden in onset, investigate the cause, posibbly obstetrical problems, treat as on.

2.4.3.8　Birth companion

- Encourage support from the chosen birth companion throughout labour.
- Describe to the birth companion what she or he should do:
→ Always be with the woman.
→ Encourage her.
→ Help her to breathe and relax.

慢慢地呼吸(不要过度地呼气, 深吸气,慢慢地吐气)。

- 为防止产妇过早地用力(屏气),教会产妇如何哈气,张口呼吸,或在一次慢慢的呼吸后,进行 2 次快速的短呼吸。
- 在胎头快要娩出时,教会产妇不要用力,张口呼吸或缓慢地呼吸。

2.4.3.7　如何缓解产痛

- 鼓励产妇改变体位。
- 鼓励产妇活动,找到感到舒适的体位。
- 鼓励陪伴人员:
→ 按摩产妇的背部,如果她感到这样舒适。
→ 握住产妇的手,在两次宫缩之间给她擦拭汗液。
- 鼓励产妇应用呼吸技术慢慢呼吸放松。
- 如果可能,提供温暖的沐浴或盆浴。
- 如果产妇紧张焦虑,找出原因。

- 如果产妇出现持续性的宫缩(在两次宫缩间隔仍然感到腹痛),或非常严重的腹痛,或在产程一开始就非常剧烈,找出原因,可能存在产科并发症,按相应情况处理。

2.4.3.8　陪伴分娩

- 鼓励产妇自己选择分娩过程中的陪同人员。
- 告之陪同人员,她要做的事情:

→ 始终要陪伴产妇。
→ 给予产妇鼓励。
→ 协助产妇呼吸和放松。

→ Rub her back, wipe her brow with a wet cloth, do other supportive actions.

→ Give support using local practices which do not disturb labour or delivery.

→ Encourage woman to move around freely as she wishes and to adopt the position of her choice.

→ Encourage her to drink fluids and eat as she wishes.

→ Assist her to the toilet when needed.

■ Ask the birth companion to call for help if:

→ The woman is bearing down with contractions.

→ There is vaginal bleeding.

→ She is suddenly in much more pain.

→ She loses consciousness.

→ There is any other concern.

■ Tell the birth companion what she or he should NOT do and explain why:

→ DO NOT encourage woman to push.

→ DO NOT give advice other than that given by the health worker.

→ DO NOT keep woman in bed if she wants to move around.

2.4.4　First stage of labour: not in active labour

Use this chart for care of the woman when not in active labour, when cervix dilated 0-3 cm and contractions are weak, less than 2 in 10 minutes. observe in clinical unit or according to local protocol.

2.4.4.1　Monitor every 4 hours

■ Cervical dilatation. Unless indicated, do not do vaginal examination more frequently than every 4 hours.

■ Temperature.

■ Pulse.

→ 按摩产妇背部,用湿毛巾擦拭汗液,给予其他的支持性行为。

→ 给予其他支持性不干涉产程进展。

→ 鼓励产妇活动,鼓励产妇选择自己感到舒适的体位。

→ 鼓励产妇根据自己的意愿饮水和进食。

→ 协助产妇排尿和排便。

■ 告之陪伴人员,如果出现以下情况,要告诉助产人员请求帮助:

→ 产妇开始屏气用力。

→ 出现阴道流血。

→ 突然出现的剧烈疼痛。

→ 失去意识或知觉。

→ 其他不适情况。

■ 告之陪伴人员,她不应当做以下事情,并解释原因:

→ 不要指导产妇用力(产妇自己想用力的时候再用力)。

→ 不要给予其他建议(不同于助产人员的建议)。

→ 如果产妇想活动,不要让产妇卧床。

2.4.4　第一产程:未进入活跃期（潜伏期）管理

本节内容是产妇未进入活跃期的处理。产妇宫口开大 1～3 cm,宫缩较弱,少于 2 次/10 min。产妇可在门诊或临产评估单元或急诊中心进行观察评估。

2.4.4.1　每4 h评估1次的内容:

■ 检查宫口开大情况,除非有异常情况(如胎心异常),不要频繁做阴道检查,不多于1次/4 h。

■ 体温;

■ 脉搏;

- Blood pressure.

2.4.4.2　Monitor every hour

- For emergency signs, using rapid assessment (RAM).
- Frequency, intensity and duration of contractions.

- Fetal heart rate.
- Mood and behaviour (distressed, anxious).

- Record findings regularly in labour record and Partograph.
- Record time of rupture of membranes and colour of amniotic fluid.
- Never leave the woman alone.

2.4.4.3　Assess progress of labour

- After 8 hours if：
→ Contractions stronger and more frequent but
→ No progress in cervical dilatation with or without membranes ruptured.

MANAGE：

- Refer the woman urgently to hospital.
- After 8 hours if：
→ no increase in contractions, and
→ membranes are not ruptured, and
→ no progress in cervical dilatation.

MANAGE：

- Discharge the woman and advise her to return if：

→ pain/discomfort increases；
→ vaginal bleeding；
→ membranes rupture.
- Cervical dilatation 4 cm or greater.

MANAGE：

　　Begin plotting the partograph and manage the woman as in active labour

- 血压。

2.4.4.2　每小时评估 1 次的内容

- 如果出现紧急情况（如阴道流血），迅速进行急诊评估。
- 观察评估宫缩情况、收缩的强度、持续时间。
- 听诊胎心。
- 评估产妇的精神状态和行为，有无紧张焦虑。
- 在产妇记录本上作记录。

- 记录破膜时间和羊水的性状。

- 一定不要让产妇独自一人在房间里。

2.4.4.3　评估产程进展

　　如果 8 h 后，宫缩变频变强，但宫口没有开大，胎膜已破或未破。

处理：

- 转送产妇到上级医院。
- 如果 8 h 后，宫缩没有变频繁，强度没有增加，胎膜未破，宫口没有开大。

处理：

- 产妇回家等待，并告知出现下列情况时，随时返回医院：
→腹痛加重，不适；
→出现阴道流血；
→胎膜破裂。
- 如果检查宫口开大 4 cm 或更大。

处理：

- 产妇入院；开始描记产程图；
- 按活跃期管理原则。

中医分娩要诀
Basic Protocols of Normal Birth in Traditional Chinese Medicine.

睡：Sleeping, waiting for spoutenous contraction, carefully observation for the on-set of labour, in labour assessement.

忍痛：Toleration of pain：free of movement during labour for pain relief.

慢临盆：Slowly delivery of the baby in natural way, including spoutenous pushing, no-supine positon delivery and waiting for shoulders technique in all birth.

2.4.5 First stage of labour：in active labour

Use this chart when the woman is in active labour (or established first stage of labour), when cervix dilated 4 cm or more to the full dilation of 10 cm.

2.4.5.1 Monitor every 4 hours

- Cervical dilatation：Unless indicated, do not do vaginal examination more frequently than every 4 hours.
- Temperature.
- Pulse.
- Blood pressure.

2.4.5.2 Monitor every 30 minutes

- For emergency signs, using rapid assessment (RAM).
- Frequency, intensity and duration of contractions.
- Fetal heart rate.
- Mood and behaviour (distressed, anxious).
- Record findings regularly in Labour record and Partograph.
- Record time of rupture of membranes and colour of amniotic fluid.
- Give Supportive care.
- Never leave the woman alone.

2.4.5 第一产程活跃期管理

本节内容为产妇进入活跃期管理，当宫口开大 4 cm 或更大时。

2.4.5.1 每 4 h 评估内容

- 检查子宫口开大情况 1 次/4 h。除非有异常情况（如胎心异常），不要频繁做阴道检查，不多于 1 次/4 h。
- 体温；
- 脉搏；
- 血压。

2.4.5.2 每 30 min 评估内容

- 如果出现紧急情况（如阴道流血），迅速进行急诊评估。
- 观察评估宫缩情况、收缩的强度、持续时间。
- 听诊胎心。
- 评估产妇的精神状态和行为，有无紧张焦虑。
- 在产妇记录本上作记录（开始描记产程图）。
- 记录破膜时间和羊水的性状。
- 给予产妇支持性照顾。
- 一定不要让产妇独自一人在房间里。

2.4.5.3　Assess progress of labour

Definition of delay in the established first stage.

A diagnosis of delay in the established first stage of labour needs to take into consideration all aspects of progress in labour and should include:

- cervical dilatation of less than 2 cm in 4 hours for first labours.
- cervical dilatation of less than 2 cm in 4 hours or a slowing in the progress of labour for second or subsequent labours.
- descent and rotation of the fetal head.
- changes in the strength, duration and frequency of uterine contractions.
- Partograph passes to the right of ALERT LINE(4 hours apart from cervical dialation of 4 cm).

MANAGE:

- Reassess woman and consider criteria for referral.

- Call senior person if available. Alert emergency transport services.
- Encourage woman to empty bladder.
- Ensure adequate hydration but omit solid foods.

- Encourage upright position and walking if woman wishes.
- Monitor intensively. Reassess in 2 hours and refer if no progress. If referral takes a long time, refer immediately (DO NOT wait to cross action line).

- Partograph passes to the right of ACTION LINE (4hours apart from alert line).

MANAGE:

- Refer urgently to hospital unless birth is imminent.
- Cervix dilated 10 cm or bulging perineum.

MANAGE:

- Manage as in Second stage of labour.

2.4.5.3　第一产程活跃期延长处理

对于活跃期产程延长的判断,需要对产妇产程进展的各个方面进行评估。

- 初产妇,宫颈口扩张速度在 4 h 内少于 2 cm。
- 经产妇,宫颈口扩张速度在 4 h 内少于 2 cm。

- 胎头的旋转与下降程度
- 子宫收缩的频率和强度的变化。
- 如果产程图接近警戒线(自宫口开大 4 cm,4 h 后宫口未开全)。

处理:

- 评估产妇情况,是否有需要转诊的情况。
- 请示高级医师,报告急诊转运部门(有可能要转院,作准备)。
- 鼓励产妇排空膀胱。
- 保持产妇水电平衡但不要吃固体食物。
- 鼓励产妇取直立体位和走动,按产妇的意愿。
- 加强观察,2 h 后再次评估,如果仍然没有进展,转到上级医院(或进行处理);如果转院需要较长时间,迅速转院(不要等待产程超过行动线(警戒线后 4 h)。
- 如果产程图接近行动线(自警戒线,4 h 后宫口未开全)。

处理:

- 转到上级医院(或进行相应处理),除非可以立即分娩。
- 如果宫口开大 10 cm,会阴开始膨胀。

处理:

按第二产程原则处理。

2.4.6　Second stage of labour

2.4.6.1　Definition of the second stage of labour

The second stage can be divided into two phases: the passive and the positive phase.

■ The passive second stage of labour

Is from the finding of full dilatation of the cervix prior to or in the absence of involuntary expulsive contractions. In a woman without epidural analgesia, full dilatation of the cervix has been diagnosed but she does not get an urge to push further assessment should take place after 1 hour.

If women and fetus condition do not show any pathological signs, no intervention should be offered (not strict to 1 hour limitition).

■ The active second stage of labour.

■ Onset of the active second stage of labour:

—the baby is visible.

—expulsive contractions with a finding of full dilatation of the cervix or other signs of full dilatation of the cervix.

—chang in the behavior of women, urge to pushing.

—the active second stage of labour in nuliparous women is often within 2 hours, and within 1 hours in parous women.

■ delay in the second stage

Nulliparous women:

• Birth would be expected to take place within 3 hours of the start of the active second stage in most women.

• A diagnosis of delay in the active second stage should be made when it has lasted 2 hours and women should be referred to a healthcare professional trained to undertake an operative

2.4.6　第二产程管理

2.4.6.1　第二产程的概念

第二产程分为两期,即被动期和主动期。

■ 第二产程的被动期

从宫口开全,到产妇不自主(不能控制的)想屏气用力的时间(宫口开全至第二产程的主动期开始的时间)。第二产程的被动期延长:在没有进行无痛麻醉的产妇,如果在宫口开全后 1 h,产妇仍然没有屏气用力的表现,可疑为第二产程被动期延长。处理:检查评估母儿情况,必要时做阴道检查。如果母亲与胎儿情况均良好,不主张在此期作干涉处理(不严格限制时间)。

■ 第二产程的主动期

指从宫口开全后,自下列表现出现,到胎儿娩出之间的时间:

—胎儿可见(拔露)。

—产妇行为的改变:出现宫缩时不能自控的屏气用力。

——一般初产妇在第二产程的主动期开始后 2 h 内结束分娩(娩出胎儿)。

一般经产妇在第二产程的主动期开始后 1 h 内结束分娩。

■ 第二产程主动期延长

初产妇:

• 大部分初产妇主动期 3 h 内完成分娩。如果第二产程的主动期开始后 2 h 内产妇没有分娩,可诊断为第二产程主动期延长。产妇应当转介到上级医院医生,如果不能在短时间内分娩,由经过专门培训的专科

vaginal birth if birth is not imminent.

Parous women:

- Birth would be expected to take place within 2 hours of the start of the active second stage in most women.

- A diagnosis of delay in the active second stage should be made when it has lasted 1 hour and women should be referred to a healthcare professional trained to undertake an evaluated their labor and birth imminent.

2.4.6.2　Monitor every 5 minutes

- For emergency signs, using rapid assessment (RAM).
- Frequency, intensity and duration of contractions.
- Fetal heart rate.
- Perineum thinning and bulging.
- Visible descent of fetal head or during contraction.
- Mood and behaviour (distressed, anxious).
- Record findings regularly in Labour record and Partograph.
- Give supportive care.
- Never leave the woman alone.
- Ensure all delivery equipment and supplies, including new born resuscitation equipment, areavailable, and place of delivery is clean and warm (25 ℃).

2.4.6.3　Ensure bladder is empty

- If unable to pass urine and bladder is full, empty bladder (do not left there).

2.4.6.4　Assist the woman into a comfortable position of her choice, as upright as possible

- DO NOT let her lie flat (horizontally) on her back.
- Up-right position include: kneel down (on hands and knees), squating, sit, stand up or with assistant.

医生进行手术助产。

经产妇：

- 如果经产妇在第二产程的主动期开始后经过 1 h 没有分娩，可诊断为第二产程活跃期延长，产妇应当转介到上级医院医生，如果不能在短时间内分娩，由经过专门培训的专科医生进行手术助产。

2.4.6.2　每 5 min 评估一次的内容

- 评估有无紧急情况发生：发热、晕厥、阴道流血等。
- 子宫收缩的频率、强度、持续时间。
- 听诊胎心率。
- 会阴是否变薄，开始膨胀。
- 胎头是否拔露。
- 产妇的情绪与行为，是否焦虑紧张。
- 记录描记产程图。
- 始终给予支持性的照料。
- 不要让产妇独自处于房间里。
- 准备分娩用品和仪器设备，包括新生儿抢救的用品。
- 分娩环境清洁、温暖（25 ℃）。

2.4.6.3　排空膀胱

- 鼓励产妇排尿，如果不能自行排出，膀胱膨胀，尿管导尿（不必留置尿管）。

2.4.6.4　协助产妇根据自己的选择，取舒适的体位，尽可能保持直立体位

- 不要让产妇平卧（仰卧）。
- 直立体位：包括跪（手膝俯卧位）、蹲、坐、站立等，上身保持直立或有支持物的体位。

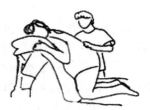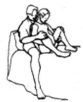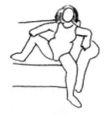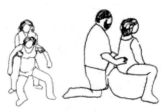

Figure 2-4-1　Up-right position and free of movement during labour

图 2-4-1　产妇直立自由体位待产

2.4.6.5 Stay with her and offer her emotional and physical support

- If the woman is distressed, encourage no pharmacy pain discomfort relief such breath technique.

2.4.6.6 Allow her to push as she wishes with contractions(spontaneous pushing)

Do not urge her to push.

- If, after 30 minutes of spontaneous expulsive efforts, the perineum does not begin to thin and stretch with contractions, do a vaginal examination to confirm full dilatation of cervix.
- If cervix is not fully dilated, await second stage. Place woman on her left side and discourage pushing. Encourage breathing technique .

2.4.6.7 Preparation of delivery

- Wait until head visible and perineum distending.

- Wash hands with clean water and soap. Put on gloves just before delivery.
- See universal precautions during labour and delivery.
- Birth would be expected to take place within 3 hours of the start of the active second stage in most nulliparous women, and within 2 hours in parous women.
- If second stage(active second stage) lasts for 2 hours (parous women lasts for 1 hours or more)or

2.4.6.5 陪伴产妇给予精神心理及生理支持

如果产妇焦虑紧张,鼓励应用非药物的镇痛技术,如呼吸放松、按摩等。

2.4.6.6 支持产妇在宫缩时根据自己的意愿用力(自主的用力方式)

- 不要指导产妇用力,产妇可以根据自身的意愿和方式,在宫缩时开始用力。
- 如果产妇出现屏气用力 30 min,未见会阴变薄和扩张现象(没有胎头拔露),行阴道检查,评估宫口是否开全。
- 如果检查宫口未开全,让产妇停止用力,侧卧位,宫缩时呼吸放松,不要用力。

2.4.6.7 准备分娩

- 等待观察直到胎头拔露和会阴扩张。
- 接产者用清水和肥皂洗手,在接产前戴(无菌)手套。
- 按照标准预防流程操作。

- 初产妇一般自开始用力 3 h 左右完成分娩(第二产程的主动期);经产妇一般 2 h 左右完成分娩。
- 如果[初产妇第二产程(第二产程的主动期)超过 2 h 或更长,

more without visible steady descent of the head, call for staff trained to use vacuum extractor or refer urgently to hospital.

- If obvious obstruction to progress (warts/scarring/keloid tissue/previous third degree tear), do a generous episiotomy.

- DO NOT perform episiotomy routinely.
- If breech or other malpresentation, manage as on.

2.4.6.8 Deliver the baby

Encourage and support mother to delivery on no-supine positon, lie on her size if she wants.

- Ensure controlled delivery of the head:
→ Keep one hand gently on the head as it advances with contractions.
→ Support perineum with other hand (hand on) or leave the perineum visible(hand off).
→ Ask the mother to breathe steadily and not to push during delivery of the head.
→ Encourage rapid breathing with mouth open.
- Discard soiled pad to prevent infection.

- Feel gently around baby's neck for the cord.

- Check if the face is clear of mucus and membranes. Gently wipe face clean with gauze or cloth, if necessary.
- If cord present and loose, deliver the baby through the loop of cord or slip the cord over the baby's head; if cord is tight(waiting for shoulders descent and emerge), then clamp and cut cord, then unwind.

经产妇用力超过 1 h 或更长〕没有见明显的胎头下降,报告上级医师,进行评估,必要时胎头吸引助产,或转到上级医院。
- 如果会阴体对分娩形成阻碍(瘢痕、结节、组织增生或有前次分娩三度裂伤史),作一个恰当的会阴侧切。
- 不要常规的会阴侧切
- 如果发现是臀位或其他异常胎位,按相关处理原则处理。

2.4.6.8 娩出胎儿

鼓励并协助产妇在非平卧位分娩。如果她想躺下,协助她取侧卧位分娩。
- 控制胎头的娩出速度:
→用一手(左手)控制胎头娩出。
→另一手垫敷料保护支持会阴体(手扶持保护法)或不用手扶持会阴(不压迫会阴法)。
→胎头着冠要娩出时,让母亲张口哈气不要用力,慢慢娩出胎头。
- 及时更换湿透的敷料以防止感染。
- 胎头娩出后,触摸颈部,判断有无脐带绕颈。
- 清洁面部,擦拭羊水(或胎膜,如果有)。

- 如果脐带绕颈但很松,沿肩部滑下或自胎儿头部松解。
如果脐带很紧,首先检查肩部是否下降并娩出,如果肩部已经能够娩出,而脐带松解困难,可结扎切断脐带,娩出胎儿。

Considser leaving cords as they are and delivering the baby "through the loop" unless the cord is extraordinarily tight if you feel you must cut it, then wait until you see the anterior shoulder. The last thing any of us wants to see is a shoulder dystocia after we have already cut the umbilical cord!

Hart G. Waiting for shoulders. Midwifery Today. 1997:32-34.

（有脐带绕颈时），尽可能不要切断脐带，试着滑下或绕过脐带娩出胎儿，除非脐带非常紧。即使你必须切断脐带，也要等待，直到确定前肩娩出。我们最不想看到的事情，就是切断脐带后，发现是肩难产！

Hart G. Waiting for shoulders. Midwifery Today. 1997:32-34.

2.4.6.9 Await spontaneous rotation of shoulders and delivery（within 1-2 minutes）

2.4.6.9 等待肩的自然旋转娩出

Waiting for a contraction after the head in all vaginal deliveries has been shown to markedly reduce shoulder dystocia incidence, as well be clinically beneficial for the fetus.

Hart G. Waiting for shoulders. Midwifery Today. 1997:32-34.

在全部的阴道分娩中（顺产和阴道助产），遵循胎头娩出后等待至少一次宫缩（胎肩自然娩出）的原则，可明显减少肩难产的发生，显示了更好的新生儿结局。

Hart G. Waiting for shoulders. Midwifery Today. 1997:32-34.

- Gentlly deliver shoulder(if the shoulder comes out too quickly, put a little counter presure to control the shoulers).
- Place baby between the thighs of mother, waiting for the pulsation of the cord till ceased before cut the cord.
- Note time of delivery.
- Thoroughly dry the baby immediately. Wipe eyes. Discard wet cloth.

DO NOT leave the baby wet-she/he will become cold.

- Assess baby's breathing while drying.
- If the baby is not crying, observe breathing:
→ breathing well (chest rising)?
→ not breathing or gasping?
- If the baby is not breathing or gasping (unless baby is dead, macerated, severely malformed):
→start new born resuscitation.

- 轻柔地娩出肩部（如果肩娩出速度很快，要适当控制一下，减缓娩出速度）。
- 新生儿娩出后，置于母亲两腿间，等待脐带搏动消失后，再断脐。
- 记录新生儿娩出时间。
- 擦干新生儿后保暖。擦拭清洁眼睛，更换掉湿的包被单。
- 注意不要让新生儿全身湿透，否则体温会很快下降。
- 评估新生儿呼吸。
- 如果新生儿没有哭，观察：呼吸是否良好（有胸部的起伏动作），有无呼吸或呻吟？
- 如果新生儿没有呼吸动作，开始新生儿复苏（除非新生儿死亡，浸软死胎，严重的畸形情况

Call for help—one person should care for the mother.

> Successful resuscitation can occur at the perineum with an intact umbilical cord. A better approach may be to keep the baby unstimulated with cord intact at the perineum, while the nasopharynx is carefully suctioned.
> Mercer, Judith S. Neonatal transitional physiology: a new paradigm. The Journal of Perinatal & Neonatal. 2002,15(4):56-75

Remain calm and explain to the woman that you need her cooperation to try

- Exclude second baby.
- Palpate mother's abdomen.
- If second baby, DO NOT give oxytocin now.
- Deliver the second baby. Manage as in *Multiple pregnancy*.
- Watch for vaginal bleeding.
- Give 10 IU oxytocin IM to the mother.
- If heavy bleeding, repeat oxytocin 10 IU, IM.

Next: If stuck shoulders

Fetal head is delivered, but shoulders are stuck and cannot be delivered.

- Awaiting for shoulders: The principle of waiting for a contraction after the head in all vaginal deliveries(spontaneous birth or assisted dilevery) has been shown to markedly reduce shoulder dystocia incidence, as well be clinically beneficial for the fetus.

HELPERR

- H: Call for additional help.
- E: Explain the problem to the woman and her companion.
- Prepare for new born resuscitation.
- L: Ask the woman to lie on her back while

下不行复苏)。

- 寻求帮助,需要有人专门照顾母亲。

> 在新生儿窒息抢救中,保留脐带不切断是重要的。更合理的做法可能是,让新生儿在产床上不切断脐带,同时完成气管吸引和插管。
> Mercer, Judith S. Neonatal transitional physiology: a new paradigm. The Journal of Perinatal & Neonatal Nursing. 2002,15(4):56-75

第一个胎儿娩出后,常规检查评估:

- 有没有第二个胎儿。
- 检查触摸母亲腹部。
- 如果有第二个胎儿,按双胎分娩处理。不要注射缩宫素。
- 观察阴道出血情况。
- 给予缩宫素 10 IU 肌内注射。
- 如果阴道出血增多,可重复给予缩宫素 10 IU 肌内注射。

附:如果肩难产

胎头娩出后,肩部不能顺利娩出。

- 等待娩肩原则:在所有的阴道分娩中(自然分娩和阴道助产),遵循在胎头娩出后,等待至少一次宫缩的原则,能够明显地降低肩难产的发生率,并对新生儿安全有利。

HELPERR

- H:寻求帮助。
- E:评估产妇,向产妇和家属解释发生的情况。
- 准备抢救新生儿。
- L:产妇双腿屈曲至胸部,陪伴

gripping her legs tightly flexed against her chest, with knees wide apart. Ask the companion or other helper to keep the legs in that position.

- P: Ask an assistant to apply continuous lateral pressure above the pubic area to help the shoulder descent to palvic and delivery.
- E: Perform an adequate episiotomy if it is necessary(not needed if the hand can enter the viginal easily).
- R: Roll the patient, assist her to adopt a kneeling on "all fours" position and ask her companion to hold her steady. This simple change of position is sometimes sufficient to dislodge the impacted shoulder and achieve delivery(the first step when alone).
- R: Introduce the right hand into the vagina along the posterior curve of the sacrum.

- Attempt to deliver the posterior shoulder the right hand to hook the posterior shoulder and arm downwards and forwards through the vagina.
- Complete the rest of delivery as normal.
- If not successful, refer urgently to hospital.
※Do not pull excessively on the head. No lateral pull on the neck!

※Never applying fundus presure at any time of the labour!

2.4.6.10　Clamp and cut the cord

- Clamp the cord close to the perineum once pulsation stops (delayed cord clamping), or after delivery of the placenta.
→ put ties tightly around the cord at 2 cm and 5 cm

人员协助保持这个体位。

- P:助手在耻骨上向腹部侧方加压,协助胎肩旋转入盆。
- E:如果需要,作会阴侧切(如果接产者的手能够容易地进入阴道,没有必要常规侧切)。
- 保持冷静,向产妇解释她可能需要更换另外的姿势(如果原来是在其他体位接产,如平卧或侧卧)。

- R:协助产妇改为手膝支持跪位,让陪伴人员协助产妇保持这个姿势。单纯这个姿势的变化,有可能让嵌顿的肩部松解,自然娩出(这可以作为首选的措施,尤其是一人急救时)。
- R:如果不成功,可尝试旋转娩出后肩。

- 肩部娩出后,常规娩出胎儿。
- 如果不成功,迅速转诊。
※在处理肩难产的过程中,任何时候都要切记:不可过度用力地牵拉胎头! 尤其不要侧向地牵拉胎头并加压!
※无论如何,不要腹部宫底部加压,以免增加新生儿产伤。

2.4.6.10　脐带钳夹和切断脐带

- 等待脐带搏动停止后或胎盘娩出后断脐(延迟脐带结扎)。

→脐带残端留 5 cm 左右,在 2 cm

from baby's abdomen.

→ cut between ties with sterile instrument.

→ observe for oozing blood.

- If blood oozing, place a second tie between the skin and the first tie.

DO NOT apply any substance to the stump. DO NOT bandage or bind the stump.

- Leave baby on the mother's chest in skin-to-skin contact.
- Place identification label.
- Cover the baby, cover the head with a hat.
- If room cool (less than 25 ℃), use additional blanket to cover the mother and baby.
- Encourage initiation of breastfeeding.
- If HIV-positive mother has chosen replacement feeding, feed accordingly.
- Check ARV treatment needed.

> CLINICAL IMPLICATIONS
> - Delayed cord clamping (*e. g.*, up to 3 minutes) after term delivery does not increase the risk of maternal hemorrhage.
> - Delayed cord clamping may improve the baby's iron status.
> - Delayed cord clamping may increase the chances of phototherapy for jaundice.
>
> McDonald SJ, Middleton P. Effect of timing of umbilical cord clamping of term infants on maternal and neonatal outcomes. Cochrane Database of Systematic Reviews, 2008, Issue 2.

和 5 cm 处用线结扎两道。

→用无菌工具(刀片或剪刀)在末端断脐。观察是否有渗血。

- 如果有出血,在皮肤与第一道结之间再次结扎脐带。
- 不要在脐带断端上面涂任何物品,不要包扎和包裹残端(暴露在空气中,或盖宽松的衣物)。
- 断脐后放置新生儿在母亲胸部作皮肤-皮肤的直接接触。
- 系好新生儿身份识别带。
- 盖好新生儿,戴帽子。
- 如果室温低于 25 ℃,增加衣物。
- 鼓励开始母乳喂养。
- 如果是 HIV 阳性,协助母亲选择哺育方法。
- 给予 ARV 抗病毒治疗。

> 临床应用
> - 晚断脐(达到或超过 3 min)在足月儿没有增加母亲产后出血危险。
> - 晚断脐能够改善新生儿的铁储备。
> - 晚断脐有可能增加新生儿光疗的概率(有争议的问题,有的研究不支持这一结论)。
>
> McDonald SJ, Middleton P. Effect of timing of umbilical cord clamping of term infants on maternal and neonatal outcomes. Cochrane Database of Systematic Reviews, 2008, Issue 2

2.4.7 Third stage of labour: deliver the placenta

Third stage of labour is from the delivery of newborn to the placenta delivery. It is ususlly completed no more than 10-15 mins, if after 1hour the placenta does not come out, suspected a delay in third stage of labour manage as on.

2.4.7.1 Controlled cord traction

- Clamp the cord once pulsation stops in new born and hold in one hand.
- Place the other hand just above the woman's pubic bone and stabilize the uterus by applying counter-pressure during controlled cord traction.
- Await a strong uterine contraction(2-3 minutes). Keep slight tension on the cord.
- With the strong uterine contraction, encourage the mother to push and very gently pull downward on the cord to deliver the placenta. Continue to apply counter-pressure to the uterus.

- If the placenta does not descend during 30-40 seconds of controlled cord traction, do not continue to pull on the cord.

　　Gently hold the cord and wait until the uterus is well contracted again;

　　With the next contraction, repeat controlled cord traction with counter-pressure.

　　※ Never apply cord traction (pull) without applying counter traction (push) above the pubic bone on a well-contracted uterus.

- As the placenta delivers, hold the placenta in two hands and gently turn it until the membranes are twisted into a rope. Slowly pull to complete the delivery.
- If the membranes tear, gently examine the upper vagina and cervix wearing sterile/disinfected gloves and use a sponge forceps to remove any pieces of membrane that are present.
- Exam the placenta carefully. If there is incompleted part or broken vessels in the membranes, be careful of accessory placenta(Figure 2-4-2).

2.4.7 第三产程管理:胎盘娩出

第三产程是自胎儿娩出,到胎盘娩出的时间。一般在 10~15 min 内完成。如果超过产后 30 min 胎盘未娩出,怀疑第三产程延长,按相应措施处理。

2.4.7.1 如何正确f 牵拉脐带娩胎盘

- 等待脐带搏动停止后断脐,用手握住脐带。
- 接产者一只手放在母亲耻骨上的腹部,固定子宫,在牵拉脐带的过程中给予反向的对抗力。
- 等待子宫收缩的增强(2~3 min),轻轻地牵拉脐带。
- 在子宫收缩时,鼓励母亲屏气用力,并轻轻地牵拉脐带娩出胎盘。在牵拉过程中,始终注意在腹部的手(固定子宫)给予反向的对抗力。
- 如果经过 30~40 s 的脐带牵拉未见胎盘娩出,不要继续牵拉脐带。轻轻地握住脐带,等待下一次子宫收缩(2~3 min),在下一次子宫收缩,继续轻轻牵拉脐带并给予腹部的反向对抗力。

　　※注意:不要单纯牵拉脐带,而没有给予腹部的反向对抗力!(有子宫内翻的危险!)

- 胎盘娩出至阴道口,用两手握住胎盘,向一个方向轻轻旋转,直到胎膜成为条索状。轻轻向外牵拉完整娩出胎盘胎膜。
- 如果胎膜断裂,戴无菌手套或用无菌卵圆钳取出残留部分。

- 仔细检查胎盘有无缺损,如果有缺失或胎膜上有断裂的血管,要注意胎盘残留(副胎盘),

If, after 30 minutes of giving oxytocin, the placenta is not delivered and the woman is not bleeding：

→Empty bladder.

→Encourage breastfeeding （ to improve uterine contraction）.

→Repeat controlled cord traction.

■ If woman is bleeding，manage as on.

■ If placents is not delivered in another 30 minutes（1 hour after delivery）：

→Remove placenta manually.

→Give appropriate IM/IV antibiotic.

■ If in 1 hour unable to remove placenta：

→Refer the woman to hospital.

→Insert an IV line and give fluids with 20 IU of oxytocin at 30 drops/min during transfer.

※Do not exert excessive traction on the cord.

※Do not squeeze or push the uterus to deliver the placenta.

※Mother and baby at delivery room at least 2 hours postpartum for observation; disposing placenta according to medical waist protocal （ or local protocal）.

报告上级医师，检查处理。副胎盘如图 2-4-2 所示。

如果经过 30 min 后（注意缩宫素后），胎盘未娩出，但产妇没有阴道流血，作如下处理：

→排空膀胱。

→开始母子接触和早吸吮（刺激子宫收缩）。

→重复轻轻地牵拉脐带（同时给予反向的对抗力）。

■ 如果出现阴道流血增多，按相关措施处理。

■ 如果经过另一个 30 min（分娩后 1 h），胎盘仍然未能娩出，尝试徒手取出胎盘，预防性应用恰当的抗生素肌内注射或静脉给药。

■ 如果 1 h 内未能娩出胎盘，则

→转诊产妇到上级医院；

→转运过程中要建立静脉通道，给予 20 IU 缩宫素，30 滴/min 持续。

※注意：切不可过度用力牵拉脐带；

※ 不要用力挤压或下推子宫试图娩出胎盘；

※产后让母亲和新生儿在产房内观察至少 2 h；按正确的方式（医疗废弃物）处理胎盘，或按当地习俗。

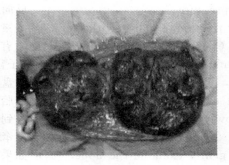

Figure 2-4-2　Succenturiate placenta

图 2-4-2　副胎盘

2.4.7.2　If heavy bleeding

■ Massage uterus to expel clots if any, until it is hard.

→ Give oxytocin 10 IU IM.

2.4.7.2　产后出血紧急处理

■ 按摩子宫排空积血，直到子宫变硬。

→给予 10 IU 缩宫素肌内注射。

→ Call for help.

→ Start an IV line, add 20 IU of oxytocin to IV fluids and give at 60 drops per minute.

→ Empty the bladder.

■ If bleeding persists and uterus is soft:

→ Continue massaging uterus until it is hard.

→ Apply bimanual or aortic compression.

→ Continue IV fluids with 20 IU of oxytocin at 30 drops per minute.

→ Refer woman urgently to hospital.

■ If third degree tear (involving rectum or anus), refer urgently to hospital.

■ For other tears: apply pressure over the tear with a sterile pad or gauze and put legs together.
DO NOT cross ankles.

■ Check after 5 minutes. If bleeding persists, repair the tear.

2.4.7.3　Care of the mother two hours after delivery of placenta

■ Monitor mother at least 2, 3 and 4 hours, then every 4 hours. For emergency signs, using rapid assessment (RAM).

■ Any emergency condition (bleeding, uncomfortable, fever et al.).

■ Feel uterus if hard and round.

■ Record findings, treatments and procedures in labour record.

■ Keep the mother and baby together.

■ Never leave the woman and newborn alone.

■ Ensure the mother has sanitary napkins or clean material to collect vaginal blood.

■ Encourage the mother to eat drink and rest. Ensure the room is warm (25 ℃).

→呼叫协助。

→建立静脉通道,另外加 20 IU 缩宫素,以 60 滴/min 速度给药。

→排空膀胱。

■ 如果阴道持续出血,子宫很软:

→继续按摩子宫直到变硬。

→应用双手加压按摩子宫(一手在阴道内),或腹主动脉加压。

→继续静脉滴注 20 IU 缩宫素,以 30 滴/min 速度给药。

→及时转诊到上级医院(或请求会诊)。

■ 如果有三度裂伤(直肠或肛门损伤),及时转诊(或请求会诊)。

■ 检查有其他裂伤(会阴或阴道):用无菌敷料或海棉压迫伤口,并起大腿(注意是两腿并行而不是交叉)。

■ 5 min 后再次检查,如果仍有出血,进行缝合止血。

2.4.7.3　产后 2 h 后产妇观察照顾

■ 自产后 1 h(产妇送出产房后到爱婴区)至少在第 2、3、4 小时观察评估 1 次。然后,至少每 4 h 评估观察一次。

■ 有无紧急情况(出血,不适,发热等)?

■ 按摩子宫,硬度和形状(硬圆子宫)。

■ 在产程图上记录。

■ 保持母婴同室。

■ 不要让母亲和新生儿单独在房间里(有陪同人员)。

■ 检查评估母亲是否有干净的卫生巾来收集阴道出血。

■ 鼓励母亲进食、饮水和休息。

■ 保持房间温暖(25 ℃)。

- Ask the mother's companion to watch her and call for help if bleeding or pain increases, if mother feels dizzy or has severe headaches, visual disturbance or epigastric distress.

- Encourage the mother to empty her bladder and ensure that she has passed urine within 6 hours after delivery.
- Check record and give any treatment or prophylaxis which is due.
- If HIV-positive: give her appropriate treatment.
- If heavy vaginal bleeding, palpate the uterus.
- → If uterus not firm, massage the fundus to make it contract and expel any clots.
- → If pad is soaked in less than 5 minutes, manage as on.
- → If bleeding is from perineal tear, repair or refer to hospital.
- If the mother cannot pass urine or the bladder is full (swelling over lower abdomen) and she is uncomfortable, help her by gently pouring water on vulva.
DO NOT catheterize unless you have to.

- If mother is on antibiotics because of rupture of membranes ＞ 18 hours but shows no signs of infection now, discontinue antibiotics.

- Advise the mother on postpartum care and nutrition.
- Counsel on birth spacing and other family planning methods.
- Advise when to seek care.
- Keep the mother at the facility for 12 hours after delivery. Never discharged mother before 12hours after delivery.
- Repeat examination of the mother.

- 指导产妇的陪伴人员,出现下列情况时及时报告医务人员:
  阴道出血增加;
  严重的疼痛;
  母亲感到头晕目眩;
  严重头痛;
  眼花或胃部不适。
- 鼓励母亲及时排空膀胱,注意产后已经排尿(产后 6 h 内)。

- 检查病历是否需要预防性应用抗生素。
- 如果 HIV 阳性,给予正规治疗。
- 如果产后出血,按摩子宫。
- →如果子宫松软,按摩子宫直到变硬,排空子宫内积血。
- →如果卫生巾在 5 min 内湿透(提示出血较多),按摩子宫。
- →如果是会阴部裂伤出血,进行缝合止血。
- 如果母亲不能自行排尿,膀胱膨胀(下腹部可触及),可用温水冲洗会阴部协助排尿。
- 如果其他方法能够诱导排尿,不要用导尿管(如果需要导尿,不要留置)。
- 如果母亲产前因为早破膜大于 18 h 而接受了预防性的抗生素,但产后没有感染的表现,停用抗生素。
- 进行产后照顾健康教育和营养指导。
- 咨询家庭避孕计划。

- 告之要返回医院的情况(见上)。
- 母亲产后至少住院 12 h 观察(不要早于 12 h 出院)。

- 出院前再次检查评估产妇。

出生时脐部处理（晚断脐，无菌结扎）	
Cleaness 清洁环境	Wash hands with clean water and soap before delivery and before cutting/tying cord 处理脐带前后洗手 Clean surface to receive baby 新生儿出生后放置到清洁的表面 Wear gloves (institutions) 操作者戴手套
When to cut/clamp the cord 断脐时机	Wait until cord stops pulsating or placenta is delivered 在脐带搏动停止后或胎盘娩出后结扎脐带
What kind of ties 结扎用品	Clean string ties, threads or narrow tapes, at least 15 cm in length, tied tightly in 2 places (infant end and maternal end) 消毒的线（或夹，橡胶圈）
Length of stump left 脐带残端的长度	2-3 cm or longer, according to local custom 脐带的长度：留 2～3 cm 或更长，推荐留 4～5 cm 过短的脐带残端会回缩至脐窝，容易存水，增加感染，不利护理
Cutting instrument 切断脐带的工具	Sterile scissors or blade 用无菌的剪刀或刀片断脐
Topical antimicrobial on stump after cutting cord 脐带断端是否需要消毒和抗生素	None unless necessary, as a temporary measure, according to local situation (*e. g.* in neonatal tetanus endemic areas, or to replace a harmful traditional substance) 不需要，除非有必要（如在破伤风高感染区域，或用来取代有害的传统包扎方法）

Postnatal Care of Cord Stump
出生后的脐带护理：清洁干燥护理法(dry and clean)

Cleanliness and protection from contamination 保持清洁 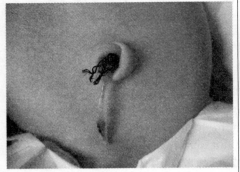	Wash hands with clean water and soap before and after care 护理新生儿前后要洗手 Keep the stump exposed to air or loosely covered with clean clothes 保持脐带暴露在空气中或覆盖宽松的清洁的衣服 Fold napkin below stump 尿布边缘折叠在脐带残端以下 Avoid applying unclean substances, touching the cord and covering it with bandages 避免涂任何不清洁的物质，不用手触摸脐带，不包扎
Beneficial practices that may decrease the risk of cord infection 有利的措施	Keep the baby with the mother (in institutions：24-hour rooming-in, no nurseries), skin-to-skin contact, early and frequent breast-feeding 保持母婴接触，24 h 的母婴同室，出生时立即母子接触，频繁多次地母乳吸吮
How to clean the cord when soiled 脐部污染时(如尿湿)如何清洁 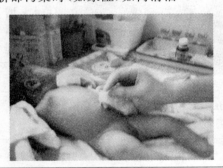	Wash with clean water and soap, dry thoroughly 用清洁的水和肥皂清洁，然后充分晾干 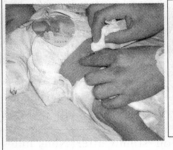脐带脱落后，仍然要注意保持干燥，每次换尿布时注意观察，有汗湿或尿湿，及时用清洁纸巾或毛巾擦干。要教会产妇及家属如何护理脐部
Topical antimicrobials on cord stump 脐带残端的局部抗菌剂	None unless necessary, according to local situation (e. g. in neonatal tetanus endemic areas, or to replace a harmful traditional substance) as a temporary measure 不需要，只在必要时应用，如在一个破伤风高发地区，或要替换有害的包扎物品时，作为一个应急的措施

Case Analysis

Nulliparas，age 24，39^{+2} weeks pregnancy，stating low abdominal pain with light viginal show for half day，being admission to inpatient unit at 16th of June in 2012. She had normal procedure during pragnancy. Check up during the admissions had no abnormal finding. Single fetues，vertical presentation.

The low abdominal pain was unregular throught the night of admission，she did not sleep well.

2012-6-17 morning round check up had found her cervical of uterus did not dialated.

At 10：00，artificial rupture of the membrane，amino fluid is clear.

（Bishop score is 5，50% afficiment，soft，at middle，the discent of presentation is S-2）

At 11：00，pethidine 50 mg im，for suspected anxiaty.

At 12：30，the woman can not pass urine，catherter is serted once.

At 14：00，cervical dialation of uterus is of 2 cm，S-2.

At 15：30，sending the woman to delivery room.

16：30 cervical dialation of uterus is of 4 cm.

17：30 cervical dialation of uterus is of 4 cm，S0. Oxtocin introvenous drip for uterus contraction augementation.

18：30 cervical dialation of uterus is of 5 cm. Clear amino fluid.

19：15 cervical dialation of uterus is of 7 cm，swelling of the cervical. Atropine 0.5mg cervical injection.

19：25 full dialation of the cervical，S+2.

19：35 fetus heart beat 100 bpm. Aminophylline 0.25 g，saline solution 20 ml，IV.

病例分析

初产妇，24 岁，39^{+2} 周下腹痛伴见红半天于 2012 年 6 月 16 日入院。孕前定期产检无殊。入院检查无异常发现。单胎，纵产式。

入院时腹痛不规则，当日晚腹痛不规则，一夜睡眠不佳。

第二日查房，宫口未开。

于上午 10 点钟给予人工破膜，羊水清（宫颈评分 5 分，宫口未开，容受 50%，宫颈软，中位，S-2）。

11 点 给予哌替啶 50 mg，肌内注射。

12：30 宫口 1.5 cm，12：45 自解小便困难，给予导尿一次。

14：00 宫口开大 2 cm，S-2。

15：30 宫口开大 3 cm，送入产房。

16：30 宫口 4 cm。

17：30 宫口 4 cm，S0。宫缩强度不足。给予滴催产素加强宫缩。

18：30 宫口 5 cm。羊水清。

19：15 宫口 7 cm，宫颈水肿，给予阿托品 0.5 mg 宫颈注射。

19：25 宫口开全，S+2。

19：35 左右胎心下降，100 bpm，持续 1 min。给予氨茶碱 0.25 g+NS 20 ml IV，上台准备接产。

19：44 delivery of the baby, weight 2920 g, Apgar score 5 at 1 min, 10 at 5 mins.

Ananysis：

（1）Is the woman in labour at admission to hospital ?

（2）Does the interventions in this case corret or not , why?

（3）If you are the doctor of this woman , what should do from the beginning?

19：44 娩一女婴，2920 g。阿普加评分 5 分，10 分。

分析：

（1）产妇入院时是否临产？

（2）产程中的处理措施是否妥当? 请提出存在的问题，并分析。

（3）如果是你接诊这位孕妇，你会如何处理？

Test

1. Which of the following is the best practice for normal labor?　　（　）
   A. Supine position in second stage of labor
   B. Routine episiotomy
   C. Routine pubic shaving
   D. Skilled attendant
   E. Pushing at the passive stage of second labor

2. Which of the followings are the harmful practices for normal labor?　　（　）
   A. Encourage free of movement during labor
   B. Pushing at active stage of labor on women's willing
   C. No pharmacy pain relief during labor
   D. Routine artifical rupture of the membrane at the first stage of labor
   E. Encourage liquid taking oral during labor

3. The active stage of labor in the first stage（established labor）is from the dilation of the uterus at：　　（　）
   A. 2 cm
   B. 3 cm
   C. 4 cm
   D. 7 cm
   E. 10 cm

4. If, women defined as delay in second stage of labor, which interventions should be encouraged and performed　　（　）
   A. Hydration
   B. Encourage position change
   C. Supine position in labor bed
   D. Routine episiotomy
   E. Amniotomy when women with intact membrane

5. When caring women in second stage of labor, which of the interventions should be forbiddend　　（　）
   A. Urge women to push when in passive stage of labaor
   B. Restrict liquid taking to void vomiting
   C. Supine position for delivery
   D. Routine episiotomy
   E. Encourage position change

6. The right timing to clamping the umbilical cord after birth are at 　　（　）
   A. 10 second after birth
   B. 30 second after birth
   C. When pulsing of the cord ceased
   D. When pulsing ceased or after the placenta delivered
   E. Waiting for placenta delivery when heavy bleeding occur

7. Skin to skin contact is defined as　　（　）

A. Wrapping baby with clothes and putting on abdomen of mother's

B. Putting baby on mother's abdomen after 10 hours after birth

C. Putting baby on mother's abdomen with 30 minute after birth Not wrapping of clothes.

D. Putting baby on mother's abdomen when baby is asphyxia

E. No skin to skin contact when baby is preterm

8. Delay in the active second stage of labor is defined as

9. What is suportive care during the labour?

10. How to care of the umbilical cord after birth when it soiled?

Reference answer

Case Analysis：

（1）The woman was not in labour when admission to hospital，the current evidence did not support this diagnosis.

（2）The following interventions in this case may not be necessary，since the woman is not actually in labour.

（3）The adquate management of this woman would be carefully assessement of the woman and fetus，if there is no situation of abnormal，the woman is better back to home and waiting for the natural onset of the labour.

病例分析：

(1)产妇入院时没有临产,目前的证据不支持产妇临产的诊断。

(2)因为产妇尚未真正临产,随后的多项措施可能都不是必须的,没有充足的理由的。

(3)该产妇在入院时应当给予详细全面的评估,如果产妇和胎儿情况良好,应当返回家休息,等待真正的自然临产过程。

Test

1. D 2. D 3. C 4. ABE
5. ABCD 6. CD 7. C
8. A diagnosis of delay in the active second stage (from 1 full dialation of the cervical and women starting spountneous pushing to the delivery of the baby) should be made when it has lasted 2 hours in Primipara，and 1 hour in parous women. women should be referred to a healthcare

1. D 2. D 3. C 4. ABE
5. ABCD 6. CD 7. C
8. 第二产程活跃期延长的诊断(从宫口开全并且产妇开始自主的屏气用力,到胎儿娩出的时间),初产妇持续超过 2 h,经产妇持续超过 1 h。产妇应当转介到有经验的产科专家,

professional trained to undertake an evaluated their labor and birth imminent.

9. Supportive care during labour is to to provide a supportive, encouraging atmosphere for birth, respectful of the woman's wishes. including the following aspect as communication, physiological and pchyological care, help of urination, eating, drinking, encourage of breathing technique, suggest change of position. Encourage mobility, as comfortable for her.

10. (1) Wash your hand before and after care of the baby.
    (2) Wash the baby's umbilical cord with clean water and soap, dry thoroughly with clean towers or toilet papers.

2.5　Normal Puerperium

Key words

1. puerperium
2. placenta
3. postpartum bleeding
4. genital tract infection
5. breast feeding
6. lochia
7. family planning
8. episiotomy
9. umbilical care
10. retained placenta

2.5.1　Puerperium

The puerperium is the period from the end of the third stage of labour until most of the patient's organs have returned to their pre-pregnant state and lasts for 6 weeks. Almost every organ undergoes change in the puerperium. These adjustments range from mild to marked. Only those changes which are

进行评估。

9. 产程中的支持性照顾,是指给予产妇生理、心理和精神支持,包括创造良好的促进顺产分娩的氛围,尊重产妇的自我意愿,包括加强交流沟通,给予生理心理支持,协助排泄,给予饮食支持,鼓励呼吸放松,鼓励产妇活动,协助取自感舒适的体位并不断改变。

10. (1) 在照顾新生儿前后洗手。
(2) 如果新生儿脐部尿湿或其他污染,用清水和肥皂清洁,然后用干净清洁的毛巾或卫生纸彻底擦拭干燥。

2.5　正常产褥

关键词

1. 产褥期
2. 胎盘
3. 产后出血
4. 生殖道感染
5. 母乳喂养
6. 恶露
7. 计划生育
8. 会阴侧切
9. 脐带护理
10. 胎盘滞留

2.5.1　产褥期

产褥期是指从胎盘娩出后,直到产妇各器官基本恢复至正常水平的一段时间,一般为6周。全身各个器官几乎都有相应的变化,下面描述的只是其中比较明显和重要的变化情况。

important in the management of the normal puerperium will be described here：

2.5.1.1　Immediately after the delivery of the placenta

- Assess whether the uterus is well contracted.
- Assess whether vaginal bleeding appears more than normal.
- Record the patient's pulse rate, blood pressure and temperature.

2.5.1.2　Care for the first hour after the delivery of the placenta

- Continuously assess whether the uterus is well contracted and that no excessive vaginal bleeding is present.
- Repeat the measurement of the pulse rate and blood pressure after 1 hour.
- If the patient's condition changes, observations must be done more frequently until the patient's condition returns to normal.
- After the placenta has been delivered the patient needs to be：
→ Washed and cleaned, kept in warm and comfortable environment.
→ Given something to drink and to eat.
→ Allowed to bond with her infant.
→ Allowed to rest for as long as she needs to.
- She should be told that if the uterine fundus rises or the uterus relaxes or if vaginal bleeding increases, she must：
→ Immediately call the midwife.
→ In the meantime rub up the uterus.

2.5.1.3　Care before discharged home after delivery

The following examinations of mother are performed before discharge：
- Pulse rate.
- Blood pressure.
- Temperature.
- Haemoglobin concentration.
- An abdominal examination, paying.

2.5.1.1　产后即刻护理

- 评估子宫收缩情况是否良好。
- 评估阴道流血是否多于正常。
- 测量记录产妇的脉搏、血压和体温。

2.5.1.2　产后第一小时照顾

- 继续评估观察子宫收缩和阴道流血情况。
- 继续观察产妇的生命体征并记录。
- 如果产妇有异常表现（如出血量增多），要增加观察次数，直到产妇病情转为正常。
- 胎盘娩出后，产妇要给予如下照顾：
→ 擦拭清洁身体并保持温暖和舒适的环境；
→ 给予饮料或食物；
→ 接触拥抱新生儿；
→ 让产妇充分的休息。
- 告知产妇，如果她发现子宫底升高或子宫很软，或阴道出血量增多，她要：
→ 立即通知报告助产士。
→ 同时要自己按摩子宫。

2.5.1.3　出院前护理

在产妇出院前，必须进行以下检查：
- 产妇脉搏。
- 血压。
- 体温。
- 血色素水平。
- 腹部触诊检查。

- Particular attention to the state of contraction and/or tenderness of the uterus.
- An inspection of the episiotomy site and the amount, colour and odour of the lochia.
- To arrange for suitable contraception before the patient is discharged home.
- Ask if the patient passes urine normally and enquire about any urinary symptoms.
- Reassure the patient if she has not passed a stool by day 5.
- Assess the condition of the patient's breasts and nipples must be assessed. Determine whether successful breast feeding has been established.

2.5.1.4　Observations on the infant

- Assess whether the infant appears well and is thriving.
- Check whether the infant is jaundiced.

- Examine the umbilical stump for.
- Signs of infection(Figure 2-5-1).
- Examine the eyes for conjunctivitis.
- Ask whether the infant has passed urine and stool.
- Assess whether the infant is feeding well and is satisfied after a feed.

- 特别注意子宫收缩情况和宫底的高度。
- 检查会阴侧切伤口情况，有无出血、血肿等。
- 与产妇及家属讨论确定适合的避孕方法。
- 评估产妇是否已经排尿，有没有排尿困难等表现。
- 评估产妇最近 5 天内是否排过大便。
- 评估产妇乳房及乳头的情况，评估产妇是否成功进行母乳喂养。

2.5.1.4　新生儿护理

- 评估新生儿的情况，是否有活力反应良好。
- 评估新生儿有无黄疸及严重程度。
- 检查脐部有无感染现象，如图 2-5-1 所示。
- 检查眼睛，有无结膜炎。
- 评估新生儿有无排尿、排便。
- 评估新生儿喂养情况，是否母乳量充足能够满足营养需要。

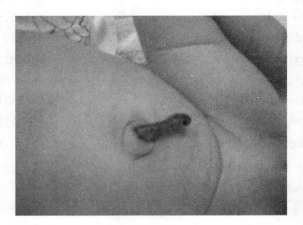

Figure 2-5-1　Normal dry umbilical cord residue

图 2-5-1　正常清洁干燥的脐带残端

2.5.1.5　Postpartum education

(1)General

■ Advise on postpartum care and hygiene.

■ Advise and explain to the woman：

→To always have someone near her for the first 24 hours to respond to any change in her condition.

→Not to insert anything into the vagina.

→To have enough rest and sleep.

■ Advise on the importance of washing to prevent infection of the mother and her baby：

→wash hands before handling baby.

→wash perineum daily and after faecal excretion.

→change perineal pads frequently if heavy lochia.

→dispose used pads safely.

→wash the body daily.

■ To avoid sexual intercourse until the perineal wound heals.

(2)Counsel on nutrition

■ Advise the woman to eat a greater amount and variety of healthy foods, such as meat, fish, oils, nuts, cereals, beans, vegetables, cheese, milk, to help her feel well and strong, give examples of types of food and how much to eat.

■ Reassure the mother that she can eat any normal foods- these will not harm the breastfeeding baby.

■ Spend more time on nutrition counselling with very thin women and adolescents.

■ Determine if there are important taboos about foods which are nutritionally healthy. Advise the woman against these taboos.

■ Talk to family members such as partner and mother-in-law, to encourage them to help ensure the woman eats enough and avoids hard physical

2.5.1.5　产褥期健康教育

(1)一般护理

■ 指导产妇产后护理及卫生清洁。

■ 指导产妇要注意以下方面：

→产后 24 h 内要有人陪伴，以免有意外情况。

→不要塞任何用品到阴道内（不要用内用的卫生巾）。

→保证足够的休息与睡眠。

■ 解释正确的洗手和清洁方法，保护母亲和新生儿，预防感染。

→抱婴儿前洗手。

→每日清洁会阴部，并在大小便后清洁。

→及时更换一次卫生垫。

→更换后的卫生垫及时丢弃。

→母亲产后每日沐浴清洁。

■ 在会阴伤口没有愈合前，避免性生活。

(2)营养咨询

■ 告之母亲要进食多样化的健康食品，例如肉类、鱼、油、干果、谷物、豆类、各种蔬菜、乳酪、奶制品，保持健康强壮的体质，告之她具体的可以进食的食物和进食的量。

■ 告知母亲她可以吃任何种类的健康食物，这不会影响到哺乳。

■ 对哪些比较瘦小的母亲和青少年妈妈要花更多的时间进行营养咨询。

■ 询问是否有关于食物的不良禁忌（哪些营养丰富但却禁忌吃的习惯，例如不吃水果等），告知母亲不要遵守这些禁忌。

■ 与家庭成员（丈夫、婆婆等）交流，鼓励她们要支持母亲保持健康足够的食物，避免重体力

work.

(3)Counsel on the importance of family planning

■ If appropriate, ask the woman if she would like her partner or another family member to be included in the counselling session.

■ Explain that after birth, if she has sex, she can become pregnant as soon as 4 weeks after delivery. Therefore it is important to start thinking early aboutwhat family planning method they will use.

■ Ask about plans for having more children. If she (and her partner) want more children, advise that waiting at least 2-3 years between pregnancies is healthier for the mother and child.

■ Councel on safer sex including use of condoms for dual protection from sexually transmitted infection (STI) or HIV and pregnancy.

■ Her partner can decide to have a vasectomy (male sterilization) at any time.

■ Lactational amenorrhoea method (LAM).

■ A breastfeeding woman is protected from pregnancy only if she is no more than 6 months postpartum, and she is breastfeeding exclusively (8 or more times a day, including at least once at night),andher menstrual cycle has not returned.

(4)Advise on danger signs

　　Advise to go to a hospital or health centre immediately, day or night, WITHOUT WAITING if any of the following signs:

■ vaginal bleeding:

→ more than 2 or 3 pads soaked in 20-30 minutes after delivery OR.

→ bleeding increases rather than decreases after delivery.

■ convulsions.

■ fast or difficult breathing.

■ fever and too weak to get out of bed.

劳动。

(3)计划生育避孕措施咨询

■ 如果可能,征求妈妈的意见,是否让丈夫或其他的家庭成员参加避孕措施的咨询。

■ 向母亲解答,如果她有正常的性生活,产后4周就可能再次怀孕,所以要及时采取有效的避孕措施。

■ 咨询是否有计划要更多的小孩,建议间隔2～3年时间,这样对母亲和孩子都有利。

■ 咨询健康性行为,避孕套的应用,有关避孕套的作用和预防性传播疾病的作用。

■ 丈夫可选择男性避孕方法,例如输精管结扎术等,没有时间性限制。

■ 关于哺乳期避孕法:产后6个月内,如果产妇完全母乳喂养(每天有8次或更多次数的哺乳,并且晚上至少哺乳1次),在月经周期未恢复之前,她可能不容易受孕,这称为哺乳期避孕法(LAM)

(4)告之产妇及家人需要产后返回医院的紧急情况

　　告知如果出现下列情况,不管是白天还是晚上,都要紧急返院处理:

■ 阴道流血

→产后20～30 min内有2～3块卫生巾被湿透。

→产后阴道出血量继续增多,而不是逐渐减少。

■ 出现抽搐。

■ 呼吸困难。

■ 发热或太虚弱而不能起床。

- severe abdominal pain.

Go to health centre as soon as possible if any of the following signs：

- fever.
- abdominal pain.
- feels ill.
- breasts swollen，red or tender breasts，or sore nipple.
- urine dribbling or pain on micturition.
- pain in the perineum or draining pus.
- foul-smelling lochia.

Discuss how to prepare for an emergency in postpartum.

- Advise to always have someone near for at least 24 hours after delivery to respond to any change incondition.
- Advise the woman to ask for help from the community，if needed.
- Advise the woman to bring her home-based maternal record to the health centre，even for an emergency visit.
- Arrangement of home visit.
- First visit Within the first week，preferably within 2-3 days.
- Second visit(4-6 weeks).

2.5.1.6　Postpartum bleeding

If heavy postpartum bleeding persists after placenta is delivered，or uterus is not well contracted (is soft)：

(1)Uterus massage

- Empty the bladder.
- Place cupped palm on uterine fundus and feel for state of contraction.
- Massage fundus in a circular motion with cupped palm until uterus is well contracted.
- When well contracted，place fingers behind fundus and push down in one swift action to expel clots.

- 严重的腹部疼痛。

出现下列情况也要及时到医院就诊：

- 发热。
- 腹痛。
- 感到不适。
- 乳头水肿，发红，触痛或乳头疼痛。
- 排尿困难或排尿疼痛。
- 会阴疼痛或有脓性分泌物排出。
- 恶露有异味、发臭。

与家人讨论如果出现异常情况，如何寻求紧急帮助。

- 在产后 24 h 内，要随时有人陪伴，以防意外情况发生。

- 如果有必要，到社区医院寻求帮助。
- 告知即使在紧急情况下，也要记得带病历卡。

- 产后随访安排。
- 产后第 1 次随访时间在产后一周，通常是第 2～3 天。
- 产后第 2 次随访(4～6 周)。

2.5.1.6　产后出血

如果胎盘娩出后持续出血，或子宫收缩不良(子宫松软)：

(1)子宫按摩

- 排空膀胱。
- 手掌弯成杯状置于宫底部，触摸感知子宫收缩状态。
- 用手掌环状按摩子宫直到子宫收缩良好。
- 当子宫收缩良好后，手指置于子宫后握住子宫(拇指在前)，轻轻挤压排出宫腔内积血。

- Collect blood in a container placed close to the vulva. Measure or estimate blood loss, and record.
- Apply bimanual uterine compression.
- If heavy postpartum bleeding persists despite uterine massage, oxytocin/ergometrine treatment and removal of placenta.

(2)bimanual compression

- Wear sterile or clean gloves.
- Introduce the right hand into the vagina, clenched fist, with the back of the hand directed posteriorly and the knuckles in the anterior fornix.
- Place the other hand on the abdomen behind the uterus and squeeze the uterus firmly between the two hands.
- Continue compression until bleeding stops (no bleeding if the compression is released).

(3)Aortic compression

　　If bleeding persists, apply aortic compression and transport woman to hospital.

- Apply aortic compression.
- Feel for femoral pulse.
- Apply pressure above the umbilicus to stop bleeding. Apply sufficient pressure until femoral pulse is not felt.
- After finding correct site, show assistant or relative how to apply pressure, if necessary.

- Continue pressure until bleeding stops. If bleeding persists, keep applying pressure while transporting woman to hospital.

(4)Give oxytocin

- If heavy postpartum bleeding Give oxytocin 10 IU IM.
- Call for help.
- Start an IV line, add 20 IU of oxytocin to IV fluids and give at 60 drops per minute.
- Continue IV fluids with 20 IU of oxytocin at 30

- 用容器收集排出血液,估计失血量,并记录。
- 必要时给予双手压迫子宫按摩。
- 如果按摩后仍然持续性子宫出血,给予缩宫素/麦角新碱,并考虑手取胎盘。

(2)双手按摩压迫子宫止血

- 戴无菌手套,常规消毒。
- 右手伸入阴道,握拳,手背朝向阴道后壁,其他指节在前方。

- 左手在腹部,从子宫后方挤压子宫在两手之间。

- 持续加压,直到阴道出血停止(如果解除按压,不再有出血)。

(3)动脉按压

　　如果出血仍然持续,给予动脉按压止血并迅速转送产妇到医院。

- 给予动脉按压。
- 触诊到股动脉的搏动。
- 在脐部上加压以减少出血,给予足够的压力直到触诊股动脉的搏动消失(不能触及)。
- 找到正确的按压部位后,示范给助手,以便助手必要时给予协助。

- 持续给予按压直到出血停止。如果出血持续,在转运产妇到上级医院的路途中要持续给予按压!

(4)缩宫素应用

- 产后出血较多时,给予缩宫素 10 IU 肌内注射。
- 寻求帮助。
- 建立静脉通路,加入缩宫素 20 IU 静滴,60 滴/min。
- 持续给予缩宫素 20 IU 维持,

drops per minute.

(5)Manually Remove placenta

If placenta not delivered 1 hour after delivery of the baby, OR If heavy vaginal bleeding continues despite massage and oxytocin and placenta cannot be delivered by controlled cord traction, or if placenta is incomplete and bleeding continues.

Preparation

- Explain to the woman the need for manual removal of the placenta and obtain her consent.
- Insert an IV line. If bleeding, give fluids rapidly. If not bleeding, give fluids slowly.

- Assist woman to get onto her back.
- Give diazepam (10mg IM/IV).

- Clean vulva and perineal area.
- Ensure the bladder is empty. Catheterize if necessary.
- Wash hands and forearms well and put on long sterile gloves (and an apron or gown if available).

Technique of manual removal of the placenta

- With the left hand hold the umbilical cord and pull the cord gently until it is horizontal.
- Insert right hand into the vagina and up into the uterus(Figure 2-5-2).
- Leave the cord and hold the fundus with the left hand in order to support the fundus of the uterus and to provide counter-traction during removal.

- Move the fingers of the right hand sideways until edge of the placenta is located.
- Detach the placenta from the implantation site by keeping the fingers tightly together and using the edge of the hand to gradually make a space between the placenta and the uterine wall.
- Proceed gradually all around the placental bed until the whole placenta is detached from the uterine wall.

30 滴/min。

(5)徒手取出胎盘及残留物

如果胎儿娩出后 1 h 胎盘未能自动娩出,或者出现较多阴道流血,给予按摩和缩宫素注射后,牵拉脐带仍然不能协助娩出胎盘,或胎盘检查时发现不全娩出,出血持续,准备手取胎盘。

准备

- 向产妇解释需要手工取胎盘,获知情同意签字。
- 建立静脉通道,快速给予液体补充;如果没有阴道流血,缓慢输液维持。
- 协助产妇取平卧位。
- 给予地西泮(安定)10 mg IM/IV。
- 清洁消毒会阴大腿内侧。
- 排空膀胱,必要时插尿管。
- 按规范洗手及前臂,戴长袖手套(和围裙或长袍,如果有准备)。

手取胎盘操作

- 左手牵拉脐带,直到脐带伸展水平位。
- 右手伸入阴道直到宫缩内。

- 放开牵拉脐带的左手,左手在腹部握住子宫底,在手取胎盘过程中支持宫底,给予反向的对抗力。
- 右手掌在宫腔内试探,找到胎盘的边缘。
- 手指并拢,用手掌的边缘分离胎盘与宫壁。

- 沿胎盘周边逐渐完整地分离胎盘与子宫壁,直到胎盘完整分离。

- Withdraw the right hand from the uterus gradually, bringing the placenta with it.
- Explore the inside of the uterine cavity to ensure all placental tissue has been removed.
- With the left hand, provide counter-traction to the fundus through the abdomen by pushing it in the opposite direction of the hand that is being withdrawn. This prevents inversion of the uterus (Figure 2-5-2).

- 慢慢地从宫腔退出右手,握住胎盘一起取出。
- 再次探查宫腔有无胎盘残留。

- 右手取胎盘退出宫腔的过程中,左手要在腹部握住子宫,给予反向的对抗力,这有助于预防子宫的翻出。操作如图 2-5-2 所示。

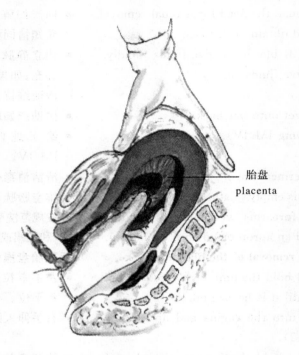

胎盘
placenta

Figure 2-5-2　Manual removal of the placenta

图 2-5-2　手取胎盘操作

- Examine the uterine surface of the placenta to ensure that lobes and membranes are complete. If any placental lobe or tissue fragments are missing, explore again the uterine cavity to remove them.
- If hours or days have passed since delivery, or if the placenta is retained due to constriction ring or closed cervix, it may not be possible to put the hand into the uterus. DO NOT persist. Referurgently to hospital.

- 检查胎盘的母体面(子宫面),小叶和胎膜是否完整,如果有残留,再次探查宫腔取出。

- 如果产妇是在分娩后数小时或数天入院(胎盘未娩出),或胎盘是因为有缩窄环或宫颈口已经关闭而不能娩出,手不能进入宫腔,不要强行进行剥离,迅速转送上级医院。

- After manual removal of the placenta Repeat oxytocin 10 IU IM/IV.
- Massage the fundus of the uterus to encourage a tonic uterine contraction.
- Give ampicillin 2 g IV/IM.

- If fever ＞38.5 ℃, foul-smelling lochia or history of rupture of membranes for 18 or more hours, also give gentamicin 80 mg IM.

If bleeding stops:
- give fluids slowly for at least 1 hour after removal of placenta.

If heavy bleeding continues:
- give ergometrine 0.2 mg IM.
- give 20 IU oxytocin in each litre of IV fluids and infuse rapidly.
- Refer urgently to hospital.

　　※ If the placenta does not separate from the uterine surface by gentle sideways movement of the fingertips at the line of cleavage, suspect placenta accreta.

　　※ DO NOT persist in efforts to remove placenta. Refer urgently to hospital.

　　During transportation, feel continuously whether uterus is well contracted (hard and round). If not,

- massage and repeat oxytocin 10 IU IM/IV.

- Provide bimanual or aortic compression.

2.5.1.7 Repair the tear or episiotomy

- Examine the tear and determine the degree:
→ The tear is small and involved only vaginal mucosa and connective tissues and underlying muscles (first or second degree tear). If the tear is not bleeding, leave the wound open.

- 手取出胎盘后,给予缩宫素 10 IU IM/IV。
- 按摩子宫,直至收缩良好。

- 预防性应用氨苄青霉素 2 g IV/IM。
- 如果有发热,恶露有异味,有超过 18 h 或更长时间的胎膜早破史,给予先锋霉素(gentamicin)80 mg IM。

如果出血停止:
- 缓慢静脉输液,手取胎盘后至少维持 1 h 以上。

如果持续阴道出血:
- 肌注麦角新碱 0.2 mg IM。
- 给予缩宫素 20 IU 静脉快速滴注。
- 迅速转诊到上级医院

　　※ 如果手取胎盘过程中手掌的轻轻剥离动作不能很好地分离胎盘,考虑胎盘植入。

　　※不要试图用力地分离胎盘。迅速转送产妇到上级医院。

　　在转运产妇到上级医院的过程中,要持续地评估按摩子宫,是否收缩良好(硬和圆的),如果收缩不好:
- 按摩子宫并重复给予缩宫素 10 IU IM/IV。
- 给予双手经阴道压迫子宫或压迫动脉止血。

2.5.1.7 修复会阴裂伤

- 检查评估裂伤程度
→一度、二度裂伤:仅有阴道黏膜和皮下组织的损伤(一度),和皮下肌肉层的损伤(二度)。如果裂伤没有活动性出血,开放

→ The tear is long and deep through the perineum and involves the anal sphincter and rectal mucosa (third and fourth degree tear). Cover it with a clean pad and refer the woman urgently to hospital.

■ If first or second degree tear and heavy bleeding persists after applying pressure over the wound:

→ Suture the tear or refer for suturing if no one is available with suturing skills.

→ Suture the tear using universal precautions, aseptic technique and sterile equipment.

→ Use a needle holder and a 21 cm, 4 gauge, curved needle.

→ Use absorbable polyglycon suture material.

→ Make sure that the apex of the tear is reached before you begin suturing.

→ Ensure that edges of the tear match up well.

■ Empty bladder.

■ If bladder is distended and the woman is unable to pass urine, Encourage the woman to urinate.

■ If she is unable to urinate, catheterize the bladder:

→ Wash hands.

→ Clean urethral area with antiseptic.

→ Put on clean gloves.

→ Spread labia. Clean area again.

→ Insert catheter up to 4 cm.

→ Measure urine and record amount.

→ Remove catheter.

※DO NOT suture if more than 12 hours since delivery. Refer woman to hospital.

伤口,不作处理。

→ 三度和四度裂伤:如果裂伤很长、很深,伤到了肛门括约肌(三度)和直肠黏膜(四度),用清洁的敷料覆盖,迅速转诊到上级医院(或请上级医生处理)。

■ 如果一度或二度裂伤,有活动性出血(在压迫止血后仍然有出血):

→ 缝合伤口(或请上级医生缝合)。

→ 注意无菌操作、消毒隔离原则,应用无菌用品。

→ 应用持针器,21 cm 敷料(长条阴道纱,带阴道外牵引线),4号圆针。

→ 应用可吸收的合成缝线。

→ 注意缝合第一针要在裂伤的最顶端。

→ 伤口边缘对合良好。

■ 排空膀胱。

■ 如果产妇不能自己排尿,鼓励产妇并协助排尿。

■ 如果不能自行排尿,必要时插尿管:

→ 洗手。

→ 消毒尿道口周围皮肤区域。

→ 戴无菌手套。

→ 分开小阴唇,再次消毒。

→ 插尿管,约深 4 cm。

→ 记录尿量。

→ 拔出尿管(不作持续尿管留置)。

※如果裂伤在 12 h 前(才到医院),不要缝合,转诊到上级医院。

Case analysis

A patient returns to a clinic for a visit 3 days after a normal first pregnancy and delivery. She complains of leaking urine when coughing or laughing, and she is also worried that she has not passed a stool since the delivery. She starts to cry and says that she should not have fallen pregnant. Her infant takes the breast well and sleeps well after each feed. On examination the patient appears well, her observations are normal, the uterus is the size of a 16 week pregnant uterus, and the lochia is red and not offensive.

Questions:

1. Is her puerperium progressing normally?
2. What should be done about the patients complaints?
3. Why is the patient regretting her pregnancy and crying for no apparent reason?

Test

1. A nurse is preparing to assess the uterine fundus of a woman in the immediate postpartum period. The uterus feels soft and boggy and she could not locate the fundus clearly. Which of the following interventions would be most appropriate one?　　　　　　　　　　　( )

   A. Massage the fundus until it is firm
   B. Elavate the mother's leg
   C. Push the uterus deep into the pelvic to expel the clotting in the uterus
   D. Encourage the mother to go toilet by self
   E. Help the mother walking aroud

2. A woman is in the postpartum period, which of the following signs indicates that the woman may be in the risk of postpartum hemorrhage?　　( )

   A. Ttemperature of 37 ℃
   B. Resperatory rate is from 18 to 22 breaths per minute
   C. Blood pressure change from 139/89 to 124/80 mmHg
   D. Pulse rate from 88 to 112 per minute
   E. Feels a round and hard uterus in low abdomen

3. Which of the following DO NOT necessary be the right interventions regarding to the retained placenta?　　　　　　　　　　　( )

   A. Give diazepam (10 mg IM/IV)
   B. Clean vulva and perineal area
   C. Empty bladder.
   D. Pull on the cord hard to separate the placenta
   E. Antibiotic therapy

4. A nurse is assessing the lochia discharge on a 1 day postpartum woman. The nurse notes that the cochia is red and had a foul-smelling odor, there is low abdominal pain. The nurse determines that this assessement finding is　　　　　　　　( )

   A. normal
   B. indicates the presence of infection
   C. indicates the need for increasing

ambulation

D. indicates the need for increasing of oral fluid

E. indicates the need for blood transfusion

5. Which of the following situations in dangerous signs that the woman should

retern to hospital immediately?（　　）

A. Nipple sore and tender

B. Pass stool at the first day of delivery

C. Pass urine at 6 hours after delivery

D. Fever and hard to get out of bed

E. Resperatory rate is from 15 to 20 per minute

Reference answer

Case analysis：

1. Yes. The patient appears healthy with normal observations，and the involution of her uterus is satisfactory.

2. Stress incontinence is common during the puerperium. Therefore，the patient must be reassured that it will improve over time. However，pelvic floor exercises must be explained to her as they will hasten improvement of her incontinence.

3. She need not be worried about not having passed a stool as this is normal during the first few days of the puerperium.

4. She probably has the "puerperal blues" which are common in the puerperium. Listen sympathetically to the patient's complaints and reassure her that she is managing well.

病例分析

1. 该产妇情况正常,属于正常产后表现,子宫恢复良好。

2. 产后短期内的尿失禁很常见,产后随时间性会逐渐恢复,告知产妇要进行产后的锻炼。产后几天不排便也很常见,属于正常范围。

3. 产褥期最初几天没有大便是正常的,产妇不必担心。

4. 该产妇可能有产后的抑郁表现,注意倾听产妇的表达,告之她这属于正常情况。

Test

1. A　2. D　3. D　4. B　5. D

Chapter 3　Diseases and Complication in Pregnancy, Fetal Medicine

第 3 章　病理产科及胎儿医学

3.1　Ectopic Pregnancy

3.1　异位妊娠

Key words

1. ectopic pregnancy
2. ampullary pregnancy
3. decidua
4. misdiagnosis
5. internal blood loss
6. pouch of douglas
7. pregnancy test
8. transvaginal sonography

关键词

1. 输卵管妊娠
2. 壶腹部妊娠
3. 蜕膜
4. 误诊
5. 内出血
6. 直肠子宫陷凹
7. 妊娠试验
8. 输卵管切除

3.1.1　Ectopic pregnancy

3.1.1　异位妊娠

Ectopic pregnancy is the occurrence of conception outside of its normal position within the uterine cavity, the most common site is within the fallopian tubes（97%）followed by the abdominal cavity, ovary, and cervix. Within the fallopian tubes, the ampulla is the most common site, followed by the isthmus and fimbria.

异位妊娠指妊娠发生在子宫腔以外的部位,最常发生的部位是输卵管内,其次是腹腔、卵巢和宫颈。输卵管内最常见的部位是壶腹部,其次是峡部和伞部。

- The fallopian tube is about 10 cm long. The diameter of the lumen varies from 1 mm in the interstitial portion to about 5 mm at the fimbriated end.

- 输卵管长约 10 cm,管腔的直径从间质部的 1 mm 到伞端的 5 mm 不等。

- The musculature is of two layer, an inner circular layer and an outer longitudinal layer, and peristaltic movements are particularly strong during and after ovulation. The mucosa is arranged in plications or folds which become much more complete and plentiful as the infundibulum is approached.

- 肌层分两层,里层为环形,外层为纵行。排卵后输卵管蠕动加强。输卵管黏膜存在很多皱褶,靠近漏斗部更多。

◆ The mucosa consists of a single layer of ciliated and secretory cells, resting on a thin basement membrane. There is little or no submucosa and no decidual reaction, so muscle is easily invaded by trophoblast.

3.1.2　Epidemiology

◆ Rate of occurrence is 2% of reported pregnancies.
◆ Carries a 7- to 13- fold increase in recurrence risk.
◆ Three to four times more common in women over age 35 compared to those in the 18- to 24-year-old age group.

3.1.3　Etiology/Risk factors

　　Ectopic implantation may be fortuitous or the result of a tubal abnormality which obstructs or delays the passage of the fertilized ovum.
◆ Preceding tubal or pelvic inflammation with residual endothelial damage or distortion by adhesions [ask about history of sexually transmitted diseases (STD)].
◆ Previous ectopic pregnancy.
◆ Previous tubal scarring (from tuberculosis or surgery, e. g. attempted sterilization, reversal of sterilization or salpingostomy).
◆ Women who conceive with an intra-uterine contraceptive device (IUCD) in situ have an increased risk of ectopic pregnancy. This may be due to infection or an effect on tubal motility.
◆ Anatomic congenital malformations of the tube such as hypoplasia, elongation or diverticulum, or of the uterus such as septate uterus.
◆ Current smoking.
◆ Assisted reproduction measures such as use of ovulation-inducing drugs and in vitro fertilization.
◆ In utero diethylstilbestrol (DES) exposure.
◆ Migration of ovum across the pelvic cavity to the fallopian tube on the side opposite to the follicle from which ovulation occurred.

◆ 黏膜层由单层纤毛和分泌细胞以及一层薄的基底膜组成,很少或没有黏膜下层,也没有蜕膜反应,所以肌层容易被滋养细胞侵犯。

3.1.2　流行病学

◆ 据报道发生率为2%。
◆ 复发风险高达7～13倍。
◆ 35岁以上妇女发生异位妊娠的概率是18～25岁妇女的3～4倍。

3.1.3　病因/危险因素

　　异位植入可为偶然发生,也可以是输卵管异常阻碍或延误受精卵运动而造成的。
◆ 之前的输卵管或盆腔炎症以及后遗的内皮损伤或粘连所致扭曲(注意询问性传播疾病史)。

◆ 既往异位妊娠史。
◆ 既往输卵管疤痕(来自结核或绝育、恢复生育以及输卵管造口等手术)。
◆ 带有宫内节育器的妇女发生异位妊娠的风险增高,这可能是因为感染或影响输卵管蠕动引起。

◆ 先天性输卵管或子宫的解剖学异常,如输卵管发育不全,延长或憩室,或子宫纵隔。
◆ 吸烟。
◆ 辅助生殖技术的实施,如诱导排卵药物的使用以及体外受精。
◆ 子宫暴露于己烯雌酚。
◆ 卵子经一侧卵巢滤泡排出后,经盆腔迁移到另一侧输卵管中。

3.1.4　Outcome

The muscle wall of the tube has no capacity of uterine muscle for hypertrophy and distension and tubal pregnancy nearly always ends in rupture and the death of the ovum.

→Rupture into lumen of tube (tubal abortion)

This is usual in ampullary pregnancy at about 8 weeks. The conceptus is extruded, complete or incomplete, towards the fimbriated end of the tube, probably by the pressure of accumulated blood.

There is a trickle of bleeding into the peritoneal cavity, and this may collect as a clot in the pouch of Douglas. It is then called a pelvic hematocele.

→Rupture into the peritoneal cavity

This occurs mainly from the narrow isthmus before 8 weeks of pregnancy, or later from the interstitial portion of the tube. Hemorrhage is likely to be severe.

Sometimes rupture is extraperitoneal between the leaves of the broad ligament—broad ligament hematoma. Hemorrhage in this site is more likely to be controlled.

→Tubal pregnancy (effect on uterus)

The uterus enlarges in the first three months almost as if the implantation was normal and may reach the size of a gravid uterus of the same maturity. This is a source of confusion in diagnosis.

The uterine decidua grows abundantly and when the embryo dies bleeding occurs as the decidua degenerates. Rarely it is expelled entire as a decidual cast.

3.1.5　Clinical manifestations

Tubal pregnancy can present in many ways and misdiagnosis is common.

→*Pain* in the lower abdomen is always present and may be either constant or cramp-like. It may be referred to the shoulder if blood tracks to the

3.1.4　结局

因为输卵管肌层不具备子宫肌层那种肥大和延展的能力，所以输卵管妊娠一般都以破裂和受精卵死亡告终。

→输卵管内妊娠破裂（输卵管妊娠流产）

通常发生在壶腹部妊娠 8 周左右。可能由于周围血块的压力，使孕体被完全或不完全挤出到输卵管伞端。

血液不断流入腹腔，可能在子宫直肠陷凹积聚形成血块，也称为盆腔血肿。

→腹膜腔内妊娠破裂

通常由于峡部妊娠在 8 周之前或间质部妊娠更晚引起。出血可能更为严重。

通常破裂发生在腹膜外阔韧带两叶之间——阔韧带血肿。这个部位的出血可能更容易被控制。

→输卵管妊娠（对子宫的影响）

妊娠前三个月中，子宫可以像正常妊娠一样增大，可能达到正常相同孕周的子宫尺寸，因此可能混淆诊断。

子宫蜕膜生长较厚，当胚胎死亡后蜕膜退化就会出血，很少完全以蜕膜管型排出。

3.1.5　临床表现

输卵管妊娠的临床表现不一，误诊比较常见。

→下腹部疼痛很常见，可以是持续性或绞痛样。如血液积聚到横膈膜，刺激膈神经而使疼痛

diaphragm and stimulates the phrenic nerve, and it may be so severe as to cause fainting. The pain is caused by distension of the gravid tube, by its efforts to contract and expel the ovum, and by irritation of the peritoneum due to leakage of blood.

→*Vaginal bleeding* occurs usually after the death of the ovum and is an effect of estrogen withdrawal. It is dark brown and scanty and its irregularity may lead the patient to confuse it with the menstrual flow and thus, inadvertently, give a misleading history. In about 25% of cases, tubal pregnancy presents without any vaginal bleeding.

→*Internal blood loss* can be severe and rapid and the usual signs of collapse and shock will appear. Acute internal bleeding is the most dramatic and dangerous consequence of tubal pregnancy, but it is less common than the condition presenting by a slow trickle of blood into the pelvic cavity.

→*Pelvic examination* in the conscious patient will demonstrate extreme tenderness over the gravid tube or in the pouch of Douglas if a hematocele has collected. If the pregnancy is sufficiently advanced and rupture has not occurred, a cystic (and very tender) mass may be felt in the fornix; but often tenderness is the only sign elicited.

→*Peritoneal irritation* may produce muscle guarding, frequency of micturition, and later a degree of fever, all leading towards a misdiagnosis of appendicitis.

→*Signs and symptoms of early pregnancy* may be present and help to distinguish the condition from other causes of lower abdominal pain. The menstrual history may be confusing, as noted above, and when implantation occurs in the isthmus, tubal rupture may occur before the patient has missed a period.

→*Abdominal examination* will demonstrate tenderness in one or other fossa. If there has been much

放射到肩部,严重时可以导致昏厥。

输卵管妊娠引起其扩张再收缩以排出受精卵,并且血液流出刺激腹膜,从而引起疼痛。

→阴道出血通常因为受精卵死亡后雌激素撤退引起。出血为少量暗褐色且不规则,导致患者误认为是月经不调。有25%的输卵管妊娠病例没有任何阴道出血。

→内出血可以非常严重和快速,常引起休克晕厥。急性内出血是输卵管妊娠最危险的后果,但没有慢性盆腔内出血的情况常见。

→对清醒患者进行盆腔检查会发现妊娠输卵管部位的明显触痛。如血肿形成,直肠子宫陷凹处也有强烈触痛。如妊娠充分发展没有破裂,可在阴道穹窿触及囊性包块(触痛明显);但通常触痛也是唯一可以引出的体征。

→腹膜刺激可导致肌卫、尿频以及之后的发热,可被误诊为阑尾炎。

→早孕症状和体征的出现,有助于与其他原因引起的下腹部疼痛相区别。患者月经史不清,如发生在峡部,可在一个月经周期未结束前就发生破裂。

→腹部检查可有局部压痛。如腹膜内出血多,可有全腹广泛触

intraperitoneal bleeding there will be general tenderness and resistance to palpation over the whole abdomen.

痛,患者疼痛拒按。

3.1.6 Diagnostic tests

→Urine pregnancy test to confirm pregnancy: Will be positive with β-hCG level > 20 mIU/ml, approximately 1 week after conception.

→β-hCG levels:

◆ Should increase by at least 66% every 48 hours in the first 6-7 weeks of gestation after day 9.

◆ Value of serial hCGs: Stable and reliable patients can be followed with serial β-hCG levels. Inadequate rise in β-hCG is suggestive of ectopic or nonviable pregnancy.

→Progesterone (results often not available immediately):

◆ >25 ng/ml: Suggests normal intrauterine pregnancy (IUP).

◆ <5 ng/ml: Suggests abnormal pregnancy (either ectopic or nonviable pregnancy).

◆ 5-25 ng/ml: unclear.

→Ultrasonography—diagnostic modality of choice:

◆ Ectopic pregnancy is suspected if there is lack of visualization of the gestational sac within the uterine cavity in the setting of a positive pregnancy test.

◆ Transvaginal sonography (TVUS) is more sensitive than transabdominal approach. The threshold for detecting an IUP on TVUS is β-hCG =1000 mIU/ml, or 4-6 weeks' gestation.

◆ Findings suggestive of ectopic pregnancy in addition to lack of the intrauterine gestational ring include ectopic gestational sac or cardiac activity, fluid or mass within the pouch of Douglas, and adnexal mass.

→Laparoscopy remains the main means of diagnosis in suspected ectopic pregnancy although the increased use of transvaginal ultrasound and better

3.1.6 诊断试验

→尿妊娠试验确定妊娠:受孕后约 1 周测 β-hCG 水平大于 20 mIU/ml。

→β-hCG 水平:

◆ 受孕 9 天以后的 6~7 周以内,每 48 h 至少升高 66%。

◆ 持续监测 hCG 值:
依从性好的患者可持续监测 β-hCG 水平。β-hCG 水平上升不足提示异位妊娠或无活力的妊娠。

→孕酮水平(结果通常需等待):

◆ >25 ng/ml:提示正常宫内妊娠(IUP)。

◆ <5 ng/ml:异常妊娠(异位妊娠或无活力妊娠)。

◆ 5~25 ng/ml:无法确定。

→超声检查—选择诊断模式:

◆ 如妊娠试验阳性,而宫腔内未见孕囊,应怀疑异位妊娠。

◆ 经阴道超声比腹部超声更敏感。经阴道超声能检测到宫内妊娠的阈值是 β-hCG 达到1 000 mIU/ml 或孕周达到 4~6 周。

◆ 除了宫腔内缺乏孕囊外,在子宫直肠陷凹发现异位妊娠囊或胎心搏动,羊水或包块以及附件区发现包块均提示异位妊娠。

→尽管更多的采用经阴道超声及更好的妊娠试验使腹腔镜的使用变得不必要,但腹腔镜仍然是

pregnancy testing may make it unnecessary.

- The laparoscope is particularly useful for identifying an unruptured tubal pregnancy which is producing equivocal symptoms，and for excluding salpingitis and bleeding from small ovarian cysts.

- Laparoscopy may also enable operative treatments using minimally invasive methods.

→Culdocentesis means passing a needle through the posterior fornix into the pouch of Douglas.

- This may be helpful if laparoscopy is not available.

- Intraperitoneal blood does not readily clot and if such blood is obtained it is an indication for laparotomy.

3.1.7　Differential diagnosis

→Salpingitis

- Swelling and pain are bilateral，fever is higher and a pregnancy test is usually negative.

- There may be a purulent discharge from the cervix.

→Miscarriage（threatened or incomplete）

- Bleeding is the dominant clinical feature and usually precedes pain.

- The bleeding is red rather than brown and the pain is crampy or colicky.

- The uterus is larger and softer and the cervix patulous or dilated.

- Products of conception may be recognized on vaginal examination.

→Appendicitis

- The area of tenderness is higher and may be localized in the right iliac fossa.

- There may be a swelling if an appendix abscess was formed but is not so deep in the pelvis as a tubal swelling.

- Fever is greater and the patient may show toxic symptoms.

诊断疑似异位妊娠的主要手段。

- 在诊断症状可疑的未破裂的输卵管妊娠，以及排除输卵管炎和卵巢小囊肿出血方面，腹腔镜尤为有用。

- 腹腔镜使运用微创方法进行手术治疗成为可能。

→后穹窿穿刺术指经阴道后穹窿穿刺进入子宫直肠陷凹。

- 如无法实施腹腔镜，该方法可能有用。

- 腹膜内出血不易凝固，所以抽取到不凝血是腹腔镜的一个适应证。

3.1.7　鉴别诊断

→输卵管炎

- 肿胀和疼痛为双侧的，发热时体温较高，妊娠试验通常阴性。

- 宫颈可有脓性分泌物。

→流产（先兆或不全）

- 出血是最主要的临床特征，通常在腹痛之前出现。

- 出血是红色的而不是褐色的，腹痛为痉挛性或疝气痛样。

- 子宫更大更软，宫颈扩张。

- 阴道检查可能发现妊娠产物。

→阑尾炎

- 疼痛部位更高，可局限在右髂窝。

- 如阑尾脓肿形成，可有肿胀，但没有输卵管肿胀部位那么深。

- 发热体温更高，患者可能表现为中毒症状。

- A pregnancy test will usually be negative although pregnancy and appendicitis can, of course, co-exist.

→ Torsion of pedicle of ovarian cyst

- The mass so formed can usually be felt separate from the uterus, while a tubal pregnancy usually feels attached.
- Tenderness may be marked, and intraperitoneal bleeding may produce fever.
- Signs and symptoms of pregnancy are absent but there is a history of repeated sudden attacks of pain which pass off.

→ Rupture of corpus luteum

- It is virtually impossible to distinguish this, by examination, from a tubal pregnancy, but such a severe reaction is rare.

3.1.8　Management

If hemorrhage and shock are present, restore the blood volume by the transfusion of red cells or a volume expander and proceed with operation. The patient's condition will improve as soon as the bleeding is controlled.

- General

→ Resuscitative measures for all but the most stable patients, including two large-bore IVs, normal saline hydration, type and crossmatch.

→ RhoGAM for all Rh-negative women.

- Medical

Candidates for medical management with intramuscular methotrexate (folic acid antagonist) include：

→ Asymtomatic women.

→ Serum β-hCG<15000 mIU/ml.

→ Ability for daily follow-up.

→ Tubal ring<3 cm.

→ Absence of cardiac activity.

→ No hypersensitivity of medical contraindications to

- 妊娠试验通常为阴性,尽管妊娠和阑尾炎可以同时存在。

→ 卵巢囊肿蒂扭转

- 肿块感觉与子宫分离,而输卵管妊娠通常感觉与子宫相连。

- 疼痛明显,腹膜内出血可能导致发热。

- 没有妊娠的症状和体征,但存在反复突然腹痛又逐渐缓解的病史。

→ 黄体破裂

- 事实上,不可能通过一般检查将其与输卵管妊娠区别开来,但情况比较少见。

3.1.8　处理

如有出血和休克,先输注浓缩红细胞或容量扩张剂补充血容量,然后再进行手术。一旦控制了出血,患者的情况就会有所恢复。

- 一般治疗

→ 虽然大多数患者病情稳定,但需为所有患者准备复苏措施,包括两支大孔径静脉导管、生理盐水输液、血型检查和交叉配血。

→ 对所有 Rh 阴性妇女使用 RhoGAM。

- 药物治疗

可肌内注射甲氨蝶呤(叶酸阻断剂)治疗的患者包括：

→ 无症状的妇女

→ 血清 β-hCG<15 000 mIU/ml

→ 能够每日复诊

→ 输卵管孕囊环直径<3 cm

→ 无胎心搏动

→ 对甲氨蝶呤治疗无过敏禁忌

methotrexate therapy.

◆ Surgical

→Immediate intervention is warranted for symptomatic women with hemodynamic instability and patients who do not meet criteria for medical management.

→Laparoscopy with salpingostomy without fallopian tube removal is the preferred treatment.

3.1.9　Case report and analysis

Case 1

≫A 23-year-old woman underwent a dilation and curettage (D & C) for an incomplete abortion 3 days previously. She complains of continued vaginal bleeding and lower abdominal cramping. Over the last 24 hr, she notes significant fever and chills. On examination, her temperature is 39.2 ℃, BP 90/40, and HR 120 bpm. The cardiac examination reveals tachycardia and the lungs are clear. There is moderately severe lower abdominal tenderness. The pelvic examination shows the cervix to be open to 1.5 cm, and there is uterine tenderness. The leukocyte count is 20 000/mm³ and the hemoglobin level is 12 g/dl. The urinalysis shows 2 WBC/hpf.

◇What is the most likely diagnosis?

◇What is the next step in management?

☑ANSWERS

Most likely diagnosis: Septic abortion (with retained products of conception).

Next step in management: Broad-spectrum antibiotics followed by dilatation and curettage of the uterus.

☑ANALYSIS

Objectives

◆ Understand the clinical presentation of septic abortion.

◆ Know that the treatment of septic abortion involves both antibiotic therapy and uterine curettage.

◆ 手术治疗

→立即手术干预适用于有症状的血流动力学不稳定的患者,以及达不到药物治疗标准的患者。

→腹腔镜手术倾向于输卵管造口,而非输卵管切除。

3.1.9　病例报道和分析

病例 1

≫23 岁女性,3 天前因不全流产行清宫术。患者主述不断阴道出血和下腹部绞痛,1 天前开始出现明显发热和寒战。查体:体温 39.2 ℃,血压 90/40 mmHg,心率 120 次/min,心肺检查示心动过速,双肺清,下腹部触痛较明显。盆腔检查:宫颈口扩张 1.5 cm,子宫触痛。化验:白细胞计数 20 000/mm³,血红蛋白 12 g/dl,尿液分析示每高倍镜视野见 2 个白细胞。

◇最可能的诊断是什么?

◇下一步处理是什么?

☑答案

最可能的诊断:流产感染(妊娠产物滞留)。

下一步处理:应用广谱抗生素控制感染后清宫。

☑分析

目的

◆ 理解流产感染的临床表现。

◆ 了解流产感染的处理,包括抗生素和清宫治疗。

Considerations

This 23-year-old woman underwent a D & C procedure for an incomplete abortion 3 days previously and now presents with lower abdominal cramping, vaginal bleeding, fever, and chills. The open cervical os, lower abdominal cramping, and vaginal bleeding suggest retained products of conception (POC). The retained POC may lead to ongoing bleeding or infection. In this case, the fever, chills, and leukocytosis point toward infection. The retained tissue serves as a nidus for infection. The most common source of the bacteria is the vagina, via an ascending infection. The best treatment is broad-spectrum antibiotics with anaerobic coverage and a uterine curettage. Usually, the surgery is delayed until antimicrobial agents are infused for 4 hr to allow for tissue levels to increase. Hemorrhage may occur with the curettage procedure. Also, the patient should be monitored for septic shock.

☑APPROACH TO SEPTIC ABORTION

Definitions

◆ **Septic abortion**: Any type of abortion associated with a uterine infection.
◆ **Septic shock**: The septic portion refers to the presence of an infection (usually bacterial), and the shock describes a process whereby the patient's cells, organs, and/or tissues are not being sufficiently supplied with nutrients and/or oxygen.

Clinical approach

◆ Septic abortion occurs in approximately 1% of all spontaneous abortions and about 0.5% of induced abortions. This risk is increased if an abortion is performed with nonsterile instrumentation. This condition is potentially fatal in 0.4 to 0.6/100 000 spontaneous abortions.
◆ Signs and symptoms of septic abortion are uterine bleeding and/or spotting in the first trimester with

病例分析

23 岁女性 3 天前因不全流产清宫,现表现为下腹部绞痛,阴道流血、发热和寒战。宫颈扩张,下腹部绞痛和阴道出血提示妊娠产物滞留宫腔。滞留的妊娠产物可导致继续出血或感染。这个病例中患者发热、寒战以及白细胞增多提示感染。滞留的组织为感染的滋生地。最常见的细菌来源是阴道的上行感染。最好的治疗是使用具有抗厌氧菌谱的广谱抗生素控制感染以及清宫。一般在输入抗感染药物 4 h 使其在组织的水平升高后再实施清宫术。术中可出现出血。同时,应监护患者,谨防感染性休克。

☑流产感染学习指导

定义

◆ 流产感染:与子宫感染有关的流产类型。
◆ 感染性休克:感染通常为细菌性,休克时患者的细胞、器官和/或组织处于一种养分和/氧气供应不足的状态。

临床处理

◆ 流产感染在所有自然流产中的发生率为 1%,人工流产中的发生率为 0.5%。如使用有菌的器械进行流产则感染的风险增高。自然流产感染的致死率为 0.4~0.6/10 万。
◆ 感染性流产表现为孕早期子宫出血和/或点滴出血伴有临床

clinical signs of infection. The mechanism is ascending infection from the vagina or cervix to the endometrium to myometrium to parametrium, and, eventually, the peritoneum. Affected women generally will have fever and leukocyte counts of greater than 10 500 cells/μl. There is usually lower abdominal tenderness, cervical motion tenderness, and a foul-smelling vaginal discharge. The infection is almost always polymicrobial, involving anaerobic streptococci, *Bacteroides* species, *Escherichia coli* and other gram-negative rods, and group B beta-hemolytic streptococci. Rarely, *Clostridium perfringens*, *Hemophilus influenza*, and *Campylobacter jejuni* may be isolated.

When patients present with signs and symptoms of septic abortion, a CBC with differential, urinalysis, and blood chemistries including electrolytes should be obtained. A specimen of cervical discharge should be sent for Gram's stain, as well as for culture and sensitivity. If the patient appears seriously ill or is hypotensive, blood cultures, a chest x-ray, and blood coagulability studies should be done. The blood pressure, oxygen saturation, heart rate, and urine output should be monitored.

◆ The treatment has four general parts: 1) maintain the blood pressure; 2) monitor the blood pressure, oxygenation, and urine output; 3) start antibiotic therapy; 4) perform a uterine curettage. Immediate therapeutic steps include intravenous isotonic fluid replacement, especially in the face of hypotension. The combination of gentamicin and clindamycin has a favorable response 95% of the time. Alternatives include beta-lactam antimicrobials (cephalosporins and extended-spectrum penicillins) or those with beta-lactamase inhibitors. Another regimen includes metronidazole plus ampicillin and an aminoglycoside. Because retained POC are common in these situations, becoming a nidus for infection to develop, evacuation of

感染体征。发生机制为从阴道或宫颈的感染上行到子宫内膜、肌层和浆膜层，甚至到腹膜。感染的患者可有发热，白细胞计数大于 10 500 细胞/μl。通常还有下腹部压痛、宫颈举痛和阴道分泌物恶臭。感染几乎都是多种微生物引起的，包括厌氧链球菌、拟杆菌属、大肠杆菌和其他革兰阴性杆菌和 B 族溶血性链球菌。少见的产气荚膜梭菌、流感嗜血杆菌和空肠弯曲杆菌也可能分离到。

当患者出现感染性流产的症状和体征时，需进行全血细胞计数、尿液分析和包括电解质在内的血液生化检查。宫颈分泌物样本应做革兰染色、培养和药敏试验。如患者病情较重或出现低血压，则需行血培养、胸片和凝血检查。还需监测血压、血氧饱和度、心率和尿量。

◆ 治疗一般分四步：1）维持血压；2）监测血压，血氧饱和度和尿量；3）开始抗生素治疗；4）行清宫术。患者出现低血压时的急救步骤为静脉输注等渗溶液。联合使用庆大霉素和克林霉素有效率达 95%。替代方案包括 β-内酰胺类抗生素（头孢菌素和广谱青霉素类）或 β-内酰胺酶抑制剂。另一种方案包括甲硝唑联合氨苄西林和一种氨基苷类抗生素。因为妊娠产物滞留于宫腔，帮助感染滋生，所以清空子宫很重要。清

the uterine contents is important. Uterine curettage is usually performed approximately 4 hr after antibiotics are begun, allowing serum levels to be achieved.

◆ Because oliguria is an early sign of septic shock, the urine output should be carefully observed. Also, for women in shock, a central venous pressure catheter may be warranted. Aggressive intravenous fluids are usually effective in maintaining the blood pressure; however, at times, vasopressor agents, such as a dopamine infusion, may be required. Other therapies include oxygen, digitalis, and steroids.

Case 2

✍ A 19-year-old G2Ab1 woman at 7 weeks' gestation by LMP complains of vaginal spotting. She denies the passage of tissue per vagina, any trauma, or recent intercourse. Her past medical history is significant for a pelvic infection approximately 3 yr ago. She had used an oral contraceptive agent 1 yr previously. Her appetite is normal. On examination, her BP is 100/60, HR 90 bpm, and temp afebrile. The abdomen is nontender with normoactive bowel sounds. On pelvic examination, the external genitalia are normal. The cervix is closed and nontender. The uterus is 4 weeks' size, and no adnexal tenderness is noted. The quantitative β-hCG is 2 300 mIU/ml. A transvaginal sonogram reveals an empty uterus and no adnexal masses.

◇ What is your next step?

◇ What is the most likely diagnosis?

☑ ANSWERS

Next step: Laparoscopy.

Most likely diagnosis: Ectopic pregnany.

☑ ANALYSIS

Objectives

◆ Understand that any woman with amenorrhea and vaginal spotting or lower abdominal pain should

---

宫术通常在使用抗生素 4 h 到达血清药物浓度后实施。

◆ 因为少尿是感染性休克的早期征象,尿量需仔细记录。对于休克的患者,应进行中心静脉置管。大量静脉输液对维持血压通常有效,但有时需要使用多巴胺等血管加压药。其他治疗包括吸氧,使用洋地黄类和甾体类药物。

病例 2

✍ 19 岁女性,孕 2 流 1,根据末次月经算孕 7 周,主述阴道点滴出血。患者否认组织物经阴道排出,外伤或最近同房史。既往史中有意义的是约 3 年前有盆腔感染史,1 年前开始使用口服避孕药。患者食欲正常。查体:血压100/60 mmHg,心率 90 次/min,体温正常。腹部无压痛,肠鸣音正常。盆腔检查:外阴正常,宫颈口闭合,无举痛,子宫如孕 4 周大小,附件区无触痛。化验:β-hCG 定量 2 300 mIU/ml。经阴道超声检查:宫腔未见孕囊,附件区未见包块。

◇ 下一步处理是什么?

◇ 最可能的诊断是什么?

☑ 答案

下一步处理:实施腹腔镜手术。

最可能的诊断:异位妊娠。

☑ 分析

目的

◆ 理解任何主述停经、阴道点滴出血或下腹部疼痛的妇女均需

have a pregnancy test to evaluate the possibility of ectopic pregnancy.

◆ Understand the role of the hCG level and the threshold for transvaginal sonogram.

◆ Know that the lack of clinical or ultrasound signs of ectopic pregnancy does not exclude the disease.

Considerations

The woman is at 7 weeks' gestation by last menstrual period and presents with vaginal spotting. Any woman with amenorrhea and vaginal spotting should have a pregnancy test. The physical examination is normal. Notably, the uterus is slightly enlarged at 4 weeks' gestational size. The enlarged uterus does not exclude the diagnosis of an ectopic pregnancy, due to the human chorionic gonadotropin (hCG) effect on the uterus. The lack of adnexal mass or tenderness on physical examination likewise does not rule out an ectopic pregnancy. The hCG level and transvaginal ultrasound are key tests in the assessment of an extrauterine pregnancy. The ultrasound is primarily used to assess for the presence or absence of an intrauterine pregnancy (IUP), because a confirmed IUP would decrease the likelihood of an ectopic pregnancy significantly (risk 1∶ 10 000 of both an intrauterine and ectopic pregnancy). Also, the presence of free fluid in the peritoneal cavity, or a complex adnexal mass, would make an extrauterine pregnancy more likely. This woman's hCG level of 2 300 mIU/ml is greater than the threshold of 1 500 mIU/ml(transvaginal sonography); thus, the patient has a high likelihood of an ectopic pregnancy. Although the risk of an extrauterine pregnancy is high, it is not 100%. Therefore, laparoscopy is indicated, but not methotrexate, since the latter would destroy any intrauterine gestation.

☑APPROACH TO POSSIBLE ECTOPIC PREGNANCY

Definitions

◆ Ectopic pregnancy∶ A gestation that exists outside of the normal endometrial implantation sites.

进行妊娠试验以评估患异位妊娠的可能性。

◆ 理解 hCG 水平的意义和经阴道超声的阈值。

◆ 了解就算缺乏异位妊娠的临床或超声征象也不能排除该疾病。

病例分析

孕 7 周(根据末次月经推算)女性,出现阴道点滴出血。任何主述停经和阴道点滴出血的女性均需进行妊娠试验。体格检查正常。值得注意的是子宫轻度增大如孕 4 周。增大的子宫不能排除异位妊娠的诊断,因为 hCG 可以作用于子宫使其增大。查体未发现附件区包块或压痛同样不能排除异位妊娠。hCG 水平和经阴道超声是评估宫腔外妊娠的关键检查。超声最初用来评估是否宫内受孕,因为确定宫内妊娠后异位妊娠的发生率明显降低(宫内外同时妊娠的概率为万分之一)。同样,如腹膜腔内探测到游离液体或附件区复合包块,异位妊娠的可能性更大。该患者 hCG 水平达 2 300 mIU/ml,高于(经阴道超声的)阈值 1 500 mIU/ml;所以,患者为异位妊娠的可能性较大。但尽管异位妊娠的可能性大,也不是 100%。因此,有腹腔镜手术而不是使用甲氨蝶呤的指征,由于后者会危害可能存在的宫腔内妊娠。

☑异位妊娠学习指导

定义

◆ 异位妊娠:发生在正常子宫内膜植入部位以外的妊娠。

- Human chorionic gonadotropin: A glycoprotein produced by syncytiotrophoblasts, which is assayed in the standard pregnancy test.
- Threshold hCG level: The serum level of hCG where a pregnancy should be seen on ultrasound examination. When the hCG exceeds the threshold and no pregnancy is seen on ultrasound, there is a high likelihood of an ectopic pregnancy.
- Laparoscopy: Surgical technique to visualize the peritoneal cavity through a rigid telescopic instrument, known as a laparoscope.

Clinical approach

- The vast majority of ectopic pregnancies involve the fallopian tube (97%), but the cervix, abdominal cavity, and ovary have also been affected.
- Hemorrhage from ectopic gestation is the most common reason for maternal mortality in the first 20 weeks of pregnancy.
- A woman with an ectopic pregnancy typically complains of abdominal pain, amenorrhea of 4 to 6 weeks' duration, and irregular vaginal spotting. If the ectopic ruptures, the pain becomes acutely worse, and may lead to syncope.

  Shoulder pain can be a prominent complaint due to the blood irritating the diaphragm. An ectopic pregnancy can lead to tachycardia, hypotension, or orthostasis. Abdominal or adnexal tenderness is common. An adnexal mass is only palpable half the time; hence, the absence of a detectable mass does not exclude an ectopic pregnancy. The uterus may be normal in size, or slightly enlarged. A hemoperitoneum can be confirmed by the aspiration of nonclotting blood with a spinal needle piecing the posterior vaginal fornix into the cul-de-sac (culdocentesis).

- The diagnosis of an ectopic pregnancy can be a clinical challenge. The usual strategy in ruling out and ectopic pregnancy is to try to prove whether an

- 人绒毛膜促性腺激素:由合体滋养层细胞产生的糖蛋白,是标准妊娠试验检测的项目。
- hCG 水平阈值:超声检查可发现妊娠的血清 hCG 水平。当 hCG 超过阈值而超声又未发现妊娠时,存在异位妊娠的可能性较大。
- 腹腔镜检查:用硬质带有微型摄像头的器械可以观察到腹膜腔情况的外科技术。

临床处理

- 大多数异位妊娠(97%)发生在输卵管,也可发生在宫颈、腹腔和卵巢。
- 异位妊娠出血是孕 20 周之前孕妇死亡最常见的原因。

- 异位妊娠患者一般主述腹痛,停经 4～6 周以及不规则阴道点滴出血。如异位妊娠破裂,疼痛加剧可能导致晕厥。

  如内出血刺激横膈膜,肩部疼痛可为突出的主述。异位妊娠还可导致心动过速、低血压和立位晕厥。腹部或附件区压痛较常见。附件区包块仅一半可被触及,但触不到包块不能排除异位妊娠。子宫大小可能正常或轻度增大。如用脊髓穿刺针在阴道后穹窿穿刺进入子宫直肠陷凹抽吸出不凝血,则可确诊腹腔积血(后穹窿穿刺术)。

- 临床上对异位妊娠的诊断具有一定难度。异位妊娠常用的诊断策略是排除法证明宫内妊娠

intrauterine pregnancy (IUP) exists. Because the likelihood of coexisting intrauterine and extrauterine (heterotopic) gestation is so low, in the range of 1 in 10 000, if a definite IUP is demonstrated, the risk of ectopic pregnancy becomes very low. Transvaginal sonography is more sensitive than transabdominal sonography, and can detect pregnancies as early as 5.5 to 6 weeks' gestational age. Hence, the demonstration of a definite IUP by crown-rump length or yolk sac is reassuring. The "identification of gestational sac" is sometimes misleading since an ectopic pregnancy can be associated with fluid in the uterus, a so-called "pseudogestational sac". Other sonographic findings of an extrauterine gestation include an embryo seen outside the uterus, or a large amount of intra-abdominal free fluid, usually indicating blood.

◆ Often, the quantitative hCG level is used in conjunction with transvaginal sonography. When the hCG level equals or exceeds 1 500 to 2 000 mIU/ml, an intrauterine gestational sac is usually seen on transvaginal ultrasound; in fact, when the hCG level meets or exceeds this threshold and no gestational sac is seen, the patient has a high likelihood of an ectopic pregnany. Laparoscopy is usually performed in this situation. When the hCG level is less than the threshold, and the patient does not have severe abdominal pain, hypotension, or adnexal tenderness and/or mass, then a repeat hCG level in 48 hr is permissible. A rise in the hCG of at least 66% above the initial level is good evidence of a normal pregnancy; in contrast, a lack of an appropriate rise of the hCG is indicative of an abnormal pregnancy, although the abnormal change does not identify whether the pregnancy is in the uterus or the tube. Some practitioners will use a progesterone level instead of serial hCG levels to assess the health of the pregnancy. A

是否存在。因为宫内宫外同时妊娠的可能性很低,仅为万分之一,所以一旦确定宫内妊娠,则异位妊娠的风险非常低。经阴道超声比腹部超声更敏感,能够检测到早在 5.5～6 周的妊娠。因此,检测到胚胎顶臀长或卵黄囊可确诊宫内妊娠。因为异位妊娠时宫腔液体可形成"假孕囊",所以"孕囊的鉴定"有时会误诊。其他宫腔外妊娠的超声表现包括子宫外可见胚胎,腹腔内大量可能为血液的游离液体。

◆ hCG 定量检查一般与经阴道超声检查结合起来使用。当 hCG 水平达到或超过 1 500 到 2 000 mIU/ml,经阴道超声检查通常可以发现宫腔内有妊娠囊;所以当 hCG 水平达到或超过阈值而宫腔内未见孕囊时,高度怀疑异位妊娠的可能性。此时可行腹腔镜检查。当 hCG 水平低于阈值而患者没有表现出明显腹痛、低血压或附件区压痛和包块时,需要在 48 h 后重复检测 hCG 水平。hCG 较原有水平至少升高 66% 提示正常妊娠;相反,hCG 水平没有相应升高提示异常妊娠,但不能区分妊娠在宫腔内或在输卵管。部分医生也用孕酮水平代替 hCG 作为评估妊娠的依据。孕酮水平大于 25 ng/ml 通常为正常宫内妊娠,

progesterone level of greater than 25 ng/ml almost always correlates with a normal intrauterine pregnancy, whereas a level of less than 5 ng/ml almost always correlates with an abnormal pregnancy.

- Treatment of an ectopic pregnancy may be surgical or medical. Salpingectomy (removal of the affected tube) is usually performed for those gestations too larger for conservative therapy, when rupture has occurred, or for those women who do not want future fertility. For a woman who wants to preserve her fertility and has an unruptured tubal pregnancy, a salpingostomy can be performed. An incision is carried out along the long axis of the tube, and the pregnancy tissue is removed. The incision on the tube is not reapproximated, because suturing may lead to stricture formation. Conservative treatment of the tube is associated with a 10% to 15% chance of persistent ectopic pregnancy. Serial hCG levels are, therefore, required with conservative surgical therapy to identify this condition.

- Methotrexate, a folic acid antagonist, is the principal form of medical therapy. It is usually given as a one-time, low dose, intramuscular injection, reserved for ectopic pregnancies less than 4 cm in diameter. Methotrexate is highly successful, leading to resolution of properly chosen ectopic pregnancies in 85% to 90% of cases. Occasionally, a second dose is required because the hCG level does not fall. Between 3 to 7 days following therapy, a patient may complain of abdominal pain, which is usually due to tubal abortion and, less commonly, rupture. Most women may be observed; however, hypotension, worsening or persistent pain, or a falling hematocrit may indicate tubal rupture and necessitate surgery. About 10% of women treated with medical therapy will require surgical intervention.

而低于 5 ng/ml 通常为异常妊娠。

- 异位妊娠的治疗包括药物和手术治疗。对于孕囊太大无法保守治疗，妊娠破裂或以后无生育要求的妇女，一般实施输卵管切除术（移除患侧输卵管）。

对于要求保留生育能力，输卵管妊娠未破裂的患者可以实施输卵管造口术。沿输卵管纵轴切开，取出妊娠组织，切口不用近接，因为缝线可导致输卵管狭窄。对输卵管的保守手术有 10%～15% 持续异位妊娠的风险，因此需持续监测 hCG 水平以明确治疗效果。

- 药物治疗主要用叶酸阻断剂甲氨蝶呤。对孕囊直径小于 4 cm 的异位妊娠，通常为单次，低剂量，肌内内注射给药。甲氨蝶呤能有效治愈 85%～90% 符合适应证的异位妊娠病例。偶尔因 hCG 水平未下降，需要再次用药。在治疗的第 3 到 7 天，患者可能出现腹痛，通常因输卵管妊娠流产或少见的破裂引起。多数患者仅需观察，无需特殊处理；但当出现低血压，疼痛加重或持续，或血细胞比容下降时，可能已发生输卵管妊娠破裂，就必须手术。约 10% 药物治疗的患者最终需要手术干预。

- Rare types of ectopic gestations such as cervical, ovarian, abdominal, or corneal（involving the portion of the tube that traverses the uterine muscle）pregnancies usually require surgical therapy.

3.2　Abortion

Key words

1. spontaneous abortion
2. threatened abortion
3. inevitable abortion
4. incomplete abortion
5. complete abortion
6. missed abortion
7. septic abortion
8. recurrent abortion

3.2.2　Differential diagnosis

- Spontaneous abortion（Miscarriage）：usually happens before 16 weeks.
- Ectopic pregnancy：6-8 weeks, decidual bleeding.
- Hydatidiform mole：usually before 16 weeks.
- Incidental causes.
- May present at any stage of pregnancy.
- Benign and malignant lesions（*i.e.*, varicosities of cervix, vagina or vulva, cervical ectopy or polyp, choriocarcinoma, cervical carcinoma）.
- Diagnostic error（*i.e.* bleeding from urinary tract or hemorrhoids）.

3.2.2　Workup

- Vital signs（rule out shock/sepsis/illness）.

- Pelvic exam（look at cervix, source of bleed）.

- β-human chorionic gonadotropin （hCG） level, complete blood count（CBC）.

- 对于少见类型的异位妊娠,如宫颈、卵巢、腹腔或子宫角(包括输卵管进入子宫肌层部位)妊娠,一般需要手术治疗。

3.2　流产

关键词

1. 自然流产
2. 先兆流产
3. 难免流产
4. 不全流产
5. 完全流产
6. 稽留流产
7. 流产感染
8. 复发性流产

3.2.1　鉴别诊断

- 自然流产:通常发生在孕 16 周以前。
- 异位妊娠:孕 6～8 周,蜕膜出血。
- 葡萄胎:通常发生在孕 16 周以前。
- 偶发原因。
- 可见于妊娠的任何阶段。
- 良性或恶性病变(如宫颈、阴道或外阴静脉曲张,宫颈柱状上皮异位或息肉,绒毛膜癌,宫颈癌)。
- 误诊(如泌尿道或痔疮出血)。

3.2.2　诊断流程

- 生命体征(排除休克/败血症/疾病)。
- 盆腔检查(观察宫颈,注意出血的来源)。
- β-人绒毛膜促性腺激素水平(hCG),全血计数(CBC)。

◆ Ultrasound (US) [assess fetal viability; abdominal US detects fetal heart motion by ≥ 7 weeks' gestational age (GA)].

3.2.3　Spontaneous abortion(Miscarriage)

Miscarriage is the expulsion, dead, of the products of conception before 28 weeks' gestation (early in first-trimester, late in second-trimester).

◆ Occurs in 30% of all pregnancies.

◆ Most are unrecognized because they occur before or at the time of the next expected menses (70%-80%).

◆ Fifteen to twenty percent of clinically diagnosed pregnancies are lost in T1 or early T2.

◆ Process are as follows:

→ Hemorrhage occurs in the decidua basalis leading to local necrosis and inflammation.

→ The ovum, partly or wholly detached, acts as a foreign body and initiates uterine contractions. The cervix begins to dilate.

→ Expulsion complete. The decidua is shed during the next few days in the lochial flow.

◆ Up to 12 weeks, before the placenta is independently developed, miscarriage may be complete as shown, but from the 12th to 28th week the gestation sac is likely to rupture leading to expulsion of the fetus, while the placenta is retained.

3.2.3.1　Etiology

In many cases the cause is unknown.

A. Abnormal development of the ovum

Of those fetuses recovered from miscarriage about half are said to be abnormal either chromosomally or structurally.

◆ Majority of abnormal karyotypes are numeric abnormalities as a result of errors during gametogenesis, fertilization, or the first division of the fertilized ovum.

◆ 超声检查（US）（评估胎儿活力；孕 7 周以上可经腹部超声探测胎心搏动）。

3.2.3　自然流产

流产指孕 28 周之前发生的妊娠丢失，即妊娠产物娩出或死亡（前三个月为早期，中三个月为晚期）。

◆ 发生在约 30% 妊娠中。

◆ 大多数（70%～80%）因为发生在预期的下次月经来潮之前或之时而不被认识到。

◆ 约 15%～20% 临床诊断的妊娠丢失发生在孕早期或早中期。

◆ 流产过程发生如下：

→ 底蜕膜出血，导致局部坏死和炎症。

→ 受精卵部分或全部脱离子宫，成为异物引起子宫收缩。宫颈开始扩张。

→ 完全娩出。在随后几天内，脱落的蜕膜随恶露排出。

◆ 在孕 12 周之前，胎盘尚未完全形成，流产可能如上述完全排出妊娠物，但在孕 12 周以后发生的流产可能只是孕囊破裂排出胎儿组织，而胎盘仍滞留在子宫内。

3.2.3.1　病因

很多情况下，流产的病因不明。

A. 受精卵形成异常

约一半以上流产的胚胎为染色体或结构异常。

◆ 大多数异常核型为染色体数目异常，主要发生在配子发生、受精或受精卵第一次分裂过程中。

◆ Frequency：

- Trisomy：50%-60%
- Monosomy（45，X）：7%-15%
- Triploidy：15%
- Tetraploidy：10%

B. Maternal condition

　　Pyrexial illness, infection, severe rhesus iso-immunisation and any chronic maternal disease have all been associated with an increased risk of pregnancy loss. A deficiency of progesterone or human chorionic gonadotrophin have both been postulated and used as a rationale for treatment though without any significant evidence of benefit.

→Infectious agents

　　Infectious agents in cervix, uterine cavity, or seminal fluid can cause abortions. These infections may be asymptomatic：

- Toxoplasma gondii
- Herpes simplex
- Ureaplasma urelyticum
- Mycoplasma hominis
- Listeria monocytogenes
- Chlamydia
- Gonorrhea

→Endocrine abnormalities

- Progesterone deficiency
- Polycystic ovarian syndrome（PCOS）—hypersecretion of luteinizing hormone（LH）
- Diabetes—uncontrolled

→Immunologic factors

- Lupus anticoagulant
- Anticardiolipin antibody（antiphospholipid syndrome）

→Environmental factors

- Tobacco：≥ 14 cigarettes/day increases abortion rates.
- Alcohol
- Irradiation
- Environmental toxin exposure
- Caffeine：> 5 cups/day

◆ 出现频率：

- 三体：50%～60%
- 单体（45，X）：7%～15%
- 三倍体：15%
- 四倍体：10%

B. 母体因素

　　发热性疾病、感染、严重恒河猴（Rh）同种免疫以及母体任何一种慢性疾病都可以增加妊娠丢失的风险。孕酮或人绒毛膜促性腺激素的缺乏被认为与流产有关，且尽管没有明显获益的证据，但两者仍被用于治疗流产。

→病原体

　　存在于宫颈、宫腔或精液中的病原体能导致流产。这些感染可能是无症状的：

- 鼠弓形虫
- 单纯疱疹
- 解脲支原体
- 人型支原体
- 单细胞增多性利斯特菌
- 衣原体
- 淋病

→内分泌异常

- 孕酮缺乏
- 多囊卵巢综合征（PCOS）——黄体生成素（LH）过度分泌
- 糖尿病——未经控制

→免疫因素

- 狼疮抗凝物
- 抗心磷脂抗体（抗心磷脂综合征）

→环境因素

- 吸烟：≥14 支烟/天增加流产率
- 酒精
- 辐射
- 环境毒素暴露
- 咖啡因：>5 杯/天

C.　Uterine causes

- *Congenital abnormality of the uterus*

  septate/bicornuate uterus （25%-30%） may interfere with the development of the growing fetus.

- *Cervical incompetence*

  Lacerations or functional incompetence may make it impossible for the uterus to contain a gestation normally. Miscarriage occurs in mid-trimester.

- *Fibroids（especially submucosal）*

  Although the majority of women with fibroids do not experience mechanical cause of pregnancy loss，a uterus distorted by fibroids may be unable to accommodate the growing fetus.

- *Intrauterine adhesions （i.e., from previous curettage）*

- *Tumor*

3.2.3.2　Classification

Classification is based on a mixture of clinical and pathological concepts，and is sufficiently flexible to suit a condition in which diagnosis is often only presumptive. Sepsis can complicate any type of abortion and，in countries with restrictive laws on abortion，must often be due to criminal interference.

Miscarriage becomes inevitable because of the amount of blood loss or dilatation of the cervix. Then it becomes either：

→*Complete miscarriage*

Uterine contractions are felt，the cervix dilates and blood loss continues. The fetus and placenta are expelled complete，the uterus contracts and bleeding stops. No further treatment is needed.

→*Incomplete miscarriage*

In spite of uterine contractions and cervical dilatation，only the fetus and some membranes are expelled. The placenta remains partly attached and bleeding continues. This miscarriage must be completed by surgical methods.

C.　子宫因素

- 先天性结构异常

  纵隔/双角子宫（25%～30%）可能阻碍胎儿生长。

- 宫颈机能不全

  宫颈撕裂伤或功能性机能不全可使子宫无法正常容纳妊娠。流产发生在孕中期。

- 子宫肌瘤（尤其位于黏膜下）

  尽管大多数患有子宫肌瘤的妇女不会经历肌瘤机械性因素导致的流产，但肌瘤可使子宫变形而无法适应正在生长的胎儿。

- 宫腔粘连（如因既往刮宫术引起）

- 肿瘤

3.2.3.2　分类

流产的分类是基于临床和病理概念的组合，能充分适应一些无法确诊的情况。任何类型的流产均可合并败血症，在一些对堕胎有严格法律控制的国家，这种情况多由性侵犯引起。

当失血过多或宫颈扩张，流产就不可避免，出现以下两种情况：

→完全流产

可触及宫缩，宫颈扩张，继续出血。当胎儿和胎盘组织完全排出，子宫停止收缩且血止。不需要进一步处理。

→不全流产

尽管子宫收缩，宫颈扩张，仅有胎儿和部分蜕膜排出。胎盘仍部分附着在子宫壁，继续出血。这种流产需要手术才能完全清理出残留组织。

3.2.3.3　Clinical features

◆ Hemorrhage is usually the first sign and may be very heavy if placental separation is incomplete.

◆ Pain is usually intermittent, "like a small labour". It ceases when the miscarriage is complete.

→ *Threatened miscarriage*

Miscarriage is said to threaten when any bleeding, usually painless, occurs before the 24th week. It may be impossible to distinguish it from partial shedding of the decidua at the time of a missed period which can occur up to 12 weeks.

Bed rest has been traditionally advised as treatment but there is no evidence that it affects the outcome. An ultrasound scan should be carried out and if the fetus is alive, the mother can be reassured.

→ *Inevitable miscarriage*

Here the bleeding may still be slight but uterine contractions have started to dilate the cervix. This can be detected on vaginal examination. Ultrasound may diagnose an inevitable miscarriage at an earlier stage by demonstrating fetal death. Treatment is by evacuation of the uterus.

3.2.3.4　Differential diagnosis

The diagnosis is not usually difficult but tubal pregnancy, hydatidiform mole and some menstrual disorders (*e. g.* oligomenorrhoea) may need to be considered.

3.2.3.5　Surgical treatment of incomplete miscarriage

◆ It must be done in operation room and with the patient anaesthetized (if necessary).

◆ The patient may bleed:
  • before admission to hospital
  • while in hospital
  • during the operation

◆ Blood loss may be large and facilities for blood transfusion must be at hand.

◆ The operator must, at all times, remember the

3.2.3.3　临床特征

◆ 阴道出血通常是第一症状,如胎盘组织与子宫壁不完全分离,出血量可能很大。

◆ 腹痛通常为间歇性,"像一个小的分娩"。当完全流产时腹痛停止。

→ 先兆流产

当开始出血就是先兆流产,通常无痛性,发生在孕24周之前。可能无法与直到孕12周发生稽留流产出现的蜕膜部分脱落出血相区别。

治疗上通常要求患者卧床休息,但没有证据显示这样能影响预后。应该行超声检查,如胎儿存活,可使孕母安心。

→ 难免流产

可能出血量仍不多,但宫缩已开始使宫颈扩张。窥检可以发现这一点。如超声检查发现胎儿死亡,可更早诊断难免流产。治疗方法为清空子宫。

3.2.3.4　鉴别诊断

诊断一般不难,但需考虑与输卵管妊娠、葡萄胎和月经失调相鉴别。

3.2.3.5　不全流产的手术治疗

◆ 必须在手术室进行,必要时可以进行麻醉。

◆ 患者出血可能发生在:
  • 入院前
  • 在医院
  • 手术中

◆ 出血量可能很大,输血设施备用。

◆ 手术过程中要随时谨记妊娠的

ease with which a gravid uterus can be perforated by a metal instrument.

- Removal of placental tissue with ovum forceps. The open blades are rotated to grasp tissue and then gently withdrawn. Before using any instrument inside the uterus an oxytocic, syntocinon 10 units or ergometrine 0.25 mg, should be given intravenously to cause contraction and hardening of the uterine wall.
- Evacuation is completed by careful exploration of the cavity with a sharp curette.

3.2.4　Threatened miscarriage

Threatened miscarriage is vaginal bleeding that occurs in the first 28 weeks of pregnancy, without the passage of products of conception（POC）or rupture of membranes. Pregnancy continues, although up to 50% results in loss of pregnancy.

3.2.4.1　Diagnosis

- Speculum exam reveals blood coming from a closed cervical os, without amniotic fluid or POC in the endocervical canal.
- Follow serial hCGs：should decrease by 65% every 48 hours（peaks at 10 weeks）.

3.2.4.2　Management

Observation.

3.2.5　Inevitable miscarriage

Inevitable miscarriage is vaginal bleeding, cramps, and cervical dilation. Expulsion of the products of conception（POC）is imminent.

3.2.5.1　Diagnosis

Speculum exam reveals blood coming from an open cervical os. Menstrual-like cramps typically occur.

3.2.5.2　Management

- Surgical evacuation of the uterus or expectant

子宫容易被金属器械穿孔。

- 用卵圆钳夹出胎盘组织。旋转张开的钳叶夹住组织，然后轻轻退出。在使用器械进入子宫操作之前，应静脉给予宫缩剂，缩宫素 10 U 或麦角新碱 0.25 mg，使子宫收缩，子宫壁变硬。

- 用锐利的刮匙小心地探索宫腔，以确保清宫完全。

3.2.4　先兆流产

先兆流产指孕 28 周之前出现阴道流血，没有妊娠产物（POC）排出或胎膜破裂。妊娠可以继续，但约 50% 导致妊娠丢失。

3.2.4.1　诊断

- 窥检发现出血来自闭合的宫颈口，无羊水流出，宫颈内管无妊娠产物。
- 动态监测 hCGs：应每 48 h 下降 65%（10 周左右为峰值）。

3.2.4.2　处理

密切观察。

3.2.5　难免流产

难免流产指阴道出血，腹痛以及宫颈扩张，妊娠产物即将排出。

3.2.5.1　诊断

窥检发现出血来自张开的宫颈口。典型时出现月经样腹部绞痛。

3.2.5.2　处理

- 手术清空子宫或期待疗法（13

management （＜13 weeks）.

◆ Rh typing-D immunoglobulin （RhoGAM） is administered to Rh-negative, unsensitized patient to prevent isoimmunization.

3.2.6　Incomplete miscarriage

Incomplete miscarriage is the passage of some, but not all POC from the cervical os.

3.2.6.1　Diagnosis

◆ Cramping and bleeding.
◆ Enlarged, boggy uterus.
◆ Dilated internal os with POC present in the endocervical canal or vagina.

3.2.6.2　Management

◆ Stabilization （i. e., IV fluids and oxytocin if heavy bleeding is present）.
◆ Blood typing and crossmatching for possible transfusion if bleeding is brisk or low hemoglobin/ patient symptomatic.
◆ RhoGAM if needed.
◆ POC are removed from the endocervical canal and uterus with ring forceps. Suction dilation and curettage （D&C） is performed after vital signs have stabilized.

Karyotyping of POC if loss is recurrent.

3.2.7　Complete miscarriage

Complete miscarriage is the complete passage of POC.

3.2.7.1　Diagnosis

◆ Uterus is well contracted.
◆ Cervical os may be closed.
◆ Pain has ceased.

3.2.7.2　Management

◆ Examination all POC for completeness and characteristics.

周以前）。

◆ 对 Rh 血型阴性,未致敏的患者,给予 RhoGAM 免疫球蛋白防止同种免疫。

3.2.6　不全流产

不全流产是指仅有部分而非全部妊娠产物从宫颈口排出。

3.2.6.1　诊断

◆ 腹部绞痛和阴道出血。
◆ 增大而柔软的子宫。
◆ 宫颈内口扩张,可见妊娠产物在宫颈内管或阴道。

3.2.6.2　处理

◆ 维持体液（如出血量大,静脉输液并给予缩宫素）。
◆ 如出血活跃或低血红蛋白/患者有症状,则需检测血型,交叉配血以备输血。
◆ 如必要,给予 RhoGAM。
◆ 用环钳从宫颈内管和宫腔夹出妊娠产物。在生命体征平稳后实施抽吸清宫。

如妊娠丢失再次发生,妊娠产物可做核型分析。

3.2.7　完全流产

完全流产指妊娠产物完全排出。

3.2.7.1　诊断

◆ 子宫收缩良好。
◆ 宫颈口可能闭合。
◆ 腹痛停止。

3.2.7.2　处理

◆ 检查所有妊娠产物,看是否完整和具有特征性。

- Between 8 and 14 weeks, curettage is often performed due to increased likelihood that the abortion was incomplete.
- Observe patient for further bleeding and fever.

3.2.8 Missed miscarriage

Missed miscarriage is when the POC are retained after the fetus has expired. The retention of a fetus, after its death, lasts for a period of several weeks.

Death of the fetus occurs unnoticed or is marked by some vaginal bleeding which is regarded as a threat to miscarry. Symptoms of pregnancy regress, however, and the uterus shrinks as liquor is absorbed. The pregnancy test will become negative and ultrasound confirms the diagnosis.

If retained long enough the gestation may end up as:

→CARNEOUS MOLE

A carneous mole is a lobulated mass of laminated blood clot. The projections into the shrunken cavity are caused by repeated hemorrhages in the chorio-decidual space.

In very early pregnancies (up to 12 weeks) complete absorption of the dead ovum may occur.

→MACERATED FETUS

The skull bones collapse, override and the spine is flexed and there is little or no amniotic fluid on ultrasound examination. The internal organs degenerate and the abdomen is filled with blood stained fluid. The skin peels very easily.

Pathological changes in the fetus such as mummification (fetus papyraceous) and calcification (lithopaedion) are exceedingly rare.

3.2.8.1 Diagnosis

- The pregnant uterus fails to grow, and symptoms of pregnancy have disappeared.
- Intermittent vaginal bleeding/spotting/brown

- 在孕 8~14 周,往往实施刮宫术,因为这个阶段流产不全的可能性增高。
- 观察患者是否继续出血或出现发热。

3.2.8 稽留流产

稽留流产指胎儿死亡后妊娠产物仍滞留于宫腔。胎儿死亡后滞留于宫腔可持续数周。

胎儿死亡时不被发现或在阴道出血时被认为是先兆流产。但是妊娠的症状退化,因为羊水被吸收,所以子宫变小。妊娠试验变为阴性以及超声检测可以确诊。

如妊娠产物滞留时间长,则妊娠可发展为:

→肉样胎块

肉样胎块是层压血块包绕胎块形成的分叶状包块,向萎缩的宫腔突出,是由于绒毛膜-蜕膜间隙反复出血造成的。

在孕早期(直至孕 12 周),死亡的卵子可能被完全吸收。

→浸软胎

死胎颅骨塌陷并重叠,脊柱屈曲,超声检查羊水很少或无羊水,胎儿内脏器官变质,腹部充满血性液体,皮肤很容易剥脱。

胎儿干尸化(薄纸样胎)和钙化(石胎)等病理改变比较罕见。

3.2.8.1 诊断

- 妊娠的子宫停止长大,妊娠的症状消失。
- 间歇性阴道出血/点滴出血/血

discharge and a firm, closed cervix.

♦ Decline in quantitative β-hCG.

♦ Ultrasound confirms lack of fetal heartbeat.

3.2.8.2　Management

If left alone most missed miscarriages will be expelled spontaneously, but during the waiting period there is a slight risk of coagulation defect and this should be investigated before embarking on evacuation of the uterus in cases of fetal death of more than four weeks.

♦ Check fibrinogen level, partial thromboplastin time (PTT), antibody screen, and ABO blood type.

♦ *Surgical*. Evacuate the uterus.

→If the uterus is not larger than the size of an eight to ten week pregnancy it may be emptied by suction D & C in first trimester. This operation requires experience and as bleeding is free until the uterus is emptied, transfusion facilities must be available.

→If the size of uterus is larger, induce labor with IV oxytocin and cervical dilators or prostaglandin E2 suppositories.

♦ *Medical*. Mifepristone, a progesterone receptor blocker may be used to "prime" the uterus for miscarriage and be followed by the use of gemeprost or misoprostol and medical management of this condition is highly effective in producing complete miscarriage.

♦ Administer RhoGAM to Rh-negative, unsensitized patients.

3.2.9　Septic miscarriage

Infection may complicate miscarriage once the cervix starts to dilate or instruments are introduced into the uterine cavity.

♦ Infected products of conception (POC) are present.

性白带,宫颈牢固、闭合。

♦ β-hCG 下降。

♦ 超声确诊没有胎心。

3.2.8.2　处理

如不加强管理,大多数稽留流产会被忽略,但在等待过程中存在出现凝血障碍的风险。因此在胎儿死亡超过 4 周的病例中,开始清空子宫之前就应做凝血相关检查。

♦ 检测纤维蛋白原水平,部分凝血活酶时间(PTT),抗体筛查和 ABO 血型检查。

♦ **手术**。清空子宫。

→如子宫不大于妊娠 8～10 周大小,可实施早孕期清宫术。该手术需要一定经验,且子宫清空前可能一直出血,所以必须备好输血设施。

→如子宫更大,需要给予静脉用缩宫素和宫颈扩张剂或前列腺素 E2 栓剂进行引产。

♦ **药物**。米非司酮是一种孕酮受体阻断剂,可用来使子宫处于准备状态。之后再使用吉美前列素或米索前列醇。经药物治疗后,对稽留流产实施的清宫术能更有效地完成。

♦ 对 Rh 阴性且未致敏的患者使用 RhoGAM。

3.2.9　流产感染

一旦宫颈开始扩张或器械进入宫腔操作,可增加流产合并感染的机会。

♦ 感染的妊娠产物存在于宫腔。

◆ The infection is usually polymicrobial often with *Staphylococcus aureus*, *Escherichia coli*, and other gram-negative organisms. These are usually the vaginal or bowel commensals.

3.2.9.1 Causes

◆ Delay in evacuation of the uterus. Either the patient delays seeking advice, or the surgical evacuation has been incomplete. Infection occurs from vaginal organisms after 48 hours.

◆ Trauma, either perforation or cervical tear. Healing is delayed and infection is more likely to be a peritonitis or cellulitis. Criminal abortions are, of course, particularly liable to sepsis.

3.2.9.2 Diagnosis

◆ Generalized pelvic discomfort, pain, and tenderness.

◆ Signs of peritonitis.

◆ Malodorous vaginal and cervical discharge.

◆ Leukocytosis.

3.2.9.3 Management

◆ This should be active to minimize the risk of septic shock.

◆ Cervical and high vaginal swabs and blood cultures are taken.

◆ Check CBC, urinalysis (UA), serum electrolytes, liver function tests (LFTs), blood urea nitrogen (BUN), creatinine, and coagulation panel.

◆ Abdominal and chest films to exclude free air in the peritoneal cavity (also helpful to look for the presence of gas-forming bacteria or foreign body).

◆ A broad spectrum antibiotic such as a cephalosporin together with an agent effective against anaerobes prescribed by IV.

◆ Curettage should be carried out as soon as possible; there is nothing to be gained by leaving infected material in utero. The septic uterus is particularly vulnerable to trauma.

◆ 通常为多种微生物感染,包括金黄色葡萄球菌、大肠杆菌以及其他革兰阴性菌等阴道或肠道正常菌群。

3.2.9.1 病因

◆ 子宫排空延迟。患者延误就诊或清宫手术不彻底。感染在 48 h 后从阴道菌群开始。

◆ 外伤,包括穿孔或宫颈裂伤。如延误治疗,感染可能加重发展为腹膜炎或蜂窝织炎。当然,犯罪所致的流产多为感染性的。

3.2.9.2 诊断

◆ 一般症状如盆腔不适、疼痛和触痛。

◆ 腹膜炎体征。

◆ 阴道和宫颈分泌物恶臭。

◆ 白细胞增多症。

3.2.9.3 处理

◆ 应尽可能降低感染性休克的风险。

◆ 应做宫颈和高位阴道拭子以及血培养检查。

◆ 全血计数,尿液分析,血电解质,肝功能,血尿素氮,肌酐和凝血检查。

◆ 拍腹部平片和胸片排除腹腔游离气体(也有助于发现产气细菌或异物)。

◆ 静脉用广谱抗生素,如头孢菌素,并合用一种有效对抗厌氧菌的药物。

◆ 应尽快实施清宫术,因为宫腔残留物无益。感染的子宫尤其容易受创。

3.2.10 Recurrent miscarriage

Three or more successive clinically recognized pregnancy losses prior to 28 weeks' GA constitutes recurrent miscarriage. Women with two successive spontaneous abortions have a recurrence risk of 25%-30%.

3.2.10.1 Etiology

- Parental chromosomal abnormalities (balanced translocation is the most common).
- Anatomic abnormalities (congenital and acquired).
- Endocrinologic abnormalities.
- Infections (*e. g.*, Chlamydia, Ureaplasma).
- Autoimmunity.
- Unexplained (majority of cases).
- Maternal state hypercoagulable.

3.2.10.2 Management

Investigate possible etiologies. Potentially useful tests include:
- Parental peripheral blood karyotypes.
- Sonohysterogram (Intrauterine structural study).
- Luteal-phase endometrial biopsy.
- Anticardiolipin and antiphosphatidyl serine antibodies.

- Lupus anticoagulant.
- Factor V Leiden.

3.3 Preterm Labour and PROM

Key words

1. preterm
2. moderately preterm
3. extremely preterm
4. fFN testing

5. cervical assessement
6. tocolysis

3.2.10 复发性流产

复发性流产指连续 3 次或以上经临床确诊孕 28 周前的妊娠丢失。有过两次连续自发性流产的妇女再次发生流产的风险为 25%～30%。

3.2.10.1 病因

- 亲代染色体异常（平衡易位最常见）。
- 解剖学异常（先天性和获得性）。
- 内分泌异常。
- 感染（如衣原体、解脲支原体）。
- 自身免疫病。
- 原因不明（大多数病例）。
- 母体血液高凝状态。

3.2.10.2 处理

查找可能的病因，以下为可能有用的检查：
- 亲代外周血核型分析。
- 子宫超声造影（宫腔内结构检查）。
- 黄体期子宫内膜活检。
- 抗心磷脂和抗磷脂酰基抗体血清学检查。
- 狼疮抗凝物。
- 凝血因子 V。

3.3 早产及胎膜早破

关键词

1. 早产
2. 中期早产
3. 极早早产
4. 胎儿纤维连接蛋白宫颈阴道分泌物检查
5. 宫颈评估
6. 宫缩抑制剂

7. corticosteroids

8. cervical cerclage

9. prelabour rupture of the membranes

10. group B streptococcal

3.3.1　Definition

■ Demonstrated progressinve dilatation of the cervix with uertine contractions between 20 and 36^{+6} completed weeks gestation(Canada).

■ An infant in classified as preterm if the delivery occurs before 37 weeks' gestation，between 28 and 37 completed weeks(China).

■ Between 24 to 37 weeks(USA).

Mild Preterm：$34-36^{+6}$ weeks.

Moderately preterm：$32-33^{+6}$ weeks.

Early preterm：28-32 weeks.

Extremely preterm：20-28 weeks.

3.3.2　Prevention measures in antenatal care

Up to 50% of preterm births are potentially preventable. Population based strategies that provide effective in reducing the rate of preterm births include：

■ Preconception preparation：nutritional status, avoidance of smoking and drug.

■ Supportive environment.

■ Providing the woman with information of avoidance of risk factors of preterm.

■ Education of early symptoms of preterm labour.

■ Treatment of symptomatic vaginal infections before 32 weeks.

■ For women with previous preterm birth，routine screening and treatment for the presence of bacterial vaginosis reduce the likelihood of preterm labour, prelabour rupture of membrances.

■ For women with a history of cervical insufficiency, cervical cerclage is effective method of prevention preterm.

3.3.1　定义

■ 孕 20 周到 36^{+6} 孕周之间,出现子宫收缩和宫口进行性的扩大现象,称为早产(加拿大)。

■ 在孕 28 周至 37 周之间出生的新生儿称为早产儿(中国)。

■ 在孕 24 周至 37 周之间出生,称为早产(美国)。

轻型早产:$34\sim36^{+6}$周之间早产;

中期早产:$32\sim33^{+6}$周之间早产;

早期早产:$28\sim32$周之间早产;

极早早产:$20\sim28$周之间早产。

3.3.2　早产的预防措施

50%的早产是可以预防的。下列在社区人群中实施的措施有助于预防早产发生:

■ 作好孕前准备:改善营养状态,戒烟,戒毒品。

■ 支持性的环境。

■ 告之产妇避免引发早产的危险因素。

■ 提供产前教育,告之早产的症状与表现。

■ 在 32 孕周前治疗无症状性阴道炎。

■ 对于有前次早产史的孕妇,常规阴道细菌学检查与治疗能够降低早产、早破膜的发生率。

■ 对于有宫颈机能不全的孕妇,预防性地宫颈结扎对预防早产有效。

■ There is no evidence supporting the use of routine hospitalization for bed rest to prevent preterm birth in women with multiple pregnancy.

3.3.3 Diagnosis

3.3.3.1 Signs

■ Low abdominal pain, cramps and/or pelvic pressure.
■ Low backache.
■ Increased vaginal discharge/Bleeding, spotting, or show.
■ Regular uterine activity accompanied by cervical effacement and dilatation.

3.3.3.2 Assessment

■ General：accuracy of gestational age , maternal vital signs.
■ Fetal heart rate assessment.
■ Sterile speculum examination to obtain.
■ Sample for fetal fibronectin test, determine status of membranes, and to obtain vaginal cultures sample.
■ Cervical assessement：transvaginal cervical measurement by B ultrasound is superior to the digital examination of the cervix in predicting preterm birth. An endovaginal ultrasound for cervical length should be obtained if possile.
■ For women idenfified to be at increased risk of preterm birth, cervical length less than 15 mm has a postive predictive value for extreme preterm (＜28 weeks).
■ And the cervical length greater than 30 mm after 24 weeks has a high negative predictive value.

■ There is no evidence to support routine prenatal transvaginal ultrasound assessment of cervical length in the absence of risk factors.
■ For preterm labour with intact membranes beyond 34 weeks, management decisions can be based on digitalexam(transvaginal ultrasound may not be done).

■ 没有证据支持双胎的孕妇常规的住院并卧床休息可以预防早产发生。

3.3.3 诊断

3.3.3.1 表现

■ 下腹部疼痛，腿麻木或骨盆内压力感。
■ 后腰背部疼痛。
■ 阴道分泌物增多，阴道流血，点滴状出血或见红。
■ 规律性的子宫收缩并伴有宫颈的扩张展开。

3.3.3.2 评估

■ 一般情况评估:准确计算判断孕周，母亲生命体征测量。
■ 胎心评估。
■ 无菌窥器检查，取胎儿纤维连接蛋白标本，评估胎膜是否破裂，并取阴道分泌物标本。
■ 宫颈的评估:对于预测早产是否会发生，利用经阴道B超评估宫颈要优于阴道内直接指检。经阴道B超测量宫颈的长度。
■ 对于有早产高危因素的孕妇，宫颈的长度小于 15 mm 有较好的阳性预测价值，有可能发生极早早产(小于 28 孕周)。
■ 24 孕周后如果宫颈长度大于 30 mm,有较好的阴性预测值不会发生早产。
■ 没有证据支持对于没有早产危险因素的产妇，做常规的B超宫颈长度评估。
■ 对于大于 34 周且胎膜完整的孕妇，可利用阴道指检评估宫颈情况(可能不需要做B超)。

- CBC，urinalysis.
- Consider ultrasound if gestational age，placental site，or fetal presentation is unknown.

※A digital exam should not be done until after the speculum exam has ruled out ROM.

3.3.4　fFN testing

3.3.4.1　Indications for fFN testing.

- 24 to 34 completed weeks.
- Threatened preterm labour：regular uterine contractions ＞6/per hour，and/or pelvic pressure.

- Intact amniotic membrane.
- CX≤3 cm dilatation.
- Established fetal wellbeing.

3.3.4.2　Contraindications for fFN testing

- EGA＜24 or ＞34 completed weeks.
- Preterm PROM.
- CX＞3 cm dilatation.
- Cervical cerclage.
- Active vaginal bleeding.
- Vaginal exam or sexual intercourse in the past 24 hours.

3.3.4.3　Specimen collectioin

- The equipment required for fFN specimen collection includes the swab，collection tube，tube cap，test cartridge and an instrument based system to perform the fFN testing.
- Perform a speculum examination before vaginal untrasound，before digital examination and without the use of lubricants. Otherwise，it should be to wait 24 hours later to obtaining the specimen.

3.3.4.4　Value if the fFN test is positive

- A positive test in association with symptoms of preterm labour and cervical change suggests a high

- 血常规,尿常规检查。
- 经腹部超声判断孕周、胎盘位置和胎方位情况（如果不明确）。

※在做无菌窥器检查之前,不要进行阴道指检。

3.3.4　胎儿纤维连接蛋白宫颈阴道分泌物检查

3.3.4.1　fFN 检查的指征

- 孕 24～34 周。
- 有先兆早产的征象:规律宫缩多于 6 次/h,或感到骨盆内压迫感。
- 胎膜完整。
- 宫颈扩张≤3 cm。
- 胎儿情况良好。

3.3.4.2　fFN 检查的负指征

- 小于 24 孕周或大于 34 孕周。
- 出现早产胎膜早破。
- 宫颈扩张大于 3 cm。
- 做过宫颈的环扎术。
- 有活动性的阴道流血。
- 在过去的 24 h 内做过阴道检查或有性生活。

3.3.4.3　标本采集

- 标本采集用物:标本采集刮片、试管、试管帽、其他试验相关的用品和 fFN 试验的仪器。

- 要在进行阴道 B 超检查、阴道指检之前进行标本采集,不能应用润滑剂,如果已经用过阴道内冲洗等,要等待 24 h 后再作采集。

3.3.4.4　fFN 检查阳性的意义

- 如果检查结果为阳性,并且伴有早产的症状和宫颈的开大变

enough risk of preterm delivery that the woman should be treated and transferred to an appropriate facility to care for a neonate of the expected gestational age.

化,提示孕妇有高度危险会发生早产,要及时转诊产妇到有抢救新生儿条件的上级医院。

- If the woman is in an urban tertiary centre, then management plans including donsideration of tocolytis, adminstration of corticosteroids, may be undertaken.

- 如果孕妇已经在一个三级医院,开始给予早产的管理,包括应用宫缩抑制药物、肾上腺皮质激素等。

3.3.4.5　Value If the fFN test is negative

3.3.4.5　fFN 检查阴性的意义

- A negative test provides greater than 95% probability that the woman will not deliver within the next 7-10 days. Consideration should be given to having her stay in her community and treatment with tocolytic therapy and corticosteroids would not be justified.

- fFN 结果阴性,提示孕妇在未来的 7～10 天内有 95% 的概率不会发生早产。建议孕妇在家中或社区内休息观察,没有必要给予宫缩抑制剂和肾上腺皮质激素。

　　※If the patient continues to have symptoms of preterm labour, reevaluation of fFN should be perfomed 5-7 days later(Figure 3-3-1).

　　※如果孕妇仍然感觉有早产的症状(如骨盆压迫感、子宫收缩等),5～7 天后可以再次检查 fFN(见图 3-3-1)。

3.3.5　Treatment of preterm labour

3.3.5　早产的治疗

3.3.5.1　General care

3.3.5.1　一般处理

- Offer support, reassurance, and attention to comfort measures.

- 给予支持、鼓励和关注,保持孕妇舒适。

- Monitor fetal heart rate and contraction frequency using electronic fetal monitoring or intermittentausculation.

- 观察胎心和宫缩频率,应用电子胎心监护设备或间断性的评估胎心。

- Always palpate the uterus to determine contraction strength.

- 始终要注意用手触摸宫缩情况,评估收缩的强度。

- There is no evidence supporting the use of intravenous hydration to prevent or arrest preterm labour. Women with evidence of dehydration my be, however, benefit from the treatment.

- 没有证据支持对于早产的孕妇要给予静脉输液。但对于有脱水症状的孕妇,输液可能有效。

- There is no evidence either supporting or refutation the use of bed rest at home or in hospital, to prevent preterm brith for women with singleton pregnancy.

- 目前没有证据支持对于早产的孕妇需要在家中或医院内卧床休息。

3.3.5.2　For suspician of preterm labour

If fFN test is negative then reassure the woman and consider：

- Transvaginal ultrasound of the cervix.
- Treatment of bacterial vaginosis(if positive).

- Discharging the woman home.
- Repeat fFN testing in 5-7 days if woman continuses to be symptomatic.

If fFN test is positive：

- Consideration should be given to transferring the woman to a care facility appropriate for her gestational age.
- Tocolysis and corticosteroids administered to accelerat lung maturity.
- In the absence of fetal fibronectin testing, consider admission tocolysis 12 hours to determine if uertine irritability felt by patient and to assess for contractions.
- Administer antibiotic therapy for GBS prophylaxis.

3.3.5.3　For diagnosis of preterm labour

- Consider maternal/fetal transfer, discuss with referral center and or call provincial transfer(120).

- Administer antibiotic therapy for GBS prophylaxis.
- Patients with PROM before 32 weeks of gestation should be cared for expectantly until 33 completed weeks of gestation if no maternal or fetal contraindications exist.
- If less than 32 weeks, consider tocolysis for 24-48 hours with Indomethacin.
- The aim of the tocolysis therapy is allow transfer to an appropriate center and to permit corticosteroids to be utilized to decrease neonatal morbidity.

3.3.5.2　先兆早产的处理

如果 fFN 检查结果是阴性，向孕妇解释并作以下处理：

- 经阴道 B 超测量宫颈长度。
- 治疗细菌性阴道炎（如果检查结果是阳性）。
- 让产妇出院回家。
- 如果产妇回家后仍然感到有早产的表现，5～7 天后再次检查 fFN。

如果 fFN 检查结果是阳性：

- 考虑让孕妇转到有抢救处理早产儿条件的上级医院。

- 考虑应用宫缩抑制药物和皮质激素促进肺成熟。
- 如果没有条件进行 fFN 检查，考虑给予孕妇 12 h 的宫缩抑制药物并观察病人是否仍然有自觉症状，评估有无子宫收缩。
- 对 B 族链球菌预防性应用抗生素治疗。

3.3.5.3　对于确诊的早产孕妇处理

- 考虑转诊母亲和新生儿，与转诊中心联系或呼叫急诊转运中心（120）。
- 应用抗链球菌药物预防治疗。
- 如果没有母亲或新生儿紧急情况，对于小于 32 周早产的孕妇应尽可能延长孕周到 33 周以上。
- 如果小于 32 孕周，考虑应用宫缩抑制剂吲哚美辛 24～48 h。
- 应用宫缩抑制剂的目的是争取时间转运到上级医院，使皮质激素有时间发挥作用促进肺成熟，降低新生儿的患病率。

3.3.5.4 Indication for indomethacin

- Gestational age <32 weeks. Not recommended for gestational age >32 weeks.
- Initial dose: 100mg rectal suppository.
- Maintenance dose: 25-50 mg orally or rectally q 4-6 h for 24-48 hours.

- Discontinue use after 48 hours, prelonged use over hours can be associated with development of ductal constriction and oligohydramnios.

  ※ Traditionallly magnesium sulfate（$MgSO_4$）therapy has been used as a tocolytic. However, there is no evidence that $MgSO_4$ is an effective tocolytic.

  The evidence suggests that $MgSO_4$ is ineffective at delaying birth or preventing preterm birth, and its use is associated with an increased mortality for the infant. $MgSO_4$ should not be used as a tocolytic medication.

  ※ There is insufficient evidence to support the routine administration of nitroglycerin in the treatment of threatened preterm labour.

3.3.5.5 Contraindications to tocolysis

- Non reassuring fetal condition.
- Lethal fetal anomaly.
- Intrauterine fetal death.
- Chorioamnionitis.
- Severe gestational hypertensioin with adverse conditions.

- Severe IUGR(<3 percentile).

3.3.5.6 Corticosteroids

- All pregnant women between 23^{+0} and 33^{+6} weeks gestation who are at risk of preterm birth within 7 days should be administered a single course of corticosteroids.
- Giving a single course of corticosteroids to

3.3.5.4 吲哚美辛应用的指征

- 只用于小于 32 孕周者。大于 32 孕周早产不建议应用。
- 首次剂量：100 mg 肛门用药。
- 维持量：25～50 mg 口服或肛门用药，1 次/4～6 h，应用 24～48 h。
- 48 h 后停药。过长时间应用有导致动脉导管闭锁和羊水过少的危险。

  ※传统应用硫酸镁（$MgSO_4$）作为宫缩抑制剂。但目前的证据不支持硫酸镁是有效的宫缩抑制剂。

  目前的研究证据显示，硫酸镁对于延迟早产分娩和预防早产是无效的。应用硫酸镁治疗早产增加新生儿的患病率。硫酸镁不能作为宫缩抑制剂应用。

  ※目前没有充分的证据支持常规应用硝酸甘油可预防早产发生。

3.3.5.5 应用宫缩抑制剂的禁忌证

- 胎儿情况不好。
- 严重的胎儿畸形。
- 宫内死胎。
- 绒毛膜羊膜炎症。
- 严重的妊娠高血压，严重的产妇并发症。
- 严重的宫内发育迟缓（小于 3%）。

3.3.5.6 皮质激素应用

- 所有在 23～33^{+6} 周之间的孕妇出现早产的症状，有可能在 7 天内发生早产危险者，应当给予皮质激素单次剂量。
- 有早产危险的孕妇给予单次剂

pregnant women at risk for preterm birth reduces the risk of death, respiratory distress syndrome, and intraventricular hemorrhage in their preterm newborns.

- Betamethasone is the drug of choice and is the only steroid medication shown in clinical trials to be effective.
- Betamethasone: 12 mg IM, 2 doses at 24 hour interval.

- Combined use of steroids in pregnancy and use of surfactant in the immediate newborn period resulted in additional improvement in outcome of newborns.

※Some practitioners still use Dexamethasone 6 mg IM, 4 doses, at 12 hour intervals, howerver, there is a lack of evidence supporting its effectiveness on the maturation of the fetal lung and recent study has shown cocerns regard to long term neurological outcomes.

3.3.5.7　Gestational age management

(1)Near term (34 weeks to 36 completed)

- Proceed to delivery, usually by induction of labor.
- Group B streptococcal prophylaxis recommended.

(2)Preterm (32 weeks to 33 completed weeks)

- Expectant management, unless fetal pulmonary maturity is documented.
- Group B streptococcal prophylaxis recommended.

- Corticosteroid—no consensus, but some experts recommend.
- Antibiotics recommended to prolong latency if there are no contraindications.

(3)Preterm (24 weeks to 31 completed weeks)

- Expectant management.
- Group B streptococcal prophylaxis recommended.

- Single-course corticosteroid use recommended.
- Tocolytics—no consensus.

量皮质激素能够降低新生儿死亡率、呼吸窘迫综合征和脑室内出血等并发症。

- 倍他米松（倍他米松二丙酸酯）是目前唯一证明有效的用于早产的皮质激素类药物。
- 应用：倍他米松 12 mg IM，24 h 内应用 2 次。
- 孕妇应用皮质激素联合新生儿出生后立即应用肺表面活性剂能够改善新生儿预后。

※目前仍有人应用地塞米松 6 mg IM，每 12 h 1 次，共 4 次。但目前没有研究证据支持这种疗法能够促进肺成熟，近期的研究发现可能有远期神经系统的影响。

3.3.5.7　不同孕周的管理原则

(1)接近足月（34～36 孕周）

- 准备分娩，通常情况是给予引产。
- 预防性应用 B 族链球菌抗生素。

(2)早产（32～33 孕周）

- 期待疗法，除非有充分的证据表明胎肺已经成熟。
- 给予预防性应用 B 族链球菌抗生素。
- 皮质激素：没有充分证据是否应用。有的专家认为需要应用。
- 预防性应用抗生素来延长孕周，如果没有其他禁忌证。

(3)早产（24～31 孕周）

- 期待疗法。
- 给予预防性应用 B 族链球菌抗生素。
- 给予皮质激素单次剂量。
- 没有证据支持应用宫缩抑制剂。

- Antibiotics recommended to prolong latency if there are no contraindications.

(4) Less than 24 weeks patient counseling

- Expectant management or induction of labor.
- Group B streptococcal prophylaxis is not recommended.
- Corticosteroids are not recommended.
- Antibiotics—there are incomplete data on use in prolonging latency.

3.3.6 Preruption of membrane

Prelabour rupture of the membrane refers to the condition of membrance ruptured before labour has initialed. It occurs in about 8% of pregnant women and more than 90% of these women go into spontaneous labour within 24 hours. Accoding to pregnant weeks, it can be divided to two groups: preterm prelabour rupture of membranes (PPROM) and term prelabour rupture of membranes.

3.3.6.1 Preterm prelabour rupture of membranes

(1) Diagnosis

- The diagnosis of spontaneous rupture of the membranes is best achieved by maternal history followed by a sterile speculum examination.
- Ultrasound examination is useful in some cases to help confirm the diagnosis.
- Digital cervical examinations should be avoided in patients with PROM unless they are in active labor or imminent delivery is anticipated.

(2) Management

- Patients with PROM before 32 weeks of gestation should be cared for expectantly until 33 completed weeks of gestation if no maternal or fetal contraindications exist.
- With PROM at 32 to 33 completed weeks of gestation, labor induction may be considered if fetal pulmonary maturity has been documented.
- A single course of antenatal corticosteroids should

预防性应用抗生素来延长孕周，如果没有其他禁忌证。

(4) 低于 24 孕周孕妇早产的处理

- 期待疗法或引产。
- 不主张预防性应用 B 族链球菌抗生素。
- 不主张应用皮质激素。
- 没有充分的依据支持预防性应用抗生素延长孕周。

3.3.6 胎膜早破

胎膜早破是指胎膜在临产前破裂。发生率大约为 8%，其中 90% 以上的孕妇在 24 h 内自然地发动宫缩临产。

根据孕周，又大体分为两类：早产胎膜早破（PPROM）和足月胎膜早破。

3.3.6.1 早产早破膜

(1) 诊断

- 诊断胎膜破裂最好的依据是产妇的自述，和应用无菌窥器检查评估。
- 某些情况下可应用 B 超来辅助检查。
- 对于早产早破膜的病人，要避免作阴道指检，除非产妇已进入活跃期或即将分娩。

(2) 处理

- 32 孕周之前的病人发生胎膜早破要给予期待疗法，尽可能延长孕周至 33 周以上，除非有异常情况不允许再延长。
- 对于 32～33 孕周之间胎膜早破病人，如果有确切证据表明肺已成熟，可以考虑行引产结束分娩。
- 孕 32 周前发生胎膜早破者要

be administered to women with PROM before 32 weeks of gestation to reduce the risks of respiratory distress syndrome（RDS），perinatal mortality，and other morbidities.

- During expectant management of preterm PROM remote from term to prolong pregnancy，a 48-hour course of intravenous ampicillin and erythromycin followed by 5 days of amoxicillin and erythromycin is recommended and to reduce infectious and gestational age-dependent neonatal morbidity.

- Tocolysis Prophylactic tocolysis in women with PPROM without uterine activity is not recommended.

（3）Delivery of the Fetus

- Delivery should be considered at 34 weeks of gestation.

- Where expectant management is considered beyond 34 weeks of gestation，women should be counselled about the increased risk of chorioamnionitis and its consequences versus the decreased risk of serious respiratory problems in the neonate，admission for neonatal intensive care，and caesarean section.

3.3.6.2　Prelabour rupture of the membranes at term

（1）Diagnosis

- Women with an uncertain history of prelabour rupture of the membranes should be offered a speculum examination to determine whether their membranes have ruptured.

- Digital vaginal examination in the absence of contractions should be avoided.

（2）Management

- Most of women with prelabour rupture of the membranes will go into labour within 24 hours.

- Induction of labour is appropriate approximately 24 hours after rupture of the membranes.

- Lower vaginal swabs and maternal C-reactive protein should not be offered until the induction is commenced or if expectant management beyond 24

给予单次皮质激素，预防新生儿肺部问题，降低患病第和病死率。

- 对于孕周很小的早产早破膜，预防性给予氨苄青霉素和红霉素 48 h 静脉给药，然后应用阿莫西林和红霉素 5 天（口服），预防感染，延长孕周，降低新生儿病死率和患病率。

- 对于早产早破膜病人，如果没有出现子宫收缩症状，不提倡应用宫缩抑制剂。

（3）分娩期处理

- 对于大于 34 孕周的早破膜孕妇，考虑结束分娩。

- 对于大于 34 周但仍然选择保守疗法的孕妇，应告知，延长孕周带来的益处（如减少肺部并发症、降低 NICU 的风险和剖宫产危险等）和增加绒毛膜羊膜炎症的危险。

3.3.6.2　足月胎膜早破

（1）诊断

- 如果发生胎膜早破，病史不明确（不能根据症状明确诊断），要进行无菌窥器评估检查。

- 如果发生了胎膜早破但病人没有宫缩，禁止进行阴道指检。

（2）处理

- 大部分孕妇发生胎膜早破后，在 24 h 内会发动宫缩临产。

- 胎膜破裂后 24 h 如果产妇没有临产，给予引产是恰当的。

- 在进行引产之前，不要给予阴道检查取标本和进行母亲 C-反应蛋白测定。如果 24 h 后

hours is chosen by the woman.

- Women should be advised to record their temperature every 4 hours during waking hours and to report immediately any change in the colour or smell of their vaginal loss.
- Women should be informed that bathing or showering are not associated with an increase in infection, but that having sexual intercourse may be.
- Assessed Fetal movement and heart rate , and the woman should be advised to report immediately any decrease in fetal movements.
- If labour has not started 24 hours after rupture of the membranes, women should be advised to give birth in hospital.
- If there are no signs of infection in the woman, antibiotics should not be given to either the woman or the baby, even if the membranes have been ruptured for over 24 hours.
- If there is evidence of infection in the woman, a full course of broad-spectrum intravenous antibiotics should be prescribed.
- Blood, cerebrospinal fluid and/or surface culture tests should not be performed in an asymptomatic baby(Figure 3-3-2).

3.3.6.3　Care of baby

- Asymptomatic term babies born to women with prelabour rupture of the membranes (more than 24 hours before labour) should be closely observed for the first 12 hours of life (at 1 hour, 2 hours and then 2-hourly for 10 hours). These observations should include:
→general wellbeing.
→chest movements and nasal flare.
→skin colour including perfusion, by testing capillary refill.
→feeding.
→muscle tone.

孕妇仍然选择保守治疗,也不要进行阴道检查。

- 告之产妇每 4 h 测量体温 1 次,并告知,如果发现阴道分泌物有异味或异常色泽要及时报告。
- 要告知产妇,她可以沐浴,并不会增加感染危险。但进行性生活可能增加感染危险。
- 评估胎心和胎动情况。告知产妇自我监护胎动,如果出现胎动减少要及时报告。
- 24 h 后,如果产妇仍然没有发动宫缩,应让产妇住院分娩。

- 对于没有出现感染征象的孕妇和新生儿,不应当给予抗生素。即使产妇破膜后超过 24 h 分娩,仍然不应当常规给药。
- 如果有感染表现,给予产妇广谱抗生素治疗。

- 对于没有感染表现的新生儿,不应当常规进行血液、脑脊液和表面细菌培养(图 3-3-2)。

3.3.6.3　新生儿护理

- 对胎膜早破超过 24 h 后出生的新生儿,即使没有异常表现,仍然要密切观察,出生后 12 h 内(1 h,2 h,然后每 2 h 1 次至 12 h)观察如下:

→一般情况。
→胸部的呼吸运动和鼻部的扇动。
→皮肤色泽和血液循环,评估微循环的再灌注情况。
→喂养情况。
→肌肉张力。

→temperature.

→heart rate and respiration.

■ A baby with any symptom of possible sepsis, or born to a woman who has evidence of chorioamnionitis, should immediately be referred to a neonatal care.

→体温。

→呼吸及心率。

■ 新生儿出现任何感染败血症现象,或母亲有确切证据有绒毛膜羊膜炎,要迅速转诊新生儿到上级医院。

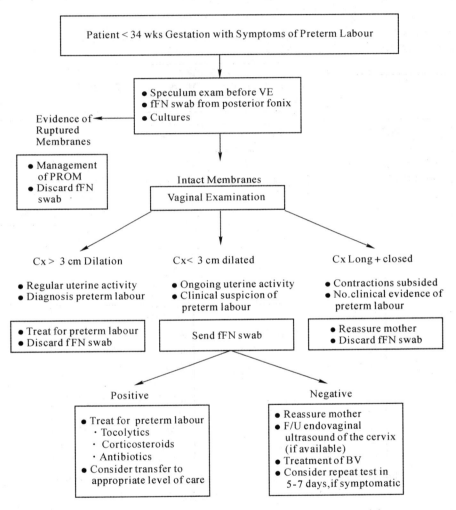

Figure 3-3-1　Fetal fibronectin testing for suspected preterm labour

图 3-3-1　先兆早产胎儿纤维连接蛋白试验流程

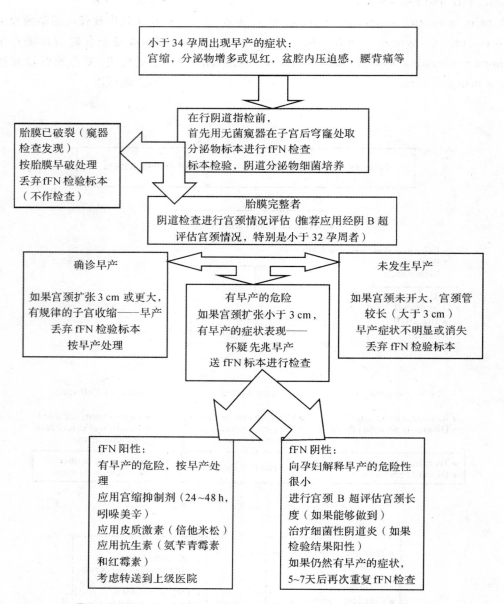

Figure 3-3-1　Fetal fibronectin testing for suspected preterm labour

图 3-3-1　先兆早产胎儿纤维连接蛋白试验流程

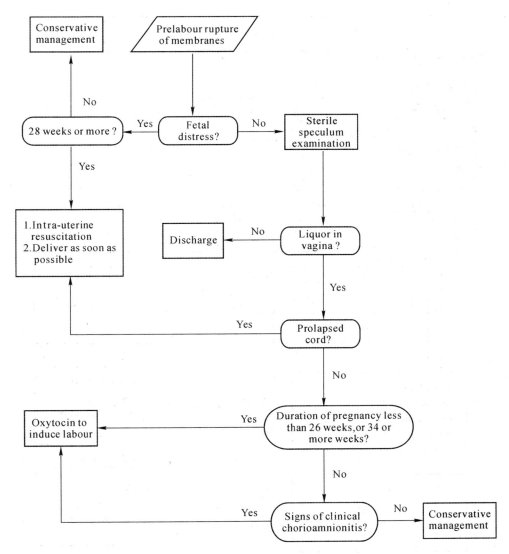

Figure 3-3-2 Management of prelabour rupture of membranes

图 3-3-2 胎膜早破的管理流程

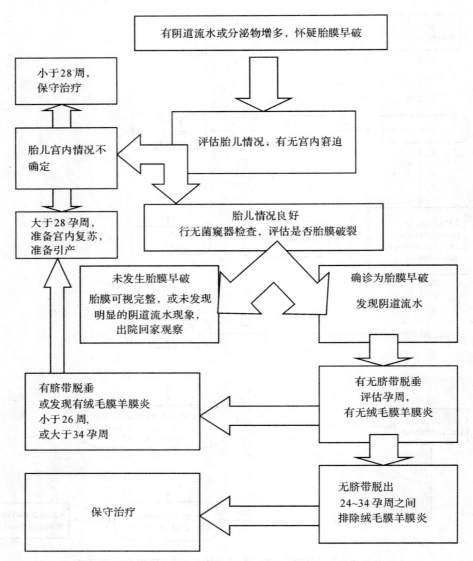

Figure 3-3-2　Management of prelabour rupture of membranes

图 3-3-2　胎膜早破的管理流程

Case analysis

Case 1

A woman is 29 weeks pregnancey, and has light show for threee day, she feels abdominal tension and back pain, the woman is urgent to hospital.

1. Which of the interventions should be a initial process?
2. If fFN result is postive, vaginal untrasound shows the length of the cervial is 15 mm, the membrane is intact, please make a plan of treatment for this patient.

Case 2

A patient, who is 36 weeks pregnant, reports that she has been draining liquor since earlier that day. The patient appears well, with normal observations, no uterine contractions and the fetal heart rate is normal.

1. Would you diagnose rupture of the membranes on the history given by the patient?
2. How would you confirm rupture of the membranes?
3. Why should you not perform a digital vaginal examination to assess whether the cervix is dilated or effaced?
4. Is this patient at high risk of having or developing chorioamnionitis?
5. Should you induce labour? Give your reasons.
6. Should you prescribe antibiotics? Give your reasons.

病例分析

病例 1

孕妇 29 孕周,有少量的见红 3 天,感下腹紧张和背痛,迅速到医院就诊。

1. 对于该病人,应当首先采取哪项措施来评估病人?
2. 如果 fFN 检查是阳性的,宫颈 B 超检查显示宫颈长度是 15 mm,应当如何处理该病人?写出一份治疗计划。

病例 2

一产妇 36 孕周,自述有阴道分泌物流出。产妇感觉良好,生命体征观察正常,没有子宫收缩,胎心正常。

1. 是否能够诊断产妇为胎膜早破?
2. 如何才能确诊是否胎膜早破?
3. 为什么要做阴道检查评估宫颈情况?
4. 这个病人有没有发生绒毛膜羊膜炎的危险?
5. 是否要开始引产? 解释原因。
6. 是否要给予抗生素? 解释理由。

Test

1. For women with history of preterm, which of the following is not of the scientific evidecce supporting to preventε preterm labour?　　（　）
   A. supportive environment
   B. education of early symptoms of preterm labour
   C. treatment of symptomatic vaginal infections before 32 weeks
   D. routine screening and treatment for the presence of bacterial vaginosis
   E. routine cervical cerclage for women with history of preterm

2. For woman with suspected preterm, which should be perfomed initially for diagnosis process?　　（　）
   A. sterile speculum examination to obtain sample for fetal fibronectin test
   B. transvaginal cervical measurement by B ultrasound
   C. digital vaginal examination
   D. antibiotic therapy
   E. tocolysis Prophylactic routinely

3. Regarding to carvical assessement, which of the following stagement indicates that the woman is at high risk of preterm?　　（　）
   A. cervis length greater than 30 mm
   B. cervical length less than 15 mm

   C. has a history of abnormal fetus
   D. blood presure 110 to 85 mmHg in the early pregnancy period
   E. fFN test is negetive

4. A woman has membrance ruptured before 32 weeks, which of the following in tervention is not necessary for the woman during expectant management of preterm PROM?　　（　）
   A. offer antibiotic therapy
   B. tocolysis Prophylactic routinely
   C. having shower daily for cleaness
   D. intercourse activity is forbidened
   E. fFN test is not recommended in prom

5. A baby born at 34 weeks with a history of prelabour rupture of membrance of 26 hours, how to treat the baby after birth?　　（　）
   A. breast feeding should not be offered to the baby
   B. a full course of broad-spectrum intravenous antibiotics should be prescribed for the baby, even there is no signs of infection
   C. routine abtibiotics for mother after birth
   D. observe closely for the vital signs of the baby
   E. separate the mother and baby for infections prevention cautions

Reference answer

Case 1

1. Fetus condition should be observed , if the fetus' condition is unsure, induction of labour will be appropriate action, if the fetus is in good conditionsl, a sterile speculum examination should

病例 1

1. 首先要评估胎儿情况。如果胎儿情况不好,可能要进行引产处理。如果胎儿情况良好,要进行无菌窥器阴道检查(在做

be performed before intraviginal untrasound or other viginal examination.

2. A postive fFN test combine with short length of the cervical (less than 20 mm) indicate the woman at high risk of preterm, chorioamnionitis should be roled out then, if it is not infected and fetus condition is well, treat as preterm according to Gestational Age Management(24-31 weeks), that include：Group B streptococcal prophylaxis, Single-course corticosteroid. But Tocolytics is not recommended for this cases.

Case 2

1. No, other causes of fluid draining from the vagina may cause confusion, *e. g.* a vaginitis or stress incontinence.

2. A sterile speculum examination should be done. If there is no clear evidence of liquor draining, the pH and ferning tests can be used to identify liquor.

3. A digital vaginal examination is contra-indicated in the presence of rupture of the membranes if the patient is not already in labour, because of the risk of introducing infection.

4. Yes. The preterm prelabour rupture of the membranes may have been caused by chorioamnionitis. In addition, all patients with ruptured membranes are at an increased risk of developing chorioamnionitis.

5. Yes. As she is more than 34 weeks pregnant, one should induce labour. As the patient does not fall into a high risk group for infection, a waiting period of 24 hours from the time of rupture can be allowed, before inducing labour. Most patients will go into labour spontaneously during this period.

6. There is no indication for giving antibiotics as there are no signs of clinical chorioamnionitis. However, a careful watch must be kept for early

阴道 B 超和其他阴道检查前进行）。

2. 如果 fFN 检查结果是阳性,同时宫颈的长度小于 15 mm,提示该病人有发生早产的高发危险,首先要排除绒毛膜炎,如果排除感染,胎儿情况良好,按相应胎龄的早产情况处理:给予预防性 B 族链球菌抗生素,单次剂量皮质激素,但宫缩抑制剂没有必要应用。

病例 2

1. 该产妇不能确诊为胎膜早破,因为有其他情况的混淆,例如阴道炎或尿失禁等情况需要排除。

2. 首先要进行无菌窥器检查,如果没有发现有明显的阴道流水,可做 pH 试验判断是否有羊水流出。

3. 不能进行阴道指检。在这种情况下若做阴道指检会增加感染机会,除非该病人已经临产接近分娩。

4. 该产妇有感染的危险,胎膜破裂增加感染机会,并且感染本身可能是胎膜早破的原因。

5. 该产妇应当进行引产,因为目前没有感染的高发危险,所以可以等待 24 h 期待宫缩发动。大部分产妇能够在这个时间内自动进入产程。

6. 该患者没有应用抗生素的指征,因为目前没有绒毛膜羊膜炎的表现,但要注意观察感染

signs of maternal infection or fetal tachycardia.

Test

1. E 2. A 3. B 4. E 5. D

3. 4 Hypertesion in Pregnancy

Key words

1. chronic hypertension during pregnancy
2. gestational hypertension
3. preeclampsia
4. severe preeclampsia
5. eclampsia

3.4.1 HELLP syndrome

Raised blood pressure in pregnancy is a common and potentially dangerous complication, associated with an increase in both maternal and fetal mortality. Blood pressure readings of 140/90 mmHg or more are generally considered abnormal. The reported overall incidence varies widely, but usually lies between 12% and 25% of all pregnancies.

The normal resting blood pressure is virtually never above 120/80 mmHg, and since the plasma volume increase averages 1 200 ml, there must be some vasodilatation to allow the peripheral pressure to remain low. If this vasodilatation is counteracted by arteriolar spasm, hypertension results and there is a reduction in the perfusion of all organs, including the uterus and thus the placental site.

3.4.1.1 Category

Hypertension in pregnancy include transient hypertension, chronic hypertension during pregnancy, and preeclampsia.

(1)Transient hypertension (most benign)
◆ A sustained or transient systolic BP≥140 mmHg

的早期表现和有无出现胎心减慢情况。

3. 4 妊娠期高血压疾病

关键词

1. 妊娠合并慢性高血压
2. 妊娠期高血压
3. 子痫前期
4. 重度子痫前期
5. 子痫

3.4.1 HELLP 综合征

妊娠期血压升高是一种常见的、具有潜在危险的并发症,与母胎死亡率增加有关。血压达到或高于 140/90 mmHg 通常为异常。妊娠期高血压疾病的发生率报道不一,占总妊娠的12%～25%。

通常妊娠期的正常血压不高于 120/80 mmHg,而妊娠血浆容量通常会增加1 200 ml,需依赖一些血管舒张因素以维持外周血管的低压力状态。如果血管舒张因素被小动脉痉挛所拮抗就会产生高血压,导致包括子宫和胎盘部位在内的所有器官血流灌注减少。

3.4.1.1 分类

妊娠期高血压疾病包括短暂性高血压、妊娠合并慢性高血压和子痫前期。

(1)短暂性高血压(大多数为良性)
◆ 妊娠 20 周以后,出现持续或短

and/or diastolic BP≥90 mmHg occurs after the 20th week of gestation without proteinuria or end-organ damage.

- Patient was normotensive prior to and during early pregnancy and become hypertensive late in pregnancy, during labor，or ≤24 hours postpartum.
- By definition，blood pressure must return to normal within 10 days after giving birth.

(2)Pre-existing or chronic hypertension during pregnancy

- In pre-existing hypertension, the hypertension begins prior to pregnancy.
- In chronic hypertension during pregnancy, a sustained systolic BP≥140 mmHg and/or diastolic BP≥90 mmHg occurs prior to the 20th week of gestation.
- Neither is associated with significant proteinuria or end-organ damage，but both persist after delivery.

(3)Preeclampsia

- Defined as proteinuria and edema in the setting of hypertension after the 20th week of gestation.
- Mild preeclampsia is defined by：
→A systolic BP≥140 mmHg or diastolic BP≥90 mmHg on two occasions >6 hours apart.

→Proteinuria（> 300 mg/24 hrs）.
- Severe preeclampsia is defined by：
→A systolic BP≥160 mmHg or diastolic BP≥110 mmHg.
→Significant proteinuria（≥5.0 g/day）.
→Evidence of end-organ damage
(e. g. visual disturbances, headache, hyperreflexia, confusion, abdominal pain, impaired liver function/hyperbilirubinemia, pulmonary edema, microangiopathic hemolytic anemia or thrombocytopenia).

(4) Preeclampsia （mild or severe） in patients with pre-existing hypertension or with chronic hypertension in pregnancy
- Patients can have hypertension prior to pregnancy and develop preeclampsia.

暂性收缩压≥140 mmHg 和（或）舒张压≥90 mmHg，但没有蛋白尿和终末器官受损。

- 患者在孕前和孕早期血压正常，孕晚期、分娩过程中或产后 24h 以内出现血压升高。
- 血压在产后 10 天内恢复正常。

(2)妊娠合并慢性高血压
- 孕前就存在高血压。

- 在妊娠合并高血压中，妊娠 20 周之前就出现持续性收缩压≥140 mmHg 和（或）舒张压≥90 mmHg。
- 与明显的蛋白尿或终末器官受损无关，产后也持续存在。

(3)子痫前期
- 孕 20 周后在高血压基础上出现蛋白尿和水肿。
- 轻度子痫前期定义为：
→相隔 6 h 以上两次测量，收缩压≥140 mmHg 或舒张压≥90 mmHg。
→蛋白尿（>300 mg/24 h）。
- 重度子痫前期定义为：
→收缩压≥160 mmHg 或舒张压≥110 mmHg。
→明显蛋白尿（≥5.0 g/d）。
→终末器官受损的证据
（如视觉障碍、头痛、反射亢进、意识模糊、腹部疼痛、肝功能受损/高胆红素血症、肺水肿、微血管病性溶血性贫血或血小板减少）。

(4)妊娠合并慢性高血压并发子痫前期（轻度或重度）

- 患者孕前和并发子痫前期之前就存在高血压。

- Patients can have seemingly benign hypertension (no proteinuria or evidence of end-organ damage) occurring during early pregnancy and develop preeclampsia.
- Proteinuria and edema in the setting of hypertension after the 20th week of gestation is preeclampsia, regardless of the timing of the onset of the hypertension.

3.4.1.2　Etiology

Preeclampsia is a multisystem disorder and in severe cases results in disturbances of liver function and the clotting system. Although the etiology remains unclear the trophoblast is causative since the condition may be seen before 20 weeks in conditions such as multiple pregnancy or hydatidiform mole, and it is cured by delivery.

The incidence is 5% to 7% of primigravid pregnancies where the disease is "primary" i. e. occurring in a patient whose blood pressure was previously normal and disappearing after pregnancy. In women with chronic hypertension and especially those with renal disease, the incidence is much higher, the preeclampsia being superimposed on the existing hypertension.

Though the cause of the condition remains unknown there is a clear pre-disposition in certain groups:

- Primigravid patients or in the first pregnancy with a given partner.
- Increased risk with age.
- Family history of preeclampsia or hypertension.
- Preexisting hypertension, especially renal disease or connective tissue disorder.
- Multiple pregnancy.
- Diabetic pregnancy.
- Hydatidiform mole.

3.4.1.3　Pathophysiology

A great mass of data has been collected and many theories propounded over the years to try to

- 在早孕期和发生子痫前期时存在的高血压可能是良性的（没有蛋白尿和终末器官受损的证据）。
- 不管高血压发生的时间，孕 20 周以后在高血压基础上出现蛋白尿和水肿即为子痫前期。

3.4.1.2　病因

子痫前期是一种多系统功能失调，严重时可导致肝功能和凝血系统的障碍。其病因尚不完全清楚，但孕 20 周之前发生的滋养层细胞功能障碍是病因之一，多发生于多胎妊娠或葡萄胎，在分娩后自愈。

子痫前期在初次妊娠中的发病率为 5%～7%，患者既往无高血压且在妊娠结束后恢复正常。在已患慢性高血压尤其并发肾脏疾病的妇女中，其发病率明显增高，此时子痫前期在原有高血压基础上叠加。

尽管子痫前期的发病原因尚不清楚，但以下群体存在明显易患病倾向：

- 初孕妇或与某一配偶的初次妊娠。
- 孕母年龄越大，患病风险越高。
- 子痫前期或高血压家族史。
- 既往高血压，尤其有肾脏疾病或结缔组织病。
- 多胎妊娠。
- 糖尿病妊娠。
- 葡萄胎。

3.4.1.3　病理生理

多年来，人们对子痫前期的病理生理过程进行了大量的研究，也

explain this much-studied disease. It is accepted that the starting point is in the placental bed. In normal pregnancy the trophoblast invades the maternal spiral arteries and converts these vessels into low resistance arteries thereby increasing perfusion. In preeclampsia this process is defective and this so-called "physiological change" does not occur.

Clinically there is evidence of widespread systemic disturbance.

A. Cardiovascular system

- The maternal hypertension results from increased peripheral resistance due possibly to imbalance of vasoactive substances such as prostanoids and local disturbances in the control of the vessel tone by substances produced by the endothelium of the vessel wall.

- In addition the normal expansion of the plasma volume is reduced in preeclampsia and there may be a fall in plasma proteins due to renal dysfunction. Together this creates a state of hypovolemia and tissue edema.

B. Renal system

- Impaired renal function has long been recognized in preeclampsia with evidence of both glomerular and tubular dysfunction.

- This is detected by the presence of protein in the urine and raised plasma urate levels:
  - Proteinuria ($>$ 300 mg per volume in a 24 hour collection)
  - Plasma urate $>$ 0.35 mmol/liter

- Urea and creatinine levels may also rise. Levels of greater than 6 mmol/liter and 100 micromoles per liter respectively are significant.

C. Clotting system

- A falling platelet count and changes in many clotting factors have been reported in preeclampsia.

- In severe cases this may proceed to disseminated intravascular coagulation with micro-angiopathic

提出了很多理论,其中认为其发病起源于胎盘着床的理论已被广泛接受。在正常妊娠中,胎盘滋养层细胞侵入母体子宫螺旋动脉,将其转化为低阻力血管以增加血流灌注。而在子痫前期中,这一过程受损,正常的生理改变没有发生。

临床上出现广泛的系统功能障碍。

A. 心血管系统

- 母体出现高血压的原因为外周血管阻力增高,可能与前列腺素等血管活性物质失衡以及局部血管壁内皮细胞产生的调节血管张力物质失衡有关。

- 此外,子痫前期中正常增加的血浆容量减少,同时可能因为肾功能不全使血浆蛋白减少,由此导致血容量不足和组织水肿。

B. 肾脏系统

- 早已证实子痫前期中存在肾功能受损,包括肾小球和肾小管功能不全。

- 检查发现尿蛋白和血尿酸增高:
  - 蛋白尿($>$300 mg/24 h)

  - 血浆尿酸$>$0.35 μmol/L

- 尿素和肌酐水平也可能增高,如分别大于 6 mmol/L 和 100 μmol/L 具有临床意义。

C. 凝血系统

- 子痫前期中可有血小板计数减少和多种凝血因子含量的改变。

- 严重时可发生弥散性血管内凝血,出现小血管阻塞继发微血

hemolysis secondary to small vessel blockage, revealed by anemia and the presence of fragmented red cells in the peripheral blood.

- Raised levels of fibrin degradation products are found.

D. Liver damage

- Post-mortem examinations of patients dying from eclampsia have long demonstrated evidence of liver damage with subcapsular hemorrhage and areas of necrosis seen microscopically in the periportal region of the liver lobules.

- Epigastric tenderness has always been described as a sign of impending eclampsia but in recent years awareness of the risk of liver damage has increased and evidence of it in the form of elevated enzymes in the mother's circulation should be sought.

- The term HELLP syndrome has been coined to emphasize the dangerous combination of disseminated intravascular coagulation and liver damage in severe preeclampsia: Hemolysis → Elevated liver enzymes→Low platelets.

E. Central nervous system—Eclampsia

- Preeclampsia is largely a disease of signs rather than symptoms. Headache, visual disturbance and abdominal pain may indicate progression towards eclampsia. The first two of these reflect the effects of hypertension on the brain in terms of hypertensive encephalopathy and the last the effect on the liver of subcapsular hemorrhage.

- The epileptiform fit, the defining aspect of eclampsia, also reflects hypertensive encephalopathy although there is no defining blood pressure at which a woman with preeclampsia will actually convulse.

- It is not clear what causes the fit but it is not solely related to the level of the blood pressure. Death may occur from cerebral hemorrhage or cardiac failure.

管病性溶血,检查可发现贫血和出现外周血破碎红细胞。

- 纤维蛋白降解产物水平增高。

D. 肝损伤

- 子痫患者死后尸检可发现肝包膜下出血,显微镜下发现门静脉周围肝小叶坏死等肝损伤迹象。

- 通常上腹部压痛被视为子痫即将发生的征兆。但近年来对肝损伤风险的认识有所提高,需注意母血中酶类的增高。

- 在严重子痫前期时同时出现弥散性血管内凝血和肝损伤,病情非常凶险,即 HELLP 综合征:溶血(H)→增高(E)的肝酶(L)→降低(L)的血小板(P)。

E. 中枢神经系统——子痫

- 子痫前期是一种体征比症状明显的疾病。头痛、视觉障碍和腹痛可能预示病程进展到子痫。前两项是高血压性脑病的效应,后一项是肝包膜下出血的效应。

- 癫痫发作,即子痫也是高血压脑病的效应,但不能确定引起子痫前期妇女发生抽搐的血压值。

- 引起子痫的原因尚不明确,但血压水平不是子痫发生的唯一相关因素。

F. Renin angiotensin system

- In normal pregnancy there is a reduction in sensitivity to the vasopressor effects of angiotensin.
- This reduction does not occur in a high proportion of cases which subsequently develop preeclampsia.

3.4.1.4　Clinical complications

- Intrauterine growth restriction — the risk is increased in cases with proteinuria.
- Fetal hypoxia and intrauterine death.
- Abruption of the placenta.
- HELLP syndrome.
- Eclampsia.
- Renal failure.
- Cerebrovascular accident.
- Cardiac failure.

3.4.1.5　Management of hypertensive pregnancy

A. Detection

- There is no established, practical screening procedure other than good antenatal care.
- Regular supervision, especially of recognized high risk groups, may be shared between the general practitioner, midwife and obstetrician.

B. Observations

Below are lists of routine observations carried out on patients in whom hypertension has been confirmed. On them are based decisions about treatment. Nowadays many hypertensive patients are assessed on an out-patient basis in a Day Care Unit with only the more severe cases being admitted. Similarly the severity of the condition would determine frequency of these observations.

- Serial blood pressure recordings.
- Quantitation of proteinuria.
- Plasma urate levels.
- Platelet counts.
- Liver enzymes if proteinuria quantitation, plasma

F. 肾素血管紧张素系统

- 正常妊娠中母体对血管紧张素的血管加压效应的敏感性下降。
- 在后续发展为子痫前期的病例中,大部分没有发生母体对血管紧张素敏感性下降的效应。

3.4.1.4　临床并发症

- 有蛋白尿的病例中,胎儿宫内发育迟缓的风险增加。
- 胎儿缺氧和宫内死亡。
- 胎盘早剥。
- HELLP 综合征。
- 子痫。
- 肾功能衰竭。
- 脑血管意外。
- 心衰。

3.4.1.5　妊娠期高血压疾病的处理

A. 发现

- 没有明确实用的筛查手段,需要依靠完善的产前检查。
- 全科医生、助产士和产科医生均需对孕妇尤其是已知的高危人群进行常规监护。

B. 观察

以下是针对已确诊高血压患者的常规监测项目,并由此决定治疗方案。目前很多高血压患者在日间病区作为门诊病例进行管理,仅病情较重的病例需要收住院。同样,病情严重程度决定以下检查的频率。

- 持续血压监测。
- 尿蛋白定量。
- 血浆尿酸水平。
- 如尿蛋白定量、血尿酸或血小板计数异常,需进行肝酶学

urate or platelet counts are abnormal.

◆ Assessment of fetal growth and well-being by kick charts, cardiotocography and ultrasound estimates of fetal weight and liquor volume.

C. Treatment

Admission to hospital

◆ This is indicated if the diastolic blood pressure remains at 100 mmHg or more.

◆ The presence of proteinuria and evidence of fetal compromise are also indications for admission.

◆ Many patients with hypertension arising late in pregnancy require no other treatment before delivery.

◆ It must always be remembered, however, that the disease can run an unpredictable course and its severity may change very quickly.

Hypotensive agents

◆ These may be used in three situations:
  • Chronic hypertension.
  • Severe pregnancy induced hypertension.
  • In the treatment of a hypertensive crisis or imminent eclampsia.

◆ Many obstetricians are still cautious about such agents in spite of the risks of hypertension because of anxieties about the effects of the drugs on placental perfusion.

◆ This is particularly the case when medication is initiated in the mid trimester of pregnancy. Most would favor medication where the mother's diastolic blood pressure remains persistently above 100 mmHg.

Termination of pregnancy

◆ Delivery is the ultimate treatment of hypertensive pregnancy and its timing depends on the observations of fetal and maternal well-being noted above.

◆ Prolongation of the pregnancy by drug therapy may reduce the risks of prematurity and improve the

检查。

◆ 通过胎动表、胎心监护以及超声估计胎儿体重和羊水量来监测胎儿生长和宫内情况。

C. 治疗

住院治疗

◆ 舒张压持续达 100 mmHg 或以上是适应证。

◆ 出现蛋白尿和胎儿窘迫的迹象也是收住院的指征。

◆ 妊娠晚期出现高血压的病例在分娩前不需其他治疗。

◆ 但需时刻谨记疾病进程不可预知且可迅速加重。

降压药物

◆ 可用在以下三种情况:
  • 慢性高血压。
  • 严重妊娠期高血压。
  • 治疗高血压危象或危急的子痫。

◆ 很多产科医生基于对药物胎盘灌注效应的忧虑,尽管存在患者血压升高的风险,但仍然对降压药物的使用持谨慎态度。

◆ 医生的这种顾虑在妊娠中期就开始药物治疗的病例中尤为明显。在孕母的舒张压持续高达 100 mmHg 以上时,大多数医生会使用降压药物。

终止妊娠

◆ 分娩是妊娠期高血压的最终治疗手段,其时机由前述对母胎安危情况的监测结果而定。

◆ 通过药物治疗延长妊娠时间可降低早产的风险并提高阴道分

chances of vaginal delivery.

◆ Epidural block for both analgesia in labor and delivery by caesarean section is excellent providing the platelet count is satisfactory.

3.4.1.6　Severe preeclampsia and eclampsia

The dangers of severe preeclampsia and eclampsia have been described. If premonitory signs are observed then the woman should be entered into a specific protocol for this situation and all institutions should have such a protocol subject to regular revision.

A. Observations and investigations

Maternal

◆ Blood pressure should be measured every 15-20 minutes (initially using a mercury sphygmomanometer to exclude cases in which automated machines underestimate pressure).

◆ Oxygen saturation should be monitored continuously.

◆ Urine output measured hourly.

◆ Urea and electrolytes, full blood count, liver function tests and coagulation screen at least every 24 hours and more often as clinically indicated.

Fetal

◆ Ultrasound biophysical assessment (Fetal maturity and estimate of fetal size if not known).

◆ Continuous cardiotocography.

B. Treatment

Use of magnesium sulphate

◆ Magnesium sulphate reduces the risk of eclampsia by around half in women with preeclampsia before delivery or presenting within 24 hours of giving birth.

◆ Intravenous access should be established as part of the admission protocol, ideally using the cannula for obtaining initial blood samples, and 4 g of magnesium sulphate should be given within 5-10 min.

◆ This should be followed by a infusion of magnesium sulphate(1 g per hour) for 24 hours after the last fit until the deep tendon reflexes

娩的机会。

◆ 如血小板计数满意,产程中实施硬膜外阻滞阵痛和剖宫产分娩是有效的手段。

3.4.1.6　重度子痫前期和子痫

重度子痫前期和子痫的危害显而易见。一旦发现征兆,就应制订一套有针对性的治疗方案,并且可供常规修订。

A. 观察和检查

母体

◆ 每 15～20 min 测量血压(用水银血压计以免电子设备低估实际血压)。

◆ 持续监测血氧饱和度。

◆ 计算每小时尿量。

◆ 至少每 24 h 监测尿素、电解质、全血计数、肝功能和凝血,视临床情况增加检查次数。

胎儿

◆ 超声生物物理评分(评估胎儿成熟度和各项指标)。

◆ 持续胎心监护。

B. 治疗

使用硫酸镁

◆ 硫酸镁可以降低一半左右子痫前期孕妇在分娩前或分娩后 24 h 内发生子痫的风险。

◆ 入院后宜从采血套管处建立静脉通道,5～10 min 内给予 4 g 硫酸镁。

◆ 之后维持输注硫酸镁,每小时 1 g,从最后一次发作开始持续 24 h,或直至深腱反射消失(每

disappear(check hourly) or the respiratory rate is below 14 per minute.

- Repeat fits may be treated by using further boluses of magnesium sulphate or diazepam.

Hypotension therapy

- Hydralazine, 5 mg over 15 min with a maximum cumulative dose of 20 mg, is an approach of choice.
- A labetalol infusion also has a role as a second line agent.

Fluid balance

- Fluid overload can occur readily and pulmonary edema develops rapidly.
- Standard fluid regimes should be used and monitored.
- A central venous pressure (CVP) line may be required to assess fluid balance and aid management.

Delivery

- For women with severe preeclampsia, the time of delivery depends on the rate of deterioration of the mother's physical conditions and maturity of the pregnancy.
- If an eclamptic fit has occurred and the baby is alive and viable, delivery should be expedited, often by caesarean section. If the cervix is favorable, induction of labor still has a role, particularly in parous women.

Prophylaxis of DVT

- Considering the coagulation status, attention should be given to prophylaxis of deep venous thrombosis (DVT). Even during the assessment period, compression stockings should be provided.

3.4.2　Case report and analysis

✎GESTATIONAL HYPERTENSION

A 19-year-old primigravida was seen in the outpatient prenatal clinic for routine visit. She was at 32 weeks of gestation, confirmed by first trimester

小时检查)或呼吸频率降至14次/min以下。

- 反复发作需加大硫酸镁剂量或使用地西泮。

降压治疗

- 可以选择15 min内给予5 mg肼屈嗪,可重复给药至累积剂量达20 mg。
- 也可以静脉给予二线药物拉贝洛尔。

体液平衡

- 体液超负荷和肺水肿发展迅速。
- 使用标准规范输液,液体出入量需记录。
- 可开放中心静脉测压通道以评估体液平衡和方便急救。

分娩

- 重度子痫前期的分娩时机由母体状况恶化程度和妊娠的成熟度决定。
- 如已发生子痫发作,而胎儿存活有生机,需尽快分娩,通常进行剖宫产。如宫颈条件成熟,特别是经产妇,可考虑引产。

预防深静脉血栓

- 考虑到凝血状态的改变,应注意预防深静脉血栓,即使在评估阶段就要给予加压袜。

3.4.2　病例报告和分析

✎妊娠期高血压

19岁初孕妇到产科门诊进行常规产检。根据早孕期超声证实为孕32周。该妇无不适主诉,否

sonogram. She had no complaints. She denied headache, epigastric pain, or visual disturbances. She had gained 2 pounds (about 0. 91 kg) since her last visit 2 weeks ago. On examination, her blood pressure (BP) was 155/95, which was persistent on repeat BP check 10 min later. She had only trace pedal edema. A spot urine dipstick was negative.

Definition：

Gestational hypertension is diagnosed with sustained elevation of BP ≥ 140/90 mmHg after 20 weeks of pregnancy without proteinuria.

◆ The BP returns to normal baseline postpartum.

Presenting Symptoms and Physical Examination：

◆ No symptoms of preeclampsia are seen, *e. g.* headache, epigastric pain, and visual disturbances.

◆ Physical findings are unremarkable for pregnancy.

Laboratory Abnormalities：

Unremarkable changes except pregnancy are observed in laboratory tests. Proteinuria is absent.

Diagnostic Tests：

The key findings are sustained elevation of BP ≥ 140/90 without proteinuria and a rapid return to baseline on repeat measurement.

Management：

◆ Conservative outpatient management is appropriate.

◆ Close observation is prudent to avoid the occurance of incipient preeclampsia.

◆ Appropriate laboratory testing should be performed to rule out preeclampsia, *e. g.* urine protein and hemoconcentration assessment.

Differential Diagnosis：

Preeclampsia should always be ruled out.

✐MILD PREECLAMPSIA

A 21-year-old primigravida was seen in the outpatient prenatal clinic for routine visit. She was at 32 weeks of gestation, confirmed by first trimester sonogram. Her only complaint was swelling in her hands and feet. She denied headache, epigastric pain, or

认头痛、上腹部疼痛或视觉模糊。距上次产检 2 周，增重 2 磅（约 0. 91 kg）。相隔 10 min 两次测量血压均为 155/95 mmHg。体检发现轻微足部水肿，尿检阴性。

定义：

◆ 孕 20 周以后出现持续性血压 ≥ 140/90 mmHg，不伴有蛋白尿，可诊断为妊娠期高血压。

◆ 产后血压恢复正常。

临床表现和体格检查：

◆ 无头痛、上腹部疼痛和视觉障碍等子痫前期的症状。

◆ 体格检查除妊娠改变，无明显发现。

实验室异常：

实验室检查除妊娠改变，无明显异常，蛋白尿阴性。

诊断试验：

关键结果为持续性血压 ≥ 140/90 mmHg 不伴有蛋白尿，且重复测量血压不恢复正常水平。

临床处理：

◆ 保守性门诊管理即可。

◆ 加强观察，谨防患者出现初期子痫前期。

◆ 进行尿蛋白和血液浓缩等实验室检查以排除子痫前期。

鉴别诊断：

通常要排除子痫前期。

✐轻度子痫前期

21 岁初孕妇到产科门诊进行常规产检。根据早孕期超声证实为孕 32 周。该妇主述手足部水肿，否认头痛、上腹部疼痛或视觉模糊。距上次产检 2 周，增重

visual disturbances. She had gained 10 pounds（about 4.54 kg）since her last visit 2 weeks ago. On examination，her BP was 155/95 and remained unchanged on repeat BP after 15 min. She has 3＋pedal edema，and her fingers appeared swollen. A spot urine dipstick showed 2＋protein.

Definition：

Preeclampsia is sustained by BP elevation in pregnancy after 20 weeks of gestation with the absence of preexisting hypertension.

Diagnostic Criteria：

- Sustained BP elevation of ≥140/90 mmHg.
- Proteinuria on dipstick of 1～2＋or ≥300 mg on a 24 h urine collection.

Risk Factors：

- Preeclampsia is found 8 times more frequently in primiparas.
- Other risk factors are multiple gestation，hydatidiform mole， diabetes mellitus， age extremes， chronic hypertension，and chronic renal diasease.

Presenting Symptoms and Physical Examination：

- The symptoms and physical findings of with mild preeclampsia are generally related to the excess weight gain and fluid retention.
- New onset of persistent headache，epigastric pain，or visual disturbances suggest mild preeclampsia becomes more severe.

Laboratory Abnormalities：

- Elevation of hemoglobin，hematocrit，blood urea nitrogen （BUN）， serum creatinine， and serum uric acid indicate hemoconcentration.
- Proteinuria is observed under diagnostic tests.
- Disseminated intravascular coagulation （DIC） or liver enzyme elevation suggest mild preeclampsia becomes more severe.

Management：

The most definitive cure is delivery and removal of all fetal-placental tissues. However， delivery strategies may be different in mild preeclampsia to

10 磅（约 4.54 kg）。相隔 15 min 两次测量血压均为155/95 mmHg。体检发现足部水肿（3＋），手指肿胀，尿检示尿蛋白（2＋）。

定义：

孕 20 周以后出现持续性血压升高，孕前无高血压病史。

诊断标准：

- 持续性血压≥140/90 mmHg。
- 尿蛋白（1～2＋）或 24 h 尿蛋白定量≥300 mg。

危险因素：

- 初产妇子痫前期的发病率高达 8 倍。
- 其他危险因素包括多胎妊娠、葡萄胎、糖尿病、高龄、慢性高血压和慢性肾脏疾病。

临床表现和体格检查：

- 轻度子痫前期的临床表现和体格检查主要与过度体重增加和体液潴留有关。
- 新出现的持续性头痛、上腹部疼痛或视觉障碍提示轻度子痫前期正往重度发展。

实验室异常：

- 血红蛋白、血细胞比容、血尿素氮、血肌酐和血尿酸的增高提示血液浓缩。
- 诊断试验发现蛋白尿。
- 如出现弥散性血管内凝血或肝酶升高的证据，提示轻度子痫前期正往重度发展。

临床处理：

最根本的治疗方法是分娩和取出所有胎儿-胎盘组织。但为了减少新生儿早产并发症，分娩

minimize neonatal complications of prematurity. Management is based on gestational age.

- ◆ Conservative inpatient. Before 36 weeks of gestation, as long as the conditions of mother and fetus are stable, mild preeclampsia should be managed in the hospital to observe possible progression to severe preeclampsia. Antihypertensive agents or MgSO₄ are not needed.

- ◆ Delivery. At ≥ 36 weeks of gestation indicating delivery, dilute oxytocin induction of labor and continuous infusion of MgSO₄ (i. v.) should be performed to prevent eclamptic seizures.

Complications：

Progression from mild to severe preeclampsia may occur.

Differential Diagnosis：

Chronic hypertension should always be ruled out.

◢SEVERE PREECLAMPSIA

A 21-year-old primigravida was seen in the outpatient prenatal clinic for routine visit. She was at 32 weeks of gestation, confirmed by first trimester sonogram. For the past 24 h, she had experienced severe unremitting occipital headache and mild epigastric pain not relieved by acetaminophen, and she also saw light flashes and spots in her vision. She had gained 10 pounds since her last visit 2 weeks ago. On examination, her BP was 165/115 mmHg. She has 3＋pedal edema, and her fingers appeared swollen. Fundal height was 29 cm. Fetal heart tones were regular at 145 beats/min. A spot urine dipstick showed 4＋ protein.

Diagnostic Tests：

The diagnosis is made on the basis of mild preeclampsia plus any one of the followings：
- ◆ Sustained BP elevation of ≥ 160/110 mmHg.
- ◆ Proteinuria on dipstick of 3-4＋ or ≥ 5 g on a 24 h urine collection.
- ◆ Evidence of maternal jeopardy. This may include：

处理与轻度子痫前期有所不同，是由孕周决定的。

- ◆ 住院保守治疗。孕周达到 36 周之前，只要母胎情况稳定，轻度子痫前期需住院监护，注意进展到重度的可能性。无需使用抗高血压药物或硫酸镁。

- ◆ 分娩。孕周≥ 36 周是分娩的指征，同时静脉内输注稀释的缩宫素引产和持续静脉用硫酸镁预防子痫发作。

并发症：

可能从轻度进展到重度子痫前期。

鉴别诊断：

要排除慢性高血压。

◢重度子痫前期

21 岁初孕妇到产科门诊进行常规产检。根据早孕期超声证实为孕 32 周。该妇主述 1 天前出现严重持续性枕部头痛、上腹部疼痛，口服乙酰氨基酚无法缓解，同时视物出现光束和光点。距上次产检 2 周，增重 10 磅（约 4.54 kg）。测量血压均为 165/115 mmHg。体检发现足部水肿（3＋），手指肿胀。宫高 29 cm，胎心搏动 145 次/min。尿检示尿蛋白（4＋）。

诊断试验：

在轻度子痫前期基础上出现以下任一项即可明确诊断：
- ◆ 持续性血压升高≥ 160/110 mmHg。
- ◆ 尿蛋白（3～4＋）或 24 h 尿蛋白定量≥ 5 g。
- ◆ 孕母病情危急的证据包括：

- symptoms (headache, epigastric pain, or visaual changes)
- thrombocytopenia (platelet count <100 000/ml)

- elevated liver enzymes
- pulmonary edema
- oliguria(<750 ml/24 h)
- cyanosis

◆ Edema may or may not be seen.

Risk Factors：

Besides the same risk factors for mild preeclampsia, small vessel diseases such as systemic lupus and longstanding over diabetes are also included.

Presenting Symptoms：

New onset of persistent headache, epigastric pain, or visual disturbances is the characteristic of severe preeclampsia.

Laboratory Abnormalities：

◆ More severe hemoconcentration.

◆ Proteinuria under diagnostic tests.

◆ Appearance of DIC and hepatocellular injury is the characteristic of severe preeclampsia.

Management：

◆ Aggressive prompt delivery is conducted for severe preeclampsia at any gestational age when maternal jeopardy or fetal jeopardy occures.

—Administer $MgSO_4$ (i. v.) to prevent convulsions. Give a 5 g loading dose followed by continue infusion of 2 g/h.

—Lower BP to diastolic values between 90 and 100 mmHg with hydralazine and labetalol(i. v.).

—Try vaginal delivery with oxytocin infusion (i. v.) if the conditions mother and fetus are stable.

◆ Conservative inpatient management may be attempted in a rare condition absence of maternal and fetal jeopardy, gestational age of 26-34 weeks, and BP that can be decreased to 160/110 mmHg. This should take place in an intensive care

- 症状（头痛，上腹疼痛，视力改变）
- 血小板减少（血小板计数<10万/ml）

- 肝酶升高
- 肺水肿
- 少尿（<750 ml/24 h）
- 发绀

◆ 水肿可有可无。

危险因素：

除与轻度子痫前期相同以外，还包括系统性红斑狼疮和长期糖尿病等小血管病变。

临床表现：

新出现的持续性头痛、上腹部疼痛或视觉障碍是重度子痫前期的特征。

实验室异常：

◆ 血液浓缩更严重。

◆ 诊断试验发现蛋白尿。

◆ 弥散性血管内凝血或肝细胞损伤的出现是重度子痫前期的特征。

临床处理：

◆ 紧急分娩是任何孕周的重度子痫前期出现母体或胎儿情况危急时的治疗方案。

—静脉输注硫酸镁防止子痫发作。用5 g负荷剂量，然后维持输注2 g/h。

—降压通过静脉用肼屈嗪和拉贝洛尔使舒张压值达90～100 mmHg。

—尝试阴道分娩，如母胎情况稳定可静脉用缩宫素。

◆ 住院保守治疗，仅在少数情况如没有出现母胎危急、孕周在26～34周，且血压可降至160/110 mmHg以下时采用，同时应在加护病房监护。需静脉持

unit (ICU) tertiary-care setting. MgSO$_4$ should be administered continually, and betamethasone should be given to mother to promote fetal lung maturity.

Complications:

Progression from severe preeclampsia to eclampsia may occur.

✎ECLAMPSIA

A 21-year-old primigravida was brought to the emergency department after suffering generalized tonic-clonic seizure at 32 weeks of gestation. The seizure was preceded by a severe headache. She lost control of her bowels and bladder. She had gained 10 pounds since her last prenatal visit 2 weeks ago. On examination, she was in a postictal unresponsive state. Her BP was 185/115 mmHg, and a spot urine dipstick showed 4+ protein.

Definition:

Eclampsia is an unexplained grand mal seizures in a hypertensive, proteinuria pregnant woman in the last half of pregnancy.

Risk Factors:

The risk factors for eclampsia are the same as those for mild and severe preeclampsia. A primary seizure disorder does not predispose to eclampsia.

Presenting Symptoms:

In addition to the symptoms of mild and severe preeclampsia, the most significant one is unexplained tonic-clonic seizures.

Laboratory Abnormalities:

These are the same as those of mild and severe preeclampsia.

Diagnosis:

The diagnosis is made clinically with unexplained grand mal seizures occurring in a hypertensive, proteinuric pregnant woman in the last half of pregnancy.

续使用硫酸镁,且母体给予倍他米松促胎儿肺成熟。

并发症:

可能从重度子痫前期进展到子痫。

✎子痫

21 岁初孕妇在孕 32 周发生全身强制性阵挛后由急诊收入院。根据早孕期超声证实。癫痫发作是在剧烈头痛后发生的,伴有大小便失禁。距上次产检 2 周,增重 10 磅(约 4.54 kg)。测量血压均为 165/115 mmHg。体检发现患者为发作后处于无反应状态,测血压为 185/115 mmHg,尿检示尿蛋白(4+)。

定义:

子痫是在妊娠后半期,患有高血压和蛋白尿的孕妇出现的一种难以解释的癫痫大发作。

危险因素:

与轻度和重度子痫前期相同。原发性癫痫发作不是造成子痫的因素。

临床表现:

除与轻度和重度子痫前期相同外,最显著的症状是难以解释的强制性阵挛发作。

实验室异常:

与轻度和重度子痫前期相同。

诊断:

临床上在妊娠后半期,患有高血压和蛋白尿的孕妇出现难以解释的癫痫大发作可诊断子痫。

Management：

- The first step is to protect the maternal airway and tongue.
- Administer $MgSO_4$ with an IV bolus of 5 g to stop seizures，continuing maintenance infusion rate of 2 g/h.
- Aggressive prompt delivery is used for eclampsia at any gestational age after stabilization of the mother and the fetus. Attempt vaginal delivery with oxytocin infusion（i. v.）if mother and fetus are stable.
- Lower diastolic BP between 90 and 100 mmHg with hydralazine and labetalol(i. v.).

Complications：

Intra-cerebral hemorrhage and even death.

CHRONIC HYPERTENSION

A 35-year-old multigravida was seen in the outpatient prenatal clinic for her first prenatal visit. She was at 12 weeks' gestation with a BP of 155/95 mmHg. Chronic hypertension was diagnosed 5 year ago for which she had been treated with oral nifedipine. A spot urine dipstick protein was 2＋. A recent 24 h urine collection showed 1. 2 g of protein and a creatinine clearance of 85 ml/min. Serum creatinine was 1. 2 mg/dl. She had no complaints of headache or visual changes.

Risk Factors：

Most chronic hypertension （HTN） is idiopathic without specific antecedents. Its risk factors are obesity, advanced maternal age, positive family history, renal disease, diabetes, and systemic lupus erythematosis.

Diagnosis：

The diagnosis of chronic HTN is made with the onset of BP $\geqslant$ 140/90 mmHg before the pregnancy or before 20 weeks' of gestation.

Prognosis of Pregnancy with Chronic HTN：

- *Good*. Favorable maternal and neonatal outcome is found in patients with BP values between 140/90 and

临床处理：

- 第一步要保护孕母的气道和舌。
- 使用硫酸镁是静脉给予 5 g 终止发作，然后持续静脉输注每小时 2 g。
- 紧急分娩是任何孕周的子痫发作后母胎情况转安时的治疗方案，如情况稳定，可尝试静脉用缩宫素经阴道分娩。
- 降压至 90～100 mmHg 可静脉用肼屈嗪和拉贝洛尔。

并发症：

颅内出血甚至死亡。

慢性高血压

35 岁经产孕妇到产科门诊进行首次产检。孕 12 周，血压 155/95 mmHg。该妇 5 年前诊断慢性高血压，口服硝苯地平治疗。尿检示尿蛋白（2＋）。最近一次尿蛋白定量为 1.2 g，血肌酐清除率 85 ml/min，血肌酐 1.2 mg/dl。该妇无头痛或视力改变等主述。

危险因素：

大多数慢性高血压为特发性，无特殊前期病变。危险因素包括肥胖、高龄、阳性家族史、肾病、糖尿病和系统性红斑狼疮。

诊断：

孕前或孕 20 周以前出现的血压升高 $\geqslant$ 140/90 mmHg 可诊断慢性高血压。

妊娠合并慢性高血压的预后：

- 良好：血压在 140/90～179/109 mmHg 之间，无终末器官

179/109 mmHg and no evidence of end-organ damage.

- *Poor*. Pregnancy complications are more common in patients with severe HTN with the following end-organ damage:
—*Renal disease*. Pregnancy loss rates increase significantly if serum creatinine value are>1.4 mg/dl.
—*Retinopathy*. Longstanding HTN is associated with retinal vascular changes including hemorrhages, exudates, and narrowing.
—*Left ventricular hypertrophy*. This is seen mostly in women with prolonged BP values of > 180/110 mmHg.
- *Worst*. Tenfold higher fetal loss rate is observed if pregnant women have uncontrolled HTN（before conception or early in pregnancy）and chronic HTN superimposed with preeclampsia.

Chronic HTN Superimposed with Preeclampsia：

- This complication occurs in 25% of patients with chronic HTN. Risk factors include renal insufficiency, HTN for previous 4 + years, and HTN in a previous pregnancy.
- Adverse pregnancy outcomes of both mother and baby and abruptio placenta incidence are markedly increased.
- The diagnosis is made on the basis of established chronic HTN along with any of the followings:
  • Documented rising BP values.
  • Demonstrated worsening proteinuria.
  • Or evidence of maternal jeopardy including headache, epigastric pain, visual changes, thrombocytopenia（platelet count < 100 000/ml），elevated liver enzymes, pulmonary edema, oliguria（<750 ml/24 h），or cyanosis.
  • Edema may or may not be seen.

Laboratory Abnormalities：

Chronic HTN patients with mild HTN and no end-organ involvement have normal laboratory tests, whereas those with renal disease may have evidences of decreased renal function including proteinuria,

损害的证据,母胎预后满意。

- **不良**:妊娠并发症多见于严重高血压合并终末器官损害:

—肾病:如血肌酐值> 1.4 mg/dl,妊娠失败率明显增加。
—视网膜病:长期高血压可导致出血、渗出、狭窄等视网膜血管病变。
—左心室肥大:在血压持续高于180/110 mmHg 的妇女中常见。

- **差**:在(受孕期或妊娠早期)未控制的高血压以及慢性高血压合并子痫前期中,妊娠失败率呈 10 倍增高。

慢性高血压合并子痫前期:

- 25%的慢性高血压患者发生该并发症。危险因素包括肾功能不全,有 4 年以上高血压病史以及既往有慢性高血压合并妊娠史。
- 不良妊娠结局和胎盘早剥的发生率明显增高。

- 诊断标准为慢性高血压基础上出现以下情况:
  • 血压值增高。
  • 蛋白尿加重。
  • 或母体情况危重的证据(头痛,上腹部疼痛,视力改变,血小板减少,即计数低于 10 万/ml,肝酶升高,肺水肿,少尿,即少于 750 ml/24 h,或发绀)。
  • 水肿可有可无。

实验室异常:

轻度高血压不伴终末器官受损者实验室检查可常,而伴有肾脏损害者可发现蛋白尿、肌酐清除率减低,尿素氮、肌酐和尿酸增

lowered creatinine clearance, and elevated BUN, creatinine, and uric acid.

Antihypertensive Drug Therapy Issues:

- Discontinue medications. This may be done in patients with mild-to-moderate HTN caused by the normal decrease in BP that occurs in pregnancy. Pharmacologic treatment in patients with diastolic BP<100 mmHg does not improve either maternal or fetal outcome.

- Maintain medications. This is necessary in patients with severe HTN. The drug of choice is methyl-dopa because of extensive experience and documented fetal safety. Labetalol and atenolol are acceptable alternatives. However, β-blocking agents should not be used because their association with intrauterine growth retardation (IUGR).

- "Never use" medications. Angiotensin-converting enzyme inhibitors are contraindicated in pregnancy. Diuretics should not be initiated during pregnancy owing to possible adverse fetal effects of associated plasma volume reduction.

- BP target range. Reduction of BP to normal levels in pregnancy may jeopardize utero-placental blood flow. Maintain diastolic values between 90 and 100 mmHg.

Management:

- *Conservative outpatient management.* This is appropriate for mild-to-moderate chronic HTN without complications.
- —*Stop drug therapy.* Attempt discontinuation of antihypertensive agents following the guideline.
- —*Serial sonograms* and antenatal testing are appropriate after 30 weeks of gestation to monitor the increased risk of IUGR.
- —*Serial BP and urine protein assessment* is indicated for early identification of superimposed preeclampsia.

- —*Induce labor at term* if the cervix is favorable.
- *Aggressive prompt delivery* is indicated for chronic

高等肾功能下降的表现。

抗高血压药物治疗相关问题:

- 中断药物治疗。在妊娠正常降压效应下的轻至中度高血压可停用降压药物。对于舒张压小于 100 mmHg 的患者使用降压药物不能改善母胎预后。

- 继续药物治疗。在重度高血压患者是必要的。可选用确证对胎儿安全的甲基多巴,拉贝洛尔和阿替洛尔为可供方案。但 β-阻断剂与胎儿宫内发育迟缓有关,不宜使用。

- 禁用药物。血管紧张素转化酶抑制剂是妊娠禁忌药物。利尿剂不应于妊娠期使用,因其可引起血浆容量下降,对胎儿产生不利影响。

- 降压目标。将妊娠期血压降至正常水平可能危害子宫胎盘血流量。维持舒张压在 90～100 mmHg 即可。

临床处理:

- 保守性门诊管理:对于无并发症的轻至中度慢性高血压适用。
- —停用降压药物:按照指南考虑停用抗高血压药物。
- —系列超声检查:通常产前检查适用于孕 30 周后监测增加的胎儿宫内发育迟缓的风险。
- —多次血压监测和尿蛋白检查:用于评估和早期发现合并的子痫前期。
- —到期引产,如宫颈条件成熟。
- 紧急分娩:适应证是任何孕周

HTN with superimposed preeclampsia at any gestational age.

—Administer IV MgSO₄ to prevent convulsions.

—Keep diastolic BP between 90 and 100 mmHg with IV hydralazine and labetalol.

—Attempt vaginal delivery with IV oxytocin infusion if the physical conditions of mother and fetus are stable.

Complications:

Progression from chronic HTN to superimposed preeclampsia can lead to maternal and fetal death.

HELLP SYNDROME

A 32-year-old multigravida was at 32 weeks of gestation. At a routine prenatal visit, her BP was noted to be 160/105 mmHg. Previous BP readings were normal. Preeclampsia workup was begun and revealed the followings: elevated total bilirubin, lactate dehydrogenase, alanine aminotransferase, and aspartate aminotransferase, as well as platelet count of 85 000/ml. She had no complaints of headache or visual changes.

Definition:

HELLP syndrome occurs in 5%-10% of preeclampsia patients and is characterized by hemolysis, elevated liver enzymes, and low platelets.

Risk Factors:

HELLP syndrome occurs twice as often in multigravidas as in primigravidas.

Differential Diagnosis:

* It is confused with thrombotic thrombocytopenic purpura and hemolytic uremic syndrome.

* It, although frequently seen in HTN cases, is not always present.

Management:

Prompt delivery is appropriate for any gestational age. Use of maternal corticosteroids may help postpartum recovery.

Complications:

Conditions that are associated with HELLP syndrome include DIC, abruptio placenta, fetal

的慢性高血压基础上出现子痫前期。

—静脉给予硫酸镁:防止子痫发作。

—静脉给予肼屈嗪和拉贝洛尔:维持舒张压在 90～100 mmHg。

—如母胎情况稳定可尝试在静滴缩宫素的条件下经阴道分娩。

并发症:

从慢性高血压发展到叠加子痫前期,可导致母胎死亡。

HELLP 综合征

32 岁经产妇,孕 32 周行常规产检测量血压为 160/105 mmHg,之前查血压正常。行子痫前期相关检查结果发现:总胆红素增高,乳酸脱氢酶、谷丙和谷草转氨酶增高,血小板计数 8.5 万/ml。该妇无头痛和视力改变等主述。

定义:

HELLP 综合征发生在 5%～10% 子痫前期患者,其特征为溶血、肝酶升高和血小板降低。

危险因素:

经产妇 HELLP 综合征发生率为初孕妇的 2 倍。

鉴别诊断:

* 可与血栓性血小板减少性紫癜和溶血性尿毒症综合征混淆。

* 尽管常见于慢性高血压,但不常合并存在。

临床处理:

立即分娩对于任何孕周都是适用的。母体使用皮质类固醇有助于产后恢复。

并发症:

与 HELLP 综合征相关的并发症包括弥散性血管内凝血、胎盘

demise, ascites, and hepatic rupture.

早剥、胎儿死亡、腹水和肝破裂。

3.5　Placental Abruption

3.5　胎盘早剥

Key words

1. placental abruption
2. revealed abruption
3. concealed abruption
4. mixed bleeding
5. uteroplacental apoplexy
6. couvelaire uterus

关键词

1. 胎盘早剥
2. 显性剥离
3. 隐性剥离
4. 混合型出血
5. 子宫胎盘卒中
6. 库弗莱尔子宫

3.5.1　Concept

Placental abruption means some or all placental tissues strip from uterine wall of placenta at normal position after 20 weeks of pregnancy or in stages of labor. Placental abruption is a serious complication of late pregnancy, with acute onset and rapid progression. If it is not dealt in a timely manner, the lives of mother and child will be threatened. The reported incidence is 0.46%-2.10% and 0.51%-2.33% in China and foreign countries, respectively. Careful examination of placenta before delivery can lower the incidence. Some light placental abruption before labor has no obvious symptoms, and only the post-natal check of placenta reveals clot pressure trace. Thus, these patients may easily be neglected.

3.5.1　概念

妊娠 20 周后或分娩期,正常位置的胎盘在胎儿娩出前,部分或全部从子宫壁剥离,称为胎盘早剥(placental abruption)。胎盘早剥是妊娠晚期的一种严重并发症,具有起病急、进展快,若处理不及时,可危及母儿生命。国内报道的发生率为 0.46% ~ 2.10%,国外的发生率为 0.51% ~ 2.33%。发生率高低与分娩前是否仔细检查胎盘有关。有些轻型胎盘早剥于临产前可无明显症状,只在产前检查胎盘时,发现早剥处有凝血块压迹,此类患者易被忽略。

3.5.2　Etiology

The pathogenesis of placental abruption has not been fully elucidated, and the incidence may be related to the following factors:

3.5.2.1　Vascular lesions

Pregnant women with placental abruption complicated by severe pregnancy induced hypertension, chronic hypertension and chronic

3.5.2　病因学

胎盘早剥的发病机制尚未完全阐明,其发病可能与以下因素有关:

3.5.2.1　血管病变

胎盘早剥孕妇并发重度妊高征、慢性高血压及慢性肾脏疾病,尤其已有全身血管病变者居多。

kidney disease, in particular, has been systemic vascular lesions are most common. When the spasm or sclerosis of the end of decidual spiral arteries, causing the distal capillary ischemic necrosis resulting in bleeding, blood flow to the end of the decidual layer of the formation of hematoma, resulting in the stripping of the placenta from the uterine wall.

3.5.2.2 Mechanical factors

Trauma (especially the abdomen directly affected by the impact or direct contact to floor, etc.), the line outside to reverse the surgery corrected the fetal position, the umbilical cord too short or cord around the neck during delivery, and decreased fetal part are likely to promote placental abruption. In addition, twin pregnancy, the baby is delivered too quickly or polyhydramnios rupture of membranes, amniotic fluid outflow excessive intrauterine pressure suddenly reduce sudden contraction of the uterus, can also lead to the placenta from the uterine wall stripping.

3.5.2.3 The uterine vein pressure suddenly increased

When late pregnancy or labor, maternal long supine position, the supine hypotensive syndrome can occur. This time due to huge pregnant uterus oppression of the inferior vena cava, and thy blood less, blood pressure, uterine venous stasis, venous hypertension, resulting in decidual venous bed bleeding or rupture, leading to some or all of the placenta from the uterine wall stripping.

3.5.3 Classification

3.5.3.1 The dominant blood type

Peel large surface, to continue bleeding, hematoma after the formation of the placenta, so that the stripped part of the placenta continues to expand, and the bleeding gradually increases, when the blood rushes to open the placental edge, along the cervical canal between the fetal membranes and uterine wall

当底蜕膜螺旋小动脉痉挛或硬化,引起远端毛细血管缺血坏死以致破裂出血,血液流至底蜕膜层形成血肿,导致胎盘自子宫壁剥离。

3.5.2.2 机械性因素

外伤(特别是腹部直接受撞击或摔倒腹部直接触地等)、行外倒转术矫正胎位、脐带过短或脐带绕颈、在分娩过程中胎先露部下降,均可能促使胎盘早剥。此外,双胎妊娠的第一胎儿娩出过快或破膜时羊水流出过快,使子宫内压骤然降低,子宫突然收缩,也可导致胎盘自子宫壁剥离。

3.5.2.3 子宫静脉压突然升高

妊娠晚期或临产后,孕产妇长时间取仰卧位时,可发生仰卧位低血压综合征。此时由于巨大的妊娠子宫压迫下腔静脉,回心血量减少,血压下降,而子宫静脉却淤血,静脉压升高,导致蜕膜静脉床淤血或破裂,导致部分或全部胎盘自子宫壁剥离。

3.5.3 分类

3.5.3.1 显性出血型

剥离面大,继续出血,形成胎盘后血肿,使胎盘的剥离部分不断扩大,出血逐渐增多,若血液冲开胎盘边缘,沿胎膜与子宫壁之间经宫颈管向外流出。

outside the outflow.

3.5.3.2　Recessive blood type

The edge of the placenta is still attached to the uterine wall, fetal membranes and uterine wall undetached, or fetal head has been fixed at the pelvic inlet. All make placental blood not drain and accumulate between the placenta and uterine wall.

3.5.3.3　Hybrid

The blood can not drain, retroplacental hemorrhage piled up, along with increased fundus. When the bleeding is excessive, the blood can still be rushed to the open edge of the placenta and fetal membranes, cervical canal outflow.

3.5.4　Case study

3.5.4.1　Mild

Other than bleeding the main placental separation surface is usually not more than 1/3 of the placenta, more common in childbirth. The main symptoms are vaginal bleeding. Bleeding is generally more and dark in color, associated with mild abdominal pain or unobvious abdominal pain, anemia signs was not significant. Occurred in the delivery and rapid progress of labor. Abdominal examination: soft uterus, intermittent contractions, uterine size in line with gestational age, clear fetal position and normal fetal heart rate. If the bleeding is more, fetal heart rate can change, and tenderness is not obvious or only mild local(position of placental abruption). Postpartum check placenta, showing that the placental maternal surface of the clot and pressure trace. Sometimes the symptoms and signs is not only in the post-natal check placenta, the placenta and maternal surface clot and pressure trace, only to find placental abruption.

3.5.4.2　Severe

To hemorrhage, placental separation of the

3.5.3.2　隐性出血型

胎盘边缘仍附着于子宫壁上,或胎膜与子宫壁未分离,或胎头已固定于骨盆入口,均能使胎盘后血液不能外流而积聚于胎盘与子宫壁之间。

3.5.3.3　混合型

血液不能外流,胎盘后积血越积越多,宫底随之升高。当内出血过多时,血液仍可冲开胎盘边缘与胎膜,经宫颈管外流。

3.5.4　案例分析

3.5.4.1　轻型

以外出血为主,胎盘剥离面通常不超过胎盘的1/3,多见于分娩期。主要症状为阴道流血,出血量一般较多,色暗红,可伴有轻度腹痛或腹痛不明显,贫血体征不显著。若发生于分娩期,则产程进展较快。腹部检查:子宫软,宫缩有间歇,子宫大小与妊娠周数相符,胎位清楚,胎心率多正常,若出血量多则胎心率可有改变,压痛不明显或仅有轻度局部(胎盘早剥处)压痛。产后检查胎盘,可见胎盘母体面上有凝血块及压迹。有时症状与体征均不明显,只在产后检查胎盘时,胎盘母体面有凝血块及压迹,才发现胎盘早剥。

3.5.4.2　重型

以内出血为主,胎盘剥离面

placenta surface more than 1/3, while the larger placenta after hematoma, more common in severe pregnancy induced hypertension. The main symptoms are sudden onset of persistent abdominal pain and (or) backache, low back pain, the extent of stripping the surface size and placental blood in the number of different blood in the more pain is more severe. Can occur in severe nausea, vomiting, as well as pale, sweating, weak pulse and decreased blood pressure and other signs of shock. Can be no vaginal bleeding or only a small amount of vaginal bleeding, the degree of anemia and to go out blood. Abdominal examination: palpation of the uterus as hard as plate, there is tenderness, especially in the placental attachment is the most obvious. If the placenta is attached to the uterine wall, uterine tenderness and more obvious. Uterus larger than gestational age, and hematoma in the placenta after increasing the fundus with an increasing tenderness is also more obvious. Occasional contractions, the uterus is in a hypertonic state, the interim period are not well relaxed fetal position touch unclear. If the placental separation surface is more than the placenta of 1/2 or more, fetal death usually caused by severe hypoxia, the fetal heart of heavy patients is more than has disappeared.

3.5.4.3　Inspection

(1) The B type ultrasound: Suspicious and light underwent B-mode ultrasound examination to determine whether placental abruption and the surface size of the estimated stripping. If so, placental hematoma, sonographic liquid dark area between the placenta and the uterine wall, not very clear boundaries. Suspicious and light. Heavy patients with B ultrasonogram is more obvious, in addition to the placenta and the Palace of intramural liquid dark area, you can still see the dark area sometimes points of light reflection (the blood in

超过胎盘的 1/3,同时有较大的胎盘后血肿,多见于重度妊高征。主要症状为突然发生的持续性腹痛和(或)腰酸、腰痛,其程度因剥离面大小及胎盘后积血多少而不同,积血越多疼痛越剧烈。严重时可出现恶心、呕吐,以至面色苍白、出汗、脉弱及血压下降等休克征象。可无阴道流血或仅有少量阴道流血,贫血程度与外出血量不相符。腹部检查:触诊子宫硬如板状,有压痛,尤以胎盘附着处最明显。若胎盘附着于子宫后壁,则子宫压痛多不明显。子宫比妊娠周数大,且随胎盘后血肿的不断增大,宫底随之升高,压痛也更明显。偶见宫缩,子宫处于高张状态,间歇期不能很好放松,因此胎位触不清楚。若胎盘剥离面超过胎盘的 1/2 或以上,胎儿多因严重缺氧而死亡,故重型患者的胎心多已消失。

3.5.4.3　检查

(1)B 型超声检查:对可疑及轻型患者行 B 型超声检查,可确定有无胎盘早剥及估计剥离面大小。若有胎盘后血肿,超声声像图显示胎盘与子宫壁之间出现液性暗区,界限不太清楚。对可疑及轻型有较大帮助。重型患者的B 超声像图则更加明显,除胎盘与宫壁间的液性暗区外,还可见到暗区内有时出现光点反射(积血机化)、胎盘绒毛板向羊膜腔凸

machine), the placenta board protruding to the amniotic cavity and fetal status (with or without fetal movement and fetal heart beat).

(2) Laboratory tests: Understand the degree of anemia in patients with coagulation. Blood test to understand the degree of anemia in patients; urine understanding of renal function, and placental abruption is often caused by severe pregnancy induced hypertension, necessary to fashion for blood urea nitrogen, uric acid and carbon dioxide combining power checks.

Severe placental abruption may be complicated by DIC, the laboratory tests, including DIC screening test (e.g., platelet count, prothrombin time, fibrinogen determination and 3P test), and fibrinolysis in the confirmatory test (Fi test, FDP immune test, thrombin time and euglobulin lysis time, etc.). A & E patients feasible platelet count, whole blood clots observed dissolution test, as a simple coagulation monitoring to facilitate early diagnosis whether concurrent coagulation disorders.

Observation and dissolution test of whole blood clots: Take 2-5 ml blood into a small test tube, the tube tilt, if the blood in 6 min is not frozen or solidification unstable melt within one hour, suggesting that abnormal blood clotting. If the blood coagulation in 6 min, the body's blood fibrinogen levels usually above 1.5 g/L; blood clotting time over six minutes, and blood clots unstable, the body's blood fibrinogen levels usually 1 to 1.5 g/L; blood over 30 minutes still condensate, the body's blood fibrinogen levels usually less than 1 g/L.

3.5.4.4 Diagnosis

Diagnosis is based on history, clinical symptoms and signs. Light placental abruption not typical

出以及胎儿的状态（有无胎动及胎心搏动）。

（2）化验检查：主要了解患者贫血程度及凝血功能。血常规检查了解患者贫血程度；尿常规了解肾功能情况，由于胎盘早剥常由重度妊高征引起，因此必要时应做血尿素氮、尿酸及二氧化碳结合力等检查。

重型胎盘早剥可能并发DIC，应进行有关实验室检查，包括DIC的筛选试验（如血小板计数、凝血酶原时间、纤维蛋白原测定和3P试验）以及纤溶确诊试验[如Fi试验（即FDP免疫试验）、凝血酶时间及优球蛋白溶解时间等]。急症患者可行血小板计数、全血凝块观察与溶解试验，作为简便的凝血功能监测，以便及早诊断是否并发凝血功能障碍。

全血凝块观察及溶解试验：取2～5 ml血液放入小试管内，将试管倾斜，若血液在6 min内不凝固，或凝固不稳定，于1 h内又溶化，提示血凝异常。若血液在6 min凝固，其体内的血纤维蛋白原含量通常在1.5 g/L以上；血液凝固时间超过6 min，且血凝块不稳定，其体内的血纤维蛋白原含量通常在1～1.5 g/L；血液超过30 min仍不凝，其体内的血纤维蛋白原含量通常少于1 g/L。

3.5.4.4 诊断

诊断主要根据病史、临床症状及体征。轻型胎盘早剥由于症

symptoms and signs, the diagnosis often will be difficult, careful observation and analysis, and by B-mode ultrasound examination to determine. Typical symptoms and signs of severe placental diagnosis, and more. The diagnosis of severe placental abruption while there should be to determine the severity, if necessary, the above-mentioned laboratory tests to determine whether the dysfunction of blood coagulation and renal function failure and other complications, in order to develop a reasonable treatment options.

3.5.4.5　Differentiation

Late pregnancy bleeding, in addition to placental abruption, there are placenta previa, uterine rupture and cervical lesions bleeding, should be identified. In particular, It should be identified with placenta previa and uterine rupture.

（1）Placenta previa：Light placental abruption can also be as painless vaginal bleeding with unobvious signs. B-type ultrasound can be used to detect placental lower edge for final diagnosis. Uterine wall, placental abruption, abdominal signs is not obvious, is not easy with placenta previa difference, B-ultrasound can also identify. The clinical manifestations of severe placental abruption is very typical, it is not difficult to be differentiated with placenta previa.

状与体征不够典型,诊断往往有一定困难,应仔细观察与分析,并借 B 型超声检查来确定。重型胎盘早剥的症状与体征比较典型,诊断多无困难。确诊重型胎盘早剥的同时,尚应判断其严重程度,必要时进行上述的实验室检查,确定有无凝血功能障碍及肾功能衰竭等并发症,以便制订合理的处理方案。

3.5.4.5　鉴别

妊娠晚期出血,除胎盘早剥外,尚有前置胎盘、子宫破裂及宫颈病变出血等,应加以鉴别,尤其应与前置胎盘及子宫破裂进行鉴别。

（1）前置胎盘:轻型胎盘早剥也可为无痛性阴道出血,体征不明显,行 B 型超声检查确定胎盘下缘,即可确诊。子宫后壁的胎盘早剥,腹部体征不明显,不易与前置胎盘区别,B 超检查亦可鉴别。重型胎盘早剥的临床表现极典型,不难与前置胎盘相鉴别。

表 3-5-1　胎盘早剥与前置胎盘的区别

	胎盘早剥	前置胎盘
定义	妊娠 20 周后或分娩期,正常位置的胎盘在胎儿娩出前,部分或全部从子宫壁剥离	孕 28 周后若胎盘附着于子宫下段,甚至胎盘下缘达到或覆盖宫颈内口处,其位置低于胎儿的先露部
发病	发病急,有诱因,常伴妊高征	慢,无诱因
腹痛	剧烈	无
阴道流血	有内出血,失血征与外出血不成正比	仅外出血,反复出现,失血征与外出血成正比
并发症	DIC,产后出血,AFR	产后出血,产后感染
子宫	硬如板状,有压痛,宫底升高,大于孕周	子宫软,无压痛,大小与孕周相符
胎位胎心	查不清	清楚

续表

	胎盘早剥	前置胎盘
阴道检查	宫口无胎盘组织	宫口有胎盘组织
B超检查	胎盘后有液性暗区	胎盘低于先露部
胎盘检查	有凝血块压迹	无凝血块压迹,胎膜破口与胎盘边缘距离小于 7 cm

（2）Threatened uterine rupture：Often occurs during delivery with strong uterine contractions, abdominal pain refused to press, irritability, a small amount of vaginal bleeding, and signs of fetal distress. The above clinical manifestations difficult to distinguish from those of severe placental apruption. Threatened uterine rupture usually has cephalopelvic disproportion, delivery obstruction or a history of cesarean section. The examination can reveal uterine pathology contractions ring, catheterization, such as gross hematuria, but placental abruption is often seen in patients with severe pregnancy induced hypertension, and the uterus is as hard as board.

3.5.5　Treatment measures

3.5.5.1　Correct shock

Patients admitted to hospital in critical condition and a state of shock should be added volume to correct the shock as soon as possible to improve the patient's condition. Transfusion must be timely, and transfuse fresh blood to add volume and supplement clotting factors.

3.5.5.2　Timely termination of pregnancy

Placental abruption endanger the lives and safety of the mother and child. The prognosis and treatment of the mother of children is closely related to a timely manner. Before delivery, the placenta may continue to peel, and it is difficult to control bleeding. The longer the duration, the more serious the condition, the greater the possibility of concurrent coagulation disorders and other

（2）先兆子宫破裂：往往发生在分娩过程中,出现强烈宫缩、下腹疼痛拒按、烦躁不安、少量阴道流血、有胎儿窘迫征象等。以上临床表现与重型胎盘早剥较难区别。但先兆子宫破裂多有头盆不称、分娩梗阻或剖宫产史,检查可发现子宫病理缩复环,导尿有肉眼血尿等,而胎盘早剥常见于重度妊娠高血压征患者,检查子宫呈板样硬。

3.5.5　治疗措施

3.5.5.1　纠正休克

患者入院时情况危重、处于休克状态者,应积极补充血容量,纠正休克,尽快改善患者状况。输血必须及时,尽量输新鲜血,既能补充血容量,又可补充凝血因子。

3.5.5.2　及时终止妊娠

胎盘早剥危及母儿的生命安全。母儿的预后与处理是否及时有密切关系。胎儿未娩出前,胎盘可能继续剥离,难以控制出血,持续时间越长,病情越严重,并发凝血功能障碍等合并症的可能性也越大。因此,一旦确诊,必须及时终止妊娠。终止妊娠的方法根

complications. Therefore, immediately after final diagnosis, the pregnancy must terminated. Termination of pregnancy should be done according to birth, severity of early stripping, fetal status and cervix and other factors.

（1）Vaginal delivery: A good general by maternal bleeding mainly to the dominant, the cervix has been opened, it is estimated that a short period of time can quickly deliveries via vaginal delivery, the first rupture of membranes, amniotic fluid slow outflow reduction in uterine volume. With cummerbund wrapped abdomen, after rupture of membranes, the oppression. The placenta so that it no longer continue to peel, and may contribute to the contraction of the uterus, if necessary, with intravenous infusion of oxytocin to shorten the production process. The delivery process, close observation of the patient's blood pressure, pulse, the height, contractions and fetal heart rate changes in the fundus. Conditions are available the electronic fetal monitor, monitoring, and better early detection of uterine contractions and fetal heart rate abnormalities.

（2）Caesarean section: Severe placental abruption, especially primipara not end in a short time deliveries, placental abruption, although light, but there are signs of fetal distress, need rescue fetus; severe placental abruption, fetal death, maternal condition deteriorated in the risk immediate delivery; no progress after the rupture of membranes, induction of labor, the birth process, shall be timely cesarean section. Surgery to remove the fetus, placenta, should be promptly palace body intramuscular uterotonics, massage the uterus, usually can make uterine contractions control the bleeding. Found for uteroplacental apoplexy, the same contractions more than improved after injection of tocolytic agents and massage actively bleeding can also be controlled. If the uterus is still shrinking,

据胎次、早剥的严重程度、胎儿宫内状况及宫口开大等情况而定。

（1）经阴道分娩：经产妇一般情况较好，出血以显性为主，宫口已开大，估计短时间内能迅速分娩者，可经阴道分娩，先行破膜，使羊水缓慢流出，缩减子宫容积。破膜后用腹带包裹腹部，压迫胎盘使之不再继续剥离，并可促进子宫收缩，必要时配合静脉滴注催产素缩短产程。在分娩过程中，密切观察患者的血压、脉搏、宫底高度、宫缩情况及胎心等的变化。有条件者可用胎儿电子监测仪进行监护，更能早期发现宫缩及胎心的异常情况。

（2）剖宫产：重型胎盘早剥，特别是初产妇不能在短时间内结束分娩者；胎盘早剥虽属轻型，但有胎儿窘迫征象，需抢救胎儿者；重型胎盘早剥，胎儿已死，产妇病情恶化，处于危险之中又不能立即分娩者；破膜引产后，产程无进展者，均应及时行剖宫产术。术中取出胎儿、胎盘后，应及时行宫体肌注宫缩剂、按摩子宫，一般均可使子宫收缩良好，控制出血。若发现为子宫胎盘卒中，同样经注射宫缩剂及按摩等积极处理后，宫缩多可好转，出血亦可得到控制。若子宫仍不收缩，出血多且血液不凝，出血不能控制，则应

bleeding and blood coagulation，uterine bleeding can not control，you should enter the new blood at the same time resection.

3.5.5.3　To prevent postpartum hemorrhage

Placental abruption in patients prone to postpartum hemorrhage，so after delivery timely application of the uterus to contract agents such as oxytocin，ergometrine alkali and massage the uterus. By a variety of measures can not control the bleeding，poor uterine contractions，it should be time for a hysterectomy. Heavy bleeding and no blood clot，should be considered as coagulation disorders，and coagulation dysfunction.

3.5.5.4　Processing of coagulation disorders

（1）Lose new blood：The timely input of sufficient quantities of fresh blood to add volume and coagulation factors. Banked blood over 4 h，platelet function is damaged，poor results. To correct the platelet reduction，conditional to lose the platelet concentrate.

（2）Transmission and fibrinogen：Fibrinogen，accompanied by active bleeding，and blood coagulation by the input of fresh blood results are poor，to lose fibrinogen 3 g. fibrinogen soluble injection water 100ml intravenous infusion. Usually a 3-6 g fibrinogen to receive better results. Every 4 g fibrinogen can increase the blood fibrinogen 1 g/L.

（3）Infusion of fresh plasma：Fresh frozen plasma effect after the new blood，despite the lack of red blood cells，but contains the clotting factors，general 1 L of fresh frozen plasma containing fibrinogen 3 g，and can be Ⅴ，factor Ⅷ to the minimum effective level. Not be able to get new blood，fresh frozen plasma can be used for emergency measures.

（4）Heparin：There is a strong anticoagulant

在输入新鲜血的同时行子宫切除术。

3.5.5.3　防止产后出血

胎盘早剥患者容易发生产后出血，故在分娩后应及时应用子宫收缩剂如催产素、麦角新碱等，并按摩子宫。若经各种措施仍不能控制出血，子宫收缩不佳时，须及时作子宫切除术。若大量出血且无凝血块，应考虑为凝血功能障碍，并按凝血功能障碍处理。

3.5.5.4　凝血功能障碍的处理

（1）输新鲜血：及时、足量输入新鲜血液是补充血容量及凝血因子的有效措施。库存血若超过4 h，血小板功能即受破坏，效果差。为纠正血小板减少，有条件可输血小板浓缩液。

（2）输纤维蛋白原：若血纤维蛋白原低，同时伴有活动出血，且血不凝，经输入新鲜血等效果不佳时，可输纤维蛋白原3 g，将纤维蛋白原溶于注射用水100 ml中静脉滴注。通常给予3～6 g纤维蛋白原即可收到较好效果。每4 g纤维蛋白原可提高血纤维蛋白原1 g/L。

（3）输新鲜血浆：新鲜冰冻血浆疗效仅次于新鲜血，尽管缺少红细胞，但含有凝血因子，一般1 L新鲜冰冻血浆中含纤维蛋白原3 g，且可将Ⅴ、Ⅷ因子提高到最低有效水平。因此，在无法及时得到新鲜血时，可选用新鲜冰冻血浆作应急措施。

（4）肝素：肝素有较强的抗凝

effect，applicable to DIC the hypercoagulable stages and can not directly remove the cause. Placental abruption in patients with DIC in addressing key to terminate the pregnancy to interrupt thromboplastin continue to enter the blood. Stage of active bleeding in the coagulation disorder，the use of heparin may aggravate the bleeding，and therefore generally do not advocate the use of heparin therapy.

（5）Anti-fiber solvent：6-aminocaproic acid and so can inhibit the activities of the fibrinolytic system，if there are still intravascular coagulation，these drugs can increase the intravascular coagulation，it is not appropriate to use. If the cause has been removed，DIC in the stage of hyperfibrinolysis，and bleeding may be applied，such as 6-amino acid 4-6 g，tranexamic acid 0. 25-0. 50 g or carboxyl benzylamine 0. 1-0. 2 g dissolved in 5％ intravenous infusion of glucose 100 ml.

3.5.5.5　Prevention of renal failure

In the process，we should pay attention to the urine output，and hourly urine output of less than 30 ml require replenish ment of blood volume；In case of less than 17 ml or no urine，you should consider the possibility of renal failure that can be used 20％ mannitol 250 ml fast intravenous furosemide 40 mg intravenous injection，if necessary，re-use，and more generally in 1 to 2 days to restore. Treated urine output in the short term but not increase，significantly higher blood urea nitrogen，creatinine，serum potassium，CO_2 binding decline prompted serious cases of renal failure，uremia，dialysis therapy，rescue the maternal life.

3.5.6　Complication

3.5.6.1　DIC and coagulation disorders

Patients with severe placental abruption，especially fetal death，may have DIC and coagulation disorders. The clinical manifestations include the

作用，适用于 DIC 高凝阶段及不能直接去除病因者。胎盘早剥患者 DIC 的处理主要是终止妊娠以中断凝血活酶继续进入血内。对于处于凝血障碍的活动性出血阶段，应用肝素可加重出血，故一般不主张应用肝素治疗。

（5）抗纤溶剂：6-氨基己酸等能抑制纤溶系统的活动，若仍有进行性血管内凝血时，用此类药物可加重血管内凝血，故不宜使用。若病因已去除，DIC 处于纤溶亢进阶段，出血不止时则可应用，如 6-氨基己酸 4～6 g、止血环酸 0. 25～0. 50 g 或对羧基苄胺 0. 1～0. 2 g 溶于 5％葡萄糖液 100 ml 内静脉滴注。

3.5.5.5　预防肾功能衰竭

在处理过程中，应随时注意尿量，若每小时尿量少于 30 ml，应及时补充血容量；少于 17 ml 或无尿时，应考虑有肾功能衰竭的可能，可用 20％甘露醇 250 ml 快速静脉滴注，或速尿 40 mg 静脉推注，必要时可重复使用，一般多能于 1～2 日内恢复。经处理尿量在短期内不见增加，血尿素氮、肌酐、血钾等明显增高，CO_2 结合力下降，提示肾功能衰竭情况严重，出现尿毒症，此时应进行透析疗法，以抢救产妇生命。

3.5.6　并发症

3.5.6.1　DIC 与凝血功能障碍

重型胎盘早剥，特别是胎死宫内的患者可能发生 DIC 与凝血功能障碍。临床表现为皮下、

skin, mucous membranes or injection site hemorrhage, uterine bleeding of non-condensable or only a relatively soft clot, and fashion phenomena such as hematuria, hemoptysis, and hematemesis. From admission to postpartum placental abruption, patients should be closely observed, combined with the test results. Pay attention to the occurrence of DIC and coagulopathy, and give prevention and treatment.

3.5.6.2 Postpartum hemorrhage

Placental abruption affects myometrium and DIC causes coagulation disorders, which increase the possibility of severe massive postpartum hemorrhage. Doctors must be vigilant.

3.5.6.3 Acute renal failure

The main reason is that heavy bleeding severely damaged, resulting in ischemic necrosis of the renal cortex or renal vascular, acute renal failure and renal perfusion. Placental abruption, mostly associated with preeclampsia, blood loss on this base, with too much shock for a long time and DIC and other factors, were severely affect renal blood flow, resulting in bilateral renal cortical or tubular ischemic necrosis, acute renal failure. Renal vasospasm also affect the renal blood flow.

3.5.6.4 Amniotic fluid embolism

Placental abruption, amniotic fluid can enter the maternal circulation dissection surface open to the uterine vessels of visible components in the amniotic fluid emboli, embolism pulmonary vascular cause amniotic fluid embolism.

3.5.7 Prevention

Strengthen prenatal care, prevention and treatment of pregnancy-induced hypertension; strengthen the management of hypertension, chronic nephritis, and other high-risk pregnancy; avoid the supine position and abdominal trauma at third

黏膜或注射部位出血,子宫出血不凝或仅有较软的凝血块,有时尚可发生尿血、咯血及呕血等现象。对胎盘早剥患者从入院到产后均应密切观察,结合化验结果,注意 DIC 的发生及凝血功能障碍的出现,并给予积极防治。

3.5.6.2 产后出血

胎盘早剥对子宫肌层的影响及发生 DIC 而致的凝血功能障碍,这些使发生产后出血的可能性大且严重,必须提高警惕。

3.5.6.3 急性肾衰竭

主要原因是大量出血使肾灌注严重受损,导致肾皮质或肾小血管缺血坏死,出现急性肾衰竭。胎盘早剥大多伴有妊高征,在此基础上加上失血过多、休克时间长及 DIC 等因素,均严重影响肾的血流量,造成双侧肾皮质或肾小管缺血坏死,出现急性肾功能衰竭。肾血管痉挛也影响肾血流量。

3.5.6.4 羊水栓塞

胎盘早剥时,羊水可经剥离面开放的子宫血管进入母血循环,羊水中有形成分形成栓子,栓塞肺血管导致羊水栓塞。

3.5.7 预防

加强产前检查,积极预防与治疗妊高征;对合并高血压病、慢性肾炎等高危妊娠应加强管理;妊娠晚期避免仰卧位及腹部外伤;胎位异常行外倒转术纠正胎

trimester of pregnancy; in the abnormal fetal position, the line external cephalic version to correct fetal position, the operator must be gentle; when handling the hydramnios or twin birth, avoid suddenly reduced intrauterine pressure.

3.5.8　Placental abruption care measures

3.5.8.1　Maintain normal blood volume

Closely observe blood pressure, pulse, pale, vaginal bleeding and abdominal pain, and pay attention to hemorrhagic shock. Establish intravenous access and ensure the liquid input. Prohibit the digital rectal examination and do, careful vaginal examination to prevent re-bleeding.

3.5.8.2　Mitigation of hypoxia

Observe contractions and the fetus to prevent fetal hypoxia, absolute bed rest, take the left lateral position, given intermittent or continuous oxygen, thus improving placental blood supply, increased fetal oxygen supply, reducing the chance of bleeding. The size of the regular measurement of fundal height and abdominal circumference, the scope and extent of the tenderness of the Palace, close observation of the fetal heart, fetal, and found the uterus plate and tenderness, fetal heart tones fetal position is unclear, prompted a serious condition should be dealt with immediately.

3.5.8.3　Treatment with care to assist in the termination of pregnancy for preventing postpartum hemorrhage

（1）Should first vaginal delivery, artificial rupture of membranes, slow outflow of amniotic fluid, reducing the volume of the uterus and cummerbund wrapped abdomen, the oppression of partial placenta no longer continue to peel, but also can promote uterine contraction to accelerate the production process to continue to monitor the production process blood pressure, pulse, fundus

位时,操作必须轻柔;处理羊水过多或双胎分娩时,避免宫腔内压骤然降低。

3.5.8　胎盘早剥护理措施

3.5.8.1　维持正常的血容量

严密观察血压、脉搏、面色、阴道出血、腹痛的情况,注意有无失血性休克。建立静脉通路,确保液体输入。禁止肛查,慎做阴道检查,以防再次大出血。

3.5.8.2　缓解缺氧

观察宫缩和胎儿,防止胎儿缺氧,绝对卧床休息,取左侧卧位,给予间断或连续性吸氧,从而改善胎盘血液供应情况,增加胎儿供氧,减少出血机会。定时测量宫底高度和腹围的大小,宫体压痛的范围和程度,密切观察胎心、胎动,若发现子宫板状并有压痛,胎心音、胎位不清,提示病情严重应立即处理。

3.5.8.3　治疗配合护理,协助终止妊娠,预防产后出血

（1）经阴道分娩者应先行人工破膜,缓慢流出羊水,缩减子宫的容积,并用腹带包裹腹部,压迫局部使胎盘不再继续剥离,也能促进子宫收缩,加速产程,产程中继续监测血压、脉搏、宫底高度、压痛、阴道出血和胎心音。

height, tenderness, vaginal bleeding and fetal heart tones.

(2) Estimates that the end of the delivery or the birth process in a short period of time can not progress. The fetus of fetal distress, should quickly cesarean section, and timely rescue.

(3) Observe the complications of coagulation disorders and postpartum hemorrhage after childbirth generated particular attention to the phenomenon of systemic bleeding tendency, vaginal bleeding and blood coagulation, and with good blood, clotting time, prothrombin time, fiber fibrinogen were determined.

(4) Of the uterus-placenta stroke, therapy, should do the hysterectomy preparations.

3.5.8.4　Prevention of infection, and psychological care

3.5.9　CASE Medical record severe placental abruption, uteroplacental apoplexy

Primigravida, 26 years old. 36^{+2} weeks of amenorrhea, headache, vertigo for 3 weeks, sudden appearance of persistent abdominal pain, backache, low back pain, with nausea, vomiting and a small amount of vaginal bleeding, sweating, pale, suffering face in 2007 September 24th morning 8:00. Then the patient was sent to the hospital in a hurry. Questioning was informed that the previous rules of the menstrual cycle, about 30 days interval. Last menstrual period was January 13, 2007, the expected date of October 20, 2007. At 40 days amenorrhea early, morning sickness was not severe, without drug treatment, one month after it was self-healing. At nearly two months pregnancy the patient visited hospital for examination, diagnosis of early pregnancy. Start conscious fetal movement by the five months, and began to conduct regular prenatal care until 28 weeks to check high blood pressure,

（2）估计在短时间内不能结束分娩者或产程无进展,胎儿有宫内窘迫者,宜迅速行剖宫产,并及时抢救。

（3）分娩后注意观察凝血功能障碍及产后大出血的并发症产生,尤其注意全身出血倾向、阴道出血及血液不凝的现象,并配合做好血常规、出凝血时间、凝血酶原时间、纤维蛋白原等测定。

（4）子宫胎盘卒中者,若经治疗无效,应做好子宫全切除手术准备工作。

3.5.8.4　预防感染、心理护理

3.5.9　病例:胎盘早剥子宫胎盘卒中

初孕妇,26 岁。因停经 36^{+2} 周,头痛、眼花 3 周,突然出现持续性腹痛、腰酸、腰背痛,伴恶心、呕吐及少量阴道流血,家人见孕妇大汗淋漓、面色苍白、痛苦面容,于 2007 年 9 月 24 日晨 8 时急送至我院。追问得知,既往月经周期规则,30 日左右来潮一次。末次月经为 2007 年 1 月 13 日,预产期为 2007 年 10 月 20 日,停经 40 余日有"早孕反应",不严重,未经药物治疗,一个月后自愈。停经近 2 个月时去医院检查,诊断为早孕。停经 5 个月时自觉胎动,并开始行定期产前检查,直至停经 28 周检查时仍称血压不高,尿中无蛋白;以后因外出办事至今未再行产前检查。3 周

urine protein; No re-prenatal care due to outside visiting after 28 weeks. Headache three weeks ago, mainly in the forehead, and sometimes appear in the occipital, who have been taking the pain killer, and sometimes vertigo, stars, did not go to hospital for treatment, returned home yesterday, suddenly persistent pain in the morning 6:00 AM a small amount of vaginal bleeding, in view of pregnant women suffering ill, and looking pale and sweat dripping, not relieved when arrived the hospital and diagnosed, by the out-patient as parity production 10, 36^{+2} weeks of gestation, the Ⅲ degree of placental abruption, severe preeclampsia.

　　Admission examination: body temperature 37.2 ℃; pulse 96 times / min, breathing 18 times/min, blood pressure 148/106 mmHg. Eye conjunctiva slightly pale, no body skin stained yellow and bleeding, no superficial lymph node enlargement. Heart rate 96 beats/minute, the apex like systolic murmur of grade Ⅱ, breath sounds clear, no smell and the wet and dry tone. Abdominal distension was full-term pregnancy abdominal, liver and spleen palpation is not satisfied, the uterus was hard, plate and around the navel and slightly above tenderness. Not listen to fetal heart, touch unclear fetal position. Pelvic measurements were normal. Check when you see a small amount of vaginal persistent bleeding. Anemia, appearance and amount of vaginal bleeding not directly proportional to, without making a gynecological examination and rectal examination: acute and line B-mode ultrasound examination, the placenta at the anterior wall of the uterus near the fundus. The edge of clear liquid hypoechoic area between the placenta and the uterine wall, abnormal thickening of the placenta, placental hematoma and placental unclear. Seen scattered in the amniotic fluid within the small points of light floating. The fetus is dead, no fetal heart rate. LOA. Laboratory tests:

前出现头痛,主要在前额,有时也出现在枕部,曾服用索米痛止痛,且有时眼花,眼冒金星,未去医院诊治,昨日返家,今晨 6 时突然持续性腹痛及少量阴道流血,鉴于孕妇痛苦病容、面色苍白和大汗淋漓,到医院后未见缓解,经门诊以"第 1 胎第 0 产妊娠 36^{+2} 周、Ⅲ度胎盘早剥、重度子痫前期"的诊断收入院。

　　入院后查体:体温 37.2℃;脉搏 96 次/min,呼吸 18 次/min,血压 148/106 mmHg。眼睑结膜稍苍白,全身皮肤无黄染及出血点,浅表淋巴结不肿大。心率 96 次/min,心尖部有Ⅱ级吹风样收缩期杂音,呼吸音清晰,未闻及干湿啰音。腹部膨隆呈妊娠足月腹型,肝脾触诊不满意,子宫呈板状硬,以脐周围及偏上方压痛最明显。未听及胎心,触不清胎位。骨盆外测量未见异常。检查时见有少量阴道持续性流血。贫血外貌与阴道流血量不成正比,未做妇科检查及肛门检查:急行 B 型超声检查,胎盘位于子宫前壁,靠近宫底。胎盘与子宫壁之间出现边缘不清的液性低回声区,胎盘异常增厚,胎盘后血肿与胎盘界限不清。羊水内可见散在漂浮的小光点。胎儿已死,无胎心,枕左前位。实验室检查:红细胞 $2.84×10^{12}$/L,血红蛋白 74 mg/L,白细胞 $12.3×10^9$/L,中性 0.72,淋巴 0.28,血小板 196

red blood cells $2.84 \times 10^{12}/L$, and hemoglobin 74 mg/L, white blood cells $12.3 \times 10^9/L$, neutral 0.72, lymph 0.28, platelets $196 \times 10^9/L$, Bleeding time 2 minutes 30 seconds, the clotting time of 3 minutes. Blood type O. Urinary protein（＋＋）, red blood cells 23/HP. Emergency preparedness of blood is 800 ml and continuous oxygen, intravenous infusion of Ringer's solution. Clinical diagnosis：0, 1 tire production 36 weeks of pregnancy, stillbirth, severe preeclampsia, Ⅲ degree of placental abruption, and secondary anemia. And family members accountable condition after being rushed to the operating room, continuous epidural anesthesia downstream of the lower uterine segment cesarean section.

Open peritoneal see the uterine anterior wall of the large areas of copper-colored ecchymosis to the placental site is even more obvious, the diagnosis of placental abruption, uteroplacental apoplexy, uterine lower segment transverse incision, as shown in the amniotic fluid was bloody, hand to take the dead fetus and placenta immediately after the uterine raised to the abdominal incision with a sponge forceps to hold the cutting edge of the uterus to stop bleeding. See at this time the uterus, copper-colored area like a leather-like, uterine contraction, the amount of bleeding; immediately palace at the bottom and the hot brine yarn hand massage pad fomentation uterus, a rapid injection of the uterine muscle wall ergometrine 0.4 mg (2 ml) and oxytocin 20 units in (2 ml); intravenous infusion of oxytocin 20 units to promote uterine contraction, and quickly lose still more than the new blood of 600 ml. After the treatment, placental separation surface bleeding, decided to bilateral uterine artery ascending branch of (uterus support) ligation, occlusion of the bilateral uterine artery ascending branch of the uterine bleeding gradually reduced until it stops uterine contractions upturn has been observed 20 minutes,

$\times 10^9/L$。出血时间 2 分 30 秒，凝血时间 3 分。血型 O 型。尿蛋白（＋＋＋），红细胞 2～3/HP。紧急备血 800 ml 并持续吸氧，静脉滴注林格液。临床诊断：第 1 胎第 0 产妊娠 36 周、死胎、重度子痫前期、Ⅲ度胎盘早剥、继发性贫血。与家属交代病情后，立即送手术室，在连续硬膜外麻醉下行子宫下段剖宫产术。

打开腹膜后，见子宫前壁大片紫铜色瘀斑，以胎盘附着部位更明显，诊断为胎盘早剥子宫胎盘卒中，行子宫下段横切口，见羊水呈血性，手取已死胎儿和胎盘后，迅即将子宫提至腹部切口外，用海绵钳夹持子宫切缘止血。此时见子宫紫铜色区犹如皮革状，子宫收缩不良，出血量多；立即用手按摩宫底部和热盐水纱垫热敷子宫，迅速注入子宫肌壁内麦角新碱 0.4 mg（2 ml）及缩宫素 20 单位（2 ml）；同时静脉滴注缩宫素 20 单位，促使子宫收缩，并快速输新鲜血 600 ml。经上述处理后，胎盘剥离面出血仍不止，决定行双侧子宫动脉上行支（子宫体支）结扎，结扎双侧子宫动脉上行支后，子宫出血逐渐减少，直至停止，子宫收缩转佳，经观察 20 min，子宫收缩良，关腹术终。术后继续输新鲜血 200 ml。术中血压平稳，尿量不少，色清。术后血压逐渐降低，至术后第 7 日，血

the contraction of the uterus to good，off abdominal surgery end. Patients continue to lose new blood 200ml. Intraoperative blood pressure was stable，a lot of urine，clear color. Postoperative blood pressure gradually decreased to the 7th day after surgery，the blood pressure dropped to 130/86 mmHg，urinary protein negative. Fundus examination，the proportion of small artery spasm caused by artery has been restored to 2∶3. Abdominal incision suture removal，a healing back to the milk，and postoperative high-dose estradiol valerate and good efficiency. October 1，2007 Discharged. Discharge diagnosis：G_1P_1 36 weeks post-cesarean，stillbirth，severe pre-eclampsia，third degree tire，uteroplacental apoplexy，the ascending branch of uterine artery ligation，secondary anemia.

压已降至 130/86 mmHg，尿蛋白阴性。眼底检查，小动脉痉挛致动脉比例已恢复至 2∶3。腹部切口拆线，一期愈合，术后用大剂量戊酸雌二醇回乳，效佳。于 2007 年 10 月 1 日出院。出院诊断：第 1 胎第 1 产妊娠 36 周剖宫产术后、死胎、重度子痫前期、Ⅲ度胎盘早剥、子宫胎盘卒中、双侧子宫动脉上行支结扎术后、继发性贫血。

3.6　Placenta Previa

Key words

1. placenta previa
2. total placenta previa
3. partial placenta previa
4. marginal placenta previa
5. lower uterine segment
6. magnetic resonance imaging
7. placenta implantation

3.6.1　Main content

3.6.1.1　Definition

In placenta previa，the placenta is located over or very near the internal os. Four degrees of this abnormality have been recognized：

1. Total placenta previa：

The internal cervical os is covered completely by placenta.

3.6　前置胎盘

关键词

1. 前置胎盘
2. 完全性前置胎盘
3. 部分性前置胎盘
4. 边缘性前置胎盘
5. 子宫下段
6. 核磁共振
7. 胎盘植入

3.6.1　主要内容

3.6.1.1　定义

前置胎盘是指胎盘覆盖或非常接近宫颈内口。这种异常情况可分为四类：

1. 完全性前置胎盘：
宫颈内口完全被胎盘覆盖。

2. Partial placenta previa：

The internal os is partially covered by placenta.

3. Marginal placenta previa：

The edge of the placenta is at the margin of the internal os.

4. Low-lying placenta：

The placenta is implanted in the lower uterine segment such that the placenta edge actually does not reach the internal os but it is approximately close to it.

3.6.1.2　Incidence

0.3%-5.0%.

3.6.1.3　Risk factors

1. Prior cesarean delivery or abortion.
2. Multiparity and advancing maternal age.

3.6.1.4　Diagnosis

1. Clinical symptoms：

The recurring, without warning and painless hemorrhage, which usually appears near the end of the second trimester or later.

2. Localization by sonography：

The simplest, most precise, and safest method of placenta localization is provided by transabdominal sonography.

3. Magnetic resonance imaging：

This technology does not use for routine evaluation.

3.6.1.5　Management

1. MgSO$_4$ is the first choice of tocolytic.

2. No vaginal examation.

3. Serial ultrasound for observing growth and changes of partial placenta previa.

4. Delivery by cesarean.

5. Hospitalization is usually after 1st bleed but depends on clinical situation.

6. Consider delivery as soon as lung maturity is documented.

2. 部分性前置胎盘：

宫颈内口部分被胎盘覆盖。

3. 边缘性前置胎盘：

胎盘边缘在宫颈内口边缘。

4. 低置胎盘：

胎盘附着于子宫下段，胎盘边缘并未达宫颈内口但却十分接近。

3.6.1.2　发病率

0.3%～5.0%。

3.6.1.3　危险因素

1. 前次剖宫产史或流产史。
2. 多胎、高龄。

3.6.1.4　诊断

1. 临床症状：

孕中期末或以后出现的反复、无先兆、无痛性出血。

2. 超声定位：

最简单、最精确、最安全的胎盘定位方法是腹部超声。

3. 磁共振成像：

不作为常规检查技术。

3.6.1.5　处理

1. 硫酸镁是首选的宫缩抑制剂。

2. 不做阴道检查。

3. 系列超声监测部分前置胎盘的生长和变化的情况。

4. 剖宫产分娩。

5. 通常1次出血后住院，但取决于临床情况。

6. 一旦证实胎肺已成熟即考虑分娩。

7. High risk for placenta accreta, hemorrhage (especially if previous cesarean section).

3.6.1.6 Evaluation

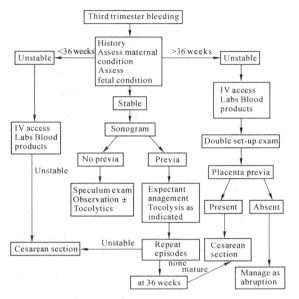

7. 有胎盘粘连为出血的高危情况(尤其有前次剖宫产史者)。

3.6.1.6 评估

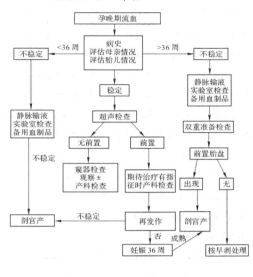

3.6.1.7 Case analysis

Maternal, 32 years old. Menopause 29 weeks, painless vaginal bleeding 2 h and admission, the patient's previous menstrual regularity, cycle 28, 5 to 6 days of menstruation, the last menstrual period October 4, 2006. Had 2 years ago, natural vaginal birth a baby girl, 2 abortion, artificial abortion at once, and the other one years ago, a medical abortion. Menopause nearly 2 months due to poor appetite, early morning vomiting go to the hospital, urine hCG tests (+), a diagnosis of early pregnancy. Fetal movement, stop by more than 4 month consciously not done regular prenatal care. The most this morning 4 am, sleep, vaginal bleeding is about 500 ml, no abdominal pain. 6 o'clock this morning sent to the hospital by ambulance, "4 child a production 29 weeks of pregnancy with placenta previa, secondary anemia" emergency income homes.

People hospitalized after the examination: body temperature 36.3 ℃, pulse 110/min, respiratory rate 20 breaths/min, blood pressure 80/50 mmHg.

3.6.1.7 案例分析和测试

经产妇,32 岁。以"停经 29 周,无痛性阴道大量流血 2 h"入院,患者既往月经规律,周期 28 日,经期 5~6 日,末次月经 2006 年 10 月 4 日。曾于 2 年前经阴道自然分娩一女婴,流产 2 次,一次行人工流产术,另一次于 1 年前药物流产。停经近 2 个月时,因食欲不佳、晨起呕吐去医院,行尿 hCG 检测(+),诊断为早孕。停经 4 月余自觉胎动,未再做过定期的产前检查。今晨 4 时许,正在睡眠中发现阴道大量流血约 500 ml,无腹痛。晨 6 时由救护车送至医院,以"第 4 胎 1 产妊娠 29 周前置胎盘、继发性贫血"急诊收入院。

入院后查体:体温 36.3 ℃,脉搏 110 次/min,呼吸 20 次/min,血压 80/50 mmHg。神志

Conscious, pale. Lung breath sounds clear, no smell and the wet and dry rales. Heart rate 110 beats/min, the apical II level of hair-like systolic murmur. Abdominal distension, liver and spleen palpation is not satisfied. Obstetric examination: uterine contractions, uterine length 28 cm, abdominal circumference 86 cm, sacral right front bits fetal heart rate of 142 bpm. Pelvic measurements were normal. Vulva how the amount of blood, a small amount of blood flow. Auxiliary examination: red blood cells 3.0 × 10^{12}/L, hemoglobin 85 g/L, platelets 105 × 10^9/L, white blood cells 10.5 × 10^9/L, neutral 0.76, lymph 0.24. Normal blood clotting. Blood type O. B-ultrasonography showed the placenta at the posterior wall of the uterus, I level. The placenta to the cervix all covered with complete placenta previa, first exposed the fetal buttocks and fetal foot fetal head biparietal diameter 7.1 cm, fetal femur length of 5.5 cm, the fetal abdominal circumference of 27 cm, the estimated weight of 1 450 g.

Treatment: people hospitalized after the immediate opening of the venous access, maintenance and blood 600 ml. Vaginal bleeding, the general practitioner to discuss and decide in continuous epidural anesthesia immediately downstream of the lower uterine segment cesarean section, hip traction delivered a 1 400 g male live births, Apgar score one minute and eight minutes, 5 minutes and 10 minutes, sent to neonatology. Hand to take the placenta smoothly, due to postpartum uterine lower segment placenta stripped surface and opening the sinuses showing activity in bleeding, gut "8"-shaped suture, and a large piece of gelatin sponge oppression stop the bleeding, followed by repair of the uterine lower segment incision, and uterine body injected shrink The official prime 20 IU, the abdomen was closed. Blood transfusion 400 ml, intraoperative blood loss of about 500 ml. Postoperative after a smooth, 7

清楚,面色苍白。双肺呼吸音清晰,未闻及干湿性啰音。心率110次/min,律齐,心尖部 II 级吹风样收缩期杂音。腹部膨隆,肝脾触诊不满意。产科检查:无宫缩,子宫长度 28 cm,腹围 86 cm,骶右前位,胎心 142 bpm。骨盆外测量未见异常。外阴有多量血迹,有少量血液流出。辅助检查:血红细胞 3.0 × 10^{12}/L,血红蛋白 85 g/L 血小板 105 × 10^9/L,白细胞 10.5 × 10^9/L,中性 0.76,淋巴 0.24。凝血四项正常。血型 O 型。B 型超声检查见胎盘位于子宫后壁,I 级。胎盘将宫颈内口全部遮盖,为完全性前置胎盘,先露为胎臀与胎足,胎头双顶径 7.1 cm,胎儿股骨长 5.5 cm,胎儿腹围 27 cm,估计体重 1 450 g。

处理:入院后立即开放静脉通路,备血 600 ml。因阴道不断流血,经全科医师讨论决定立即在持续硬膜外麻醉下行子宫下段剖宫产术,臀牵引娩出 1 400 g 男活婴,新生儿 Apgar 评分 1 min 8 分,5 min 10 分,送至新生儿科。手取胎盘顺利,因产后子宫下段胎盘剥离面开放的血窦呈活跃性出血,用肠线"8"字形缝合,并用大块明胶海绵压迫止血,随后缝合子宫下段切口,并在子宫体部注入缩宫素 20 IU,关腹。术中输血 400 ml,术中出血约 500 ml。术后经过顺利,术后第 7 日腹部切口拆线,愈合良好。术后第 8 日出院。早产儿在新生儿科住院 1 个月出院。

days after abdominal incision stitches healed well. After surgery and discharged on the 8th day. Preterm children hospitalized in neonatology a discharged.

Test

1. In antepartum haemorrhate：（　　）
   A. Maternal deaths are caused equally by placental abruption and placenta praevia
   B. Cervical carcinoma can be excluded if there is a history of a negative smear test in the past year
   C. Management can be conservative at 41 weeks as it is likely to be due to a "show"
   D. Fetal mortality is unusual with a placenta praevia
   E. Ultrasound is helpful in deciding the cause
2. With regard to placenta praevia：（　　）
   A. It is described as minor if vaginal bleeding has not occurred
   B. Intercourse should be avoided to reduce the risk of further bleeding
   C. Diagnosis is more difficult if the placenta is posterior
   D. Investigation with vaginal ultrasound is generally safe
   E. Bleeding from a placenta praevia does not require anti-D administration as there is never any fetomaternal haemorrhage

Reference answer

1. ADE
2. BCD

3.7 Amniotic Fluid Embolism

Key words

amniotic fluid embolism，AFE

测试

1. 关于产前出血：（　　）
   A. 前置胎盘与胎盘早剥的孕产妇死亡率相等
   B. 如果既往宫颈筛查阴性即可排除宫颈癌
   C. 孕 41 周产前出血可能是见红，可以保守治疗
   D. 胎儿死亡率与前置胎盘有关
   E. 超声有助于确诊病例
2. 关于前置胎盘：（　　）
   A. 如无出血，则为轻度
   B. 避免性生活以防出血
   C. 后壁胎盘时诊断困难
   D. 阴道超声是安全的
   E. 前置胎盘出血无需使用抗 D 注射，因为不存在母胎间出血

参考答案

1. ADE
2. BCD

3.7 羊水栓塞

关键词

羊水栓塞

3.7.1　Definition

Amniotic fluid embolism（AFE）is a rare and incompletely understood obstetric emergency in which amniotic fluid, fetal cells, hair, or other debris enters the mother's blood stream via the placental bed of the uterus and trigger an allergic reaction. This reaction then results in cardiorespiratory（heart and lung）collapse and coagulopathy. It was first formally characterized in 1941. It is estimated to be the fifth most common cause of maternal mortality in the world.

The condition is so rare（between 1 in 8 000 and 1 in 80 000 deliveries, although more recent studies show 1 in 20 464 deliveries for a more precise number）that most doctors will never encounter it in their professional careers, and as a result the exact process is poorly understood.

It is believed that once the fluid and fetal cells enter the maternal pulmonary circulation in general terms, there will be profound respiratory failure with deep cyanosis and cardiovascular shock followed by convulsions and profound coma, however this does occur in two phases detailed below:

First phase

The patient experiences acute shortness of breath and hypotension. This rapidly progresses to cardiac arrest leading to a reduction of perfusion to the heart and lungs. No longer after that stage, the patient will lapse into a coma. It was previously believed to have a maternal mortality rate of 60%-80%, it has been reported at 26.4% more recently.

Second phase

Although many women do not survive beyond the first stage, about 40% of the initial survivors will pass onto the second phase. This is known as the

3.7.1　定义

羊水栓塞是一种罕见及未被完全了解的产科紧急症候,指在分娩过程中,羊水、胎儿细胞、胎发、胎粪、皮屑等物,透过子宫基底的胎盘进入母体血液循环而诱发母体之炎性反应。这将引致心肺衰竭及凝血异常。此病最早在1941年被描述说明。在母体致死率的列表中羊水栓塞排列第五位。

羊水栓塞十分罕见(机会为8 000至80 000次分娩中出现一次,然而最新的研究给予更准确的数字为20 464次分娩中出现一次)。大部分产科医生在整个职业生涯中可能从未经历过。因此,这种状况的发生过程是很少被了解。

一般认为,羊水及胎儿细胞进入母体肺循环(此可能使产妇心肺衰竭而亡)后将发生下列两个阶段:

第一阶段

产妇症状为呼吸困难及低血压,肺动脉高压,迅速变成心脏停搏,出现缺氧,不久进入昏迷状态。一半以上病人在症状出现的首个小时内死亡。

第二阶段

40%的病人经过第一阶段生还,进入第二阶段。在此阶段内病人出现大量出血,出现颤抖、咳

hemorrhagic phase and may be accompanied by severe shivering，coughing，vomiting，and the sensation of a bad taste in the mouth. This is also accompanied by excessive bleeding as the blood loses its ability to clot. Collapse of the cardiovascular system leads to fetal distress and death unless the child is delivered swiftly.

3.7.2 Presentation

1. Postpartum haemorrhage of undue severity or without apparent explanation.

2. Sudden maternal collapse either during or after labour.

3. Disseminated intravascular coagulation during labour or within hours of delivery.

4. Respiratory problems such as adult respkatory distress syndrome， haemoptysis， pulmonary oedema and cyanosis.

5. Convulsions appears to be associated with caesarean delivery but this is not to say that the mode of delivery is causative，though it may go through leakage of amniotic fluid into uterine veins in some instances. The characteristic finding on autopsy examination is fetal squames or hair in the maternal lungs.

In cases of collapse which are successfully resuscitated，diagnose is impossible on these criteria. Therefore the extent to which this condition causes morbidity is unknown.

Squames might potentially be detectable in sputum or blood collected from a central line.

3.7.3 Causes

It is mostly agreed that this condition results from amniotic fluid entering the uterine veins and in order for this to occur there are three prerequisites：

1. Ruptured membranes（a term used to define the rupture of the amniotic sac）.

2. Ruptured uterine or cervical veins.

嗽,血液凝固障碍伴随大量失血。在此情况下胎儿必须被尽速分娩,否则心血管系统的崩溃会造成胎儿窘迫及死亡。

3.7.2 临床表现

1.过度严重的或者没有明显原因的产后出血。

2.分娩期间或之后母亲突然衰竭。

3.分娩期间或几个小时内出现 DIC。

4.呼吸障碍,比如成人呼吸窘迫综合征、咯血,肺水肿以及发绀。

5.抽搐,其发生与剖宫产有关但并不是说分娩方式是其发生的原因,尽管在某些情况下它可能透过羊膜进入子宫静脉。

其解剖检查的特点是在产妇肺中发现胎儿鳞屑或毛发。

如果衰竭后成功恢复,这些诊断标准不成立。所以在这种情况下引起的发病是未知的。

鳞状细胞可能从采痰液或血液中检测出来。

3.7.3 病因

多数认为羊水等物进入子宫颈是由于下列三个先决条件发生所造成的:

1.薄膜破裂(一般通称羊膜破裂)。

2.子宫或子宫颈破裂。

3. A pressure gradient from uterus to vein.

Although exposure to fetal tissue is common, and finding fetal tissue within the maternal circulation is not significant. In a small percentage of women, this exposure leads to a complex chain of events resulting in collapse and death.

There is some evidence that AFE may be associated with abdominal trauma or amniocentesis. Cervical laceration or uterine rupture, placenta previa or abruption, eclampsia, and fetal distress were also associated with an increased risk.

3.7.4　Treatment

1. Anti-allergy：dexamethasone 20-40 mg drip or hydrogenated exam to loose 300-400 mg intravenous drip.

2. Remove pulmonary hypertension：papaverine 30-90 mg vein into the pot.

Atropine 1-2 mg vein into the blood.

Aminophylline 250-500 mg intravenous drip.

3. Oxygen supply.

4. Correct shock：added blood volume, blood transfusion, fluid infusion, dopamine 20-80 mg, alamine 20-80 mg, phentolamine 20-40 mg intravenous drip.

5. Treat heart failure and nutrition myocardial：west the ground orchid 0.4 mg intravenous drip, and ATP, coenzyme A, cytochrome C.

6. Correct DIC.

7. Correct renal failure：furosemide 40 mg static push, the uric acid 50-100 mg static push, mannitol 250 ml intravenous drip.

8. Choose broad spectrum antibiotics：The first choice is cephalosporins.

9. Obstetric treatment：The first process：inhibition contractions, quickly termination of gestation cesarean section.

The second process：birth, shorten the second

3. 子宫与静脉间的压力程度。

其实在母体(孕妇)找到胎儿组织是很常见的，因此在母体血液循环中发现胎儿组织来证实羊水栓塞并没有意义。只有很少比例的妇女是在一连串复杂的事件中造成心血管崩溃及死亡。

一些证据显示羊水栓塞患者伴随有腹部的外伤。使用催生素催生，造成宫颈破裂，产妇较易发生羊水栓塞；剖宫产创伤面大，产妇也易发生羊水栓塞。

3.7.4　处置

1. 抗过敏：地塞米松 20～40 mg 静脉滴注或氢化考的松 300～400 mg 静脉滴注。

2. 解除肺动脉高压：罂粟碱 30～90 mg 静脉入壶，阿托品 1～2 mg静脉入血，氨茶碱 250～500 mg 静脉滴注。

3. 加压给氧。

4. 纠正休克：补充血容量、输血、输液，多巴胺 20～80 mg、阿拉明 20～80 mg、酚妥拉明 20～40 mg 静脉滴注。

5. 抗心衰，营养心肌：西地兰 0.4 mg 静脉滴注，ATP、辅酶 A、细胞色素 C。

6. 纠正 DIC。

7. 纠正肾衰：呋塞米(速尿) 40 mg 静推，利尿酸 50～100 mg 静推，甘露醇 250 ml 静脉滴注。

8. 选用广谱抗生素：首选头孢类。

9. 产科处理：第一产程：抑制宫缩，迅速剖宫产终止妊娠。

第二产程：助产，缩短第二

stages of labor, disable contractions agent.　　　　　　　程,禁用宫缩剂。

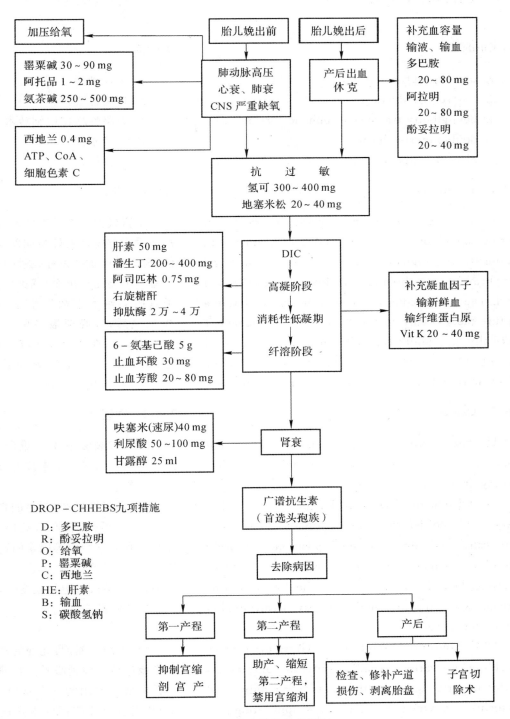

图 3-7-1　羊水栓塞抢救规程

3.8　Uterine Rupture

Key words

    1. uterine rupture
    2. obstructive dystocia
    3. negligibility transverse cephalic version
    4. double uterine horn
    5. placenta implantation

3.8.1　Definition

Uterine rupture means laceration occurs in uterine body or the lower uterine segment in childbirth or pregnancy. It is a serious obstetric complication and threaten the lives of mother and child. Died of bleeding, infection or shock. Uterine rupture most occurs in the 28 weeks of pregnancy, especially in childbirth. The incidence of control below 0.1%, the maternal mortality rate is 5%, the infant mortality rate is 50% to 75% or even higher.

3.8.2　Causes

Uterine rupture mostly occurs in a difficult labor, senior citizens, productive and uterus had surgery or had damage maternal.

(1) Obstructive dystocia：The pelvis of the first basin, said the deformity pelvic tumors of the soft birth canal and abnormal fetal position and other factors hinder fetal loss, uterine overcome resistance to strengthen the contraction of the lower uterine segment was forced to lengthen the eventual thinning of the uterine rupture.

(2) Abuse of uterotonics：Here uterotonics should include various stimulates uterine contractions in the material such as the most commonly used oxytocin (oxytocin) and the application of misoprostol only in recent years. The reported misoprostol leads more and more cases of uterine

3.8　子宫破裂

关键词

    1. 子宫破裂
    2. 梗阻性难产
    3. 忽略性横位内倒转术
    4. 双角子宫
    5. 胎盘植入

3.8.1　定义

子宫破裂是指子宫体部或子宫下段于分娩期或妊娠期发生裂伤,为产科严重并发症,威胁母儿生命。主要死于出血、感染休克。子宫破裂绝大多数发生于妊娠28周之后,分娩期最多见,目前发生率控制在1‰以下,产妇病死率为5%,婴儿病死率高达50%～75%,甚至更高。

3.8.2　病因

子宫破裂多发生于难产、高龄多产和子宫曾经手术或有过损伤的产妇。

(1)梗阻性难产:明显的骨盆狭窄、头盆不称、软产道畸形、盆腔肿瘤和异常胎位等因素阻碍胎先露下降,子宫为克服阻力加强收缩,子宫下段被迫拉长变薄,最终发生子宫破裂。

(2)滥用宫缩剂:此处的宫缩剂应该包括各种刺激子宫收缩的物质包括最常用的缩宫素(催产素)和近些年才应用的米索前列醇,报道的米索前列醇导致子宫破裂的病例越来越多。原因主要

rupture, mainly due to drug overdose or too fast drug delivery in cervical immatures, abnormal fetal obstructive dystocia, and medication during the observation of the birth process is not carefully.

（3）Vaginal delivery surgical injury: The cervix is not open, forcibly the Forceps hip traction lead to cervical severe laceration on the extension to the lower uterine segment. The negligibility transverse cephalic version, destroy fetal part of the manual stripping placental surgery due to improper operation, can cause uterine rupture.

（4）Poor uterine malformations and uterine wall development: The most common is the double uterine horn or uterine horn.

（5）Lesions of the uterus itself: Maternal history of repeated curettage, septic abortion history of intrauterine infection, manual removal of placenta, the history of hydatidiform mole history. These factors have led to the endometrium as well as damage to the muscle wall, and after pregnancy placenta accreta or penetration, and ultimately lead to uterine rupture.

3.8.3　Classification

The classification of uterine rupture is mainly based on the causes, rupture time, rupture location, rupture degree and other factors.

（1）Based on causes:

①Spontaneous uterine rupture occurred in the prenatal, common in poor scar the uterus and uterine development, like double uterine horn.

②Traumatic uterine rupture occurred in production.

（2）Based on rupture time:

①Uterine rupture is common in poor scar uterus and uterine development.

②Intrapartum uterine rupture more common in the maternal, mostly due to obstructive dystocia surgical trauma or oxytocin improper use, and the

包括药物剂量过大或给药速度过快、子宫颈不成熟、胎位不正、梗阻性难产、用药期间对产程观察不仔细等。

（3）阴道助产手术损伤：宫口未开全，强行产钳术或臀牵引术导致子宫颈严重裂伤并上延到子宫下段。忽略性横位内倒转术、毁胎术、部分人工剥离胎盘术等由于操作不当，均可以造成子宫破裂。

（4）子宫畸形和子宫壁发育不良：最常见的是双角子宫或单角子宫。

（5）子宫本身病变：多产妇多次刮宫史、感染性流产史、宫腔感染史、人工剥离胎盘史、葡萄胎史等。由于上述因素导致子宫内膜乃至肌壁受损，妊娠后胎盘植入或穿透，最终导致子宫破裂。

3.8.3　分类

子宫破裂的分类主要根据破裂原因、破裂时间、破裂部位和破裂程度等因素进行。

（1）按破裂原因分类：

①自发性子宫破裂多发生于产前，常见于瘢痕子宫和子宫发育不良，如双角子宫等。

②创伤性子宫破裂多发生于产时。

（2）按破裂发生时间分类：

①妊娠期子宫破裂常见于瘢痕子宫和子宫发育不良。

②分娩期子宫破裂多见于经产妇，原因多为梗阻性难产或手术创伤或缩宫素（催产素）使用不

majority of uterine rupture occurred in the period.

(3) Based on the site of uterine rupture:

① Uterine body burst prevalent in the Palace scar, placenta accreta and the uterine hypoplasia.

② Uterine segment rupture common cause cervical laceration, and on the extension of obstructive dystocia inappropriate vaginal delivery.

(4) Based on levels in uterine rupture:

①Complete rupture of the uterus: Uterine wall layer split, the same uterine cavity and the abdominal cavity, fetus and placenta can be incarcerated in the uterine rupture of the mouth, into the abdominal cavity, if the gestational age, small placenta, amniotic sac completely wrapped the fetus into the abdominal cavity.

②In complete uterine rupture: Uterine muscle wall part or full-thickness rupture, complete serosa. Common uterine rupture, the formation of the broad ligament hematoma, also known as uterine rupture within the broad ligament.

3.8.4 Pathogenesis

Factors for uterine rupture included

1. A bleeding uterine rupture often bleed. Bleeding is divided into internal bleeding, external bleeding or mixed bleeding. Internal bleeding that blood accumulation in the broad ligament or abdominal cavity, resulting in the broad ligament hematoma or hemoperitoneum; external bleeding that blood from the vaginal discharge.

Uterine rupture bleeding site is usually including the uterus and lower congenital tract hemorrage from the around surface of placenta. The rupture and placenta peeling surface bleeding; uterus and soft birth canal bleeding usually need to damage the site where the large blood vessels passes. If the soft birth canal injury did not hurt the great vessels which usually did not performance as bleeding or activities

当,多数子宫破裂发生于该时期。

(3)按子宫破裂的部位分类：

①子宫体部破裂多见于宫体部瘢痕、胎盘植入和子宫发育不良。

②子宫下段破裂多见于梗阻性难产，不恰当的阴道助产，导致子宫颈裂伤并上延。

(4)按子宫破裂程度分类：

①完全性子宫破裂：子宫壁全层裂开，子宫腔与腹腔相通，胎儿和胎盘可嵌顿于子宫破裂口处，也可以进入腹腔。

②不完全子宫破裂：子宫肌壁部分或全层破裂，浆膜层完整。常见子宫下段破裂，形成阔韧带内血肿，又称阔韧带内子宫破裂。

3.8.4 发病机制

子宫破裂的影响因素包括：

1. 出血子宫破裂通常表现为大出血，出血分为内出血、外出血或混合出血。内出血指出血积聚于阔韧带内或腹腔内，导致阔韧带血肿或腹腔积血；外出血指出血自阴道排出。

子宫破裂的出血部位通常包括子宫及软产道破裂口和胎盘剥离面出血；子宫和软产道出血通常需要损伤所在部位的大血管，如果软产道损伤未伤及大血管，通常不表现为大出血或活动性出血。胎盘剥离面的出血与胎盘剥离的程度与子宫收缩强度有关，

of sex bleeding do. Placental separation, the degree of surface bleeding, placental separation and uterine contraction intensity, if the placenta is not completely stripped or not discharge the uterine cavity after stripping, the impact of uterine contractions, manifested as bleeding. The contrary, if the placenta completely stripped and has discharged the uterine cavity, uterine contraction well, placental separation surface a small amount of active bleeding. The above-mentioned bleeding preoperative bleeding, postoperative bleeding, wound bleeding after the main reasons for the broad ligament hematoma clearance or DIC bleeding, or conservative treatment of uterine bleeding.

Bleeding in addition to causing hemorrhagic shock, but also due to maternal hypercoagulable state, excessive bleeding, shock too long, the emergence of DIC.

2. The site of infection of uterine rupture prone to infection after pelvic, abdominal, pelvic peritoneum, and soft birth canal. Main causes of infection: abdominal cavity or the broad ligament connected with the uterine cavity and vagina, the same after the bacteria have entered; uterine rupture after bleeding, severe anemia, or DIC, decreased resistance to susceptible; within the abdominal or pelvic hemorrhage or the blood of the extraperitoneal the plot, easy to infections; hysterectomy after uterine rupture or repair in bacteria; diagnosis during the rupture of the uterus may have more vaginal operations; longer uterine rupture more easily leads to a variety of infections at multiple sites.

Also worth mentioning infections are respiratory tract infections which are caused by many factors, shock too long expectoration of the normal respiratory defense mechanism relating thereto, except for aspiration and other factors.

3. Result in the birth canal and the injury of other abdominal and pelvic organs and tissues of

如果胎盘未完全剥离或剥离后未排出宫腔,影响子宫收缩,表现为大出血;反之,如果胎盘完全剥离并已经排出宫腔,子宫收缩很好,则胎盘剥离面少量活动性出血。上述出血指术前出血,术后亦可以出血,原因主要为阔韧带血肿清除后创面出血或 DIC 出血,或保守治疗子宫出血。

出血除引起失血性休克外,还由于产妇高凝状态,出血过多,休克时间过长,出现 DIC。

2.感染子宫破裂后容易出现感染的部位主要有盆腔、腹腔、盆腔腹膜后和软产道。造成感染的原因主要有:盆腹腔或阔韧带内与子宫腔和阴道相通,相通后有细菌进入;子宫破裂后大出血,严重贫血或 DIC,抵抗力下降容易感染;腹腔或盆腔内的积血或腹膜外的积血,容易感染;子宫破裂后的子宫切除或修补,在有菌条件下进行;子宫破裂后诊断期间可能有较多的阴道操作;时间较久的子宫破裂更容易导致多部位的各种感染。

另外值得提出的感染是呼吸道感染,引起感染的因素很多,休克时间过长正常呼吸道的排痰和防御机制受损与之有关,同时不能除外误吸等因素。

3.导致产道、其他腹腔和盆腔组织器官损伤及子宫破裂的损

uterine rupture injury to injury, including surgical intervention before and after surgical intervention. Injury before surgical intervention, including the uterus, the lower uterine segment, cervix and vagina of a variety of injuries, but also may have a primary bladder injury caused by fetal head oppression. Uterine rupture injury in patients with the diagnostic process and surgical course of treatment, and sometimes even more than the primary injury. Vaginal operation or inspection of an excessive number of unnecessary diagnostic process result in the birth canal injuries were aggravated; laparotomy, clean up the blood clots, or clean up the fetus, placenta and fetal membranes, improper operation, resulting in intestinal or retinal damage; clean up the broad ligament hematoma, causing pelvic vascular ureter and bladder damage; uterine rupture time is too long, heavier damage to abdominal organs.

4. After the rupture of the fetal uterus effects on the fetus at different times and varying degrees of bleeding caused by injury, the majority of fetal death. Viable fetus Perinatal child morbidity and mortality was significantly higher long-term complications was significantly higher.

3.8.5　Case study

In our hospital, two cases of full-term pregnant uterus rupture patients are reported below. A medical record cases of 1, 34-year-old pregnant 2 production, menopause 42+ weeks was hospitalized on February 4, 2010. Years ago in the hospital had to line the lower uterine segment cesarean section. examination: pillows left front bit, the fetal heart rate 160/min, the membranes are not broken, no contractions and Palace tenderness. B super show amniotic fluid 2 cm, placental function Ⅲ. Fetal heart guardianship stress test (NST) non-reactive. hospitalized after row of the lower uterine segment cesarean section. Surgery see a complete uterine

伤包括手术干预前和手术干预后的损伤。手术干预前的损伤包括子宫体、子宫下段、子宫颈和阴道的各种损伤,同时也可能有原发的由于胎头压迫造成的膀胱损伤。子宫破裂患者诊断过程和手术治疗过程中的损伤很多,有时甚至超过原发损伤。诊断过程中过多的不必要的阴道操作或检查导致产道损伤加重;开腹探查术,清理积血或清理胎儿、胎盘和胎膜,操作不当,导致肠道或大网膜损伤;清理阔韧带血肿,引起盆底血管、输尿管和膀胱损伤;子宫破裂时间过长,对腹腔器官的损伤更重。

4. 子宫破裂后对胎儿的影响主要是不同时间和不同程度的出血造成的损伤,多数胎儿死亡。存活胎儿的围生儿发病率和病死率明显增高,远期并发症也明显增高。

3.8.5　案例分析

我院收治 2 例足月妊娠子宫破裂患者,现报道如下:病历摘要 1,34 岁,孕 2 产 1,因停经 42+1 周于 2010 年 2 月 4 日入院。3 年前在我院曾行子宫下段剖宫产术。查体:枕左前位,胎心率 160/min,胎膜未破,无宫缩及宫体压痛。B 超示羊水 2 cm,胎盘功能Ⅲ级。胎心监护无应激试验(NST)无反应型。入院后即行子宫下段剖宫产术。术中见子宫浆膜面完整,子宫下段肌壁见长 9.5 cm 破裂口,边缘整齐,无出

serosa, the lower uterine segment muscle wall is known for a 9.5 cm rupture, neat edge, no bleeding, fetal membranes swelling, rupture and delivery and a daughter to be rupture, 3 100 g of body weight, Apgar score of 8 points. Conventional suture the uterus and the abdominal incision suture removal after 7 days. Grade healing was recovered.

3.8.6　Diagnosis

The diagnosis of complete uterine rupture generally is not difficult, based on history, childbirth after the clinical manifestations and signs may make a diagnosis. Incomplete uterine rupture, and only under close observation before being discovered. Individual in late pregnancy rupture, only the signs and symptoms of uterine rupture before being diagnosed.

After repeated vaginal examination, individual dystocia cases may be infected with peritonitis and show disease similar to the uterine rupture. Ministry of fetal remains high when the vaginal examination, the lower uterine segment was thin. Bimanual hands refers to touch as if separated by only the abdominal wall is sometimes easy to be misdiagnosed as uterine rupture. This case the matrix will not enter the abdominal cavity, and the pregnant uterus will not be reduced in the carcass flanking.

3.8.7　Diagnosis basis

3.8.7.1　Threatened uterine rupture

1. History and childbirth after the birth process, abnormal fetal position, pelvis, cephalopelvic disproportion factors, the birth process too slow or stagnant, obstructive dystocia or oxytocin application caused by improper contractions those are too strong.

2. Maternal irritability, unbearable contractions pains, call endless.

3. The lower uterine segment is bulgy, elongated,

血,胎膜于破裂口处膨出,于破裂处娩一女婴,体重 3100 g,Apgar 评分 8 分。常规缝合子宫,术后 7 天腹部切口拆线,甲级愈合,痊愈出院。

3.8.6　诊断

诊断完全性子宫破裂一般困难不大,根据病史、分娩经过、临床表现及体征可作出诊断。不完全性子宫破裂只有在严密观察下方能发现。个别晚期妊娠破裂者,只有出现子宫破裂的症状和体征时方能确诊。

个别难产病例经多次阴道检查,可能感染出现腹膜炎而表现为类似子宫破裂征象。阴道检查时由于胎先露部仍高、子宫下段菲薄,双合诊时双手指相触犹如只隔腹壁,有时容易误诊为子宫破裂,这种情况胎体不会进入腹腔,而妊娠子宫也不会缩小而位于胎体旁侧。

3.8.7　诊断依据

3.8.7.1　先兆子宫破裂

1.病史和分娩经过:产程中有异常胎位、骨盆狭窄等头盆不称因素,有产程进展过缓或停滞等情况,即阻塞性难产的表现,或缩宫素应用不当致宫缩过强。

2.产妇烦躁,宫缩阵痛难以忍受,呼叫不已。

3.子宫下段膨隆、拉长,压痛

and obviously susceptible to tenderness (intermittent contractions also tenderness.)

　　4. Pathological temper complex ring contractions.

　　5. Hematuria.

　　6. Round ligament tension and tenderness.

The first four must be essential.

3.8.7.2　Uterine rupture

　　1. History and childbirth: Uterine rupture is more common in the obstructive dystocia and may also occur in the use of oxytocin. Labor often stagnation or prolong the birth process. Or pregnant women scarred uterus or forceps delivery.

　　2. Clinical manifestations of the production process for a long time (uterine contractions), but progress is slow; maternal irritability, abdominal pain, drama, bloody urine. Severe abdominal pain, sudden pain in the temporary relief, but soon the whole abdominal tenderness, and then into the state of human hemorrhagic shock.

　　3. Abdominal examination abdominal wall clearly palpable carcass and fetal heart tones often disappeared or very weak.

　　4. Vaginal examination has dropped the first exposed part of recovery and retraction of the cervix.

　　5. B ultrasound shows the relationship between the fetus and the uterus and determines the presence of hematoma formation to estimate intra-abdominal hemorrhage.

3.8.8　Differential diagnosis

　　1. Placental abruption. Abdominal pain and internal bleeding should be identified with uterine rupture. Placental abruption is common in late pregnancy, high blood pressure or a history of trauma. Abdominal examination the uterus hard, intermittent contractions of the uterus is also the same soft, but clear uterine contour matrix in intrauterine, vaginal examination, the Ministry of fetal clear. These signs are distinguished from uterine

明显(宫缩间歇亦压痛)。

　　4.病理性子宫缩复环出现。

　　5.血尿。

　　6.圆韧带紧张、触痛。

　　其中前4条必须具备。

3.8.7.2　子宫破裂

　　1.病史及分娩经过:多见于阻塞性难产,也可发生在使用缩宫素时。临产后常有产程停滞或延长。或孕妇为瘢痕子宫者或产钳助产后。

　　2.临床表现:产程时间长,宫缩好,但进展慢;产妇烦躁、腹痛剧,小便血性。剧烈腹痛后突然疼痛暂时缓解,但很快出现全腹压痛,继而进入失血性休克状态。

　　3.腹部检查:腹壁下清楚地扪及胎体,胎心音常消失或很弱。

　　4.阴道检查:已下降的先露部又回升,宫口回缩。

　　5.B超检查:显示胎儿与子宫的关系及确定有无血肿形成,估计腹腔内出血。

3.8.8　鉴别诊断

　　1.胎盘早期剥离:有腹痛及内出血应与子宫破裂鉴别。胎盘早剥常见于妊娠晚期,有血压高或外伤史。腹部检查子宫体硬,宫缩间歇期子宫也不变软,但子宫轮廓清楚,胎体在宫腔内,阴道检查胎先露部清楚。这些体征均区别于子宫破裂,B超见有胎盘

rupture, B ultrasound to see the placenta after hematoma audio and video to help confirm the diagnosis.

2. Spastic contraction of the uterus ring. Not as pathological temper to contractions complex ring as increased gradually with the birth process. Position.

3. Pregnant women with ovarian cyst torsion or rupture during pregnancy and sudden abdominal pain should be differentiated from uterine rupture. But the disease before pregnancy or early pregnancy are known to have history of cancer, occur more time in the pregnancy for three to four months or postpartum, sudden onset of persistent abdominal pain, abdominal pain and position. Check the uterine outline is clear, the carcass in the uterine cavity, clear fetal position, fetal existence. Uterine tenderness, attachment side of the tenderness. If the tumor rupture, peritonitis symptoms, internal bleeding symptoms are not obvious. By B ultrasound can help diagnose.

4. Intrauterine infection produced intrauterine infection is more common to premature rupture of membranes, with the exception of uterine tenderness, vaginal secretions often purulent, smelly, accompanied by fever, leukocytes and neutrophils increased. But no bleeding signs of the fetus within the uterine cavity.

3.8.9　Principles of treatment

1. Threatened uterine rupture: Cesarean section should be performed as soon as possible after contraction has been inhibited by sedatives.

2. Uterine rupture in a correct shock, infection prevention, while laparotomy principles and strive to be simple, fast, and can achieve hemostasis purposes. The extent and location of uterine rupture, surgery distance to rupture length of time, and the presence of serious infection and a different surgical approach.

后血肿声像有助于明确诊断。

2. 痉挛性子宫收缩环。不会像病理性子宫缩复环那样随着产程而位置逐渐上升。

3. 妊娠合并卵巢囊肿蒂扭转或破裂：妊娠期突发腹痛应与子宫破裂相鉴别。但本病孕前或孕早期有的已知有肿瘤病史，发生时间多在妊娠 3～4 个月或产后，突然发生持续性腹痛，腹痛发生与体位有关。检查子宫轮廓清楚，胎体在宫腔内，胎位清，胎心存在。子宫多无压痛，而附件一侧有压痛。若肿瘤破裂，以腹膜炎症状为主，内出血症状不明显。通过 B 超可协助诊断。

4. 宫内感染：产时宫内感染以胎膜早破为多见，除子宫体有压痛外，阴道分泌物常为脓性，有臭味，伴发热，白细胞总数及中性粒细胞升高。但没有内出血征象，胎儿在宫腔内。

3.8.9　治疗原则

1. 先兆子宫破裂：应用镇静剂抑制宫缩后尽快剖宫产。

2. 子宫破裂在纠正休克、防治感染的同时行剖腹探查手术，原则是力求简单、迅速，能达到止血目的。根据子宫破裂的程度与部位，手术距离发生破裂的时间长短，以及有无严重感染而定不同的手术方式。

3.8.10　Treatment measures

1. General treatment: Transfusion, blood transfusion, oxygen inhalation to rescue shock. And large-dose antibiotics are given to prevent infection.

2. Surgical treatment:

（1）Threatened uterine rupture: Immediately threatened uterine rupture give inhibition of uterine contraction drugs to inhaled or intravenous general anesthesia. Intramuscular injection or intravenous sedatives such as pethidine 100 mg as soon as possible cesarean section. Such as fetal heart exists as soon as possible cesarean section, expected to be live births.

（2）Surgical treatment of uterine rupture:

① Uterine rupture in the gap edge and tidy within 12 h, and no obvious infection, the need to preserve fertility in, could be considered to repair the suture lacerations.

② Rupture of the mouth of large or irregular tearing and infection may consider a hysterectomy and subtotal hysterectomy.

③Uterine gap not only in the next paragraph, and consider the line segment extension and cervix hysterectomy.

④ Previous cesarean scar dehiscence, uterine body or the lower uterine segment, has been live births, such as maternal line cleft suture, bilateral tubal ligation.

⑤In the broad ligament, the existence of a huge hematoma in order to avoid damage to surrounding organs, must be open to the broad ligament, the free uterine artery ascending branch of its accompanying vein, the ureter and bladder from the organization will have to clamp bundles pushed, in order to avoid damage ureter or bladder. Still active bleeding, such as surgery, may be provided through the ipsilateral internal iliac artery ligation to control bleeding.

⑥ Laparotomy attention should be carefully examined the site of uterine rupture, bladder,

3.8.10　治疗措施

1. 一般治疗:输液、输血、氧气吸入等抗休克,并给予大剂量抗生素预防感染。

2. 手术治疗:

（1）先兆子宫破裂:发现先兆子宫破裂时立即给予抑制子宫收缩的药物如吸入或静脉全身麻醉,肌内注射或静脉注射镇静剂如哌替啶 100 mg 等,并尽快行剖宫产术。如胎心存在,则尽快剖宫产,可望获得活婴。

（2）子宫破裂的手术治疗:

①子宫破裂时间在 12 h 以内,裂口边缘整齐,无明显感染,需保留生育功能者,可考虑修补缝合破口。

②破裂口较大或撕裂不整齐且有感染可能者,考虑行子宫次全切除术。

③子宫裂口不仅在下段,且自下段延及宫颈口考虑行子宫全切术。

④前次剖宫产瘢痕裂开,包括子宫体或子宫下段的,如产妇已有活婴应行裂口缝合术,同时行双侧输卵管结扎术。

⑤在阔韧带内有巨大血肿存在时为避免损伤周围脏器,必须打开阔韧带,游离子宫动脉的上行支及其伴随静脉,将输尿管与膀胱从将要钳扎的组织推开,以避免损伤输尿管或膀胱。如术时仍有活跃出血,可先行同侧髂内动脉结扎术以控制出血。

⑥开腹探查时注意子宫破裂的部位,应仔细检查膀胱、输尿

ureter, cervix and vagina, if there is injury, should also line the organ repair.

⑦ Individual production process long, serious cases of infection, should try to shorten the operation time for the rescue of maternal life, surgery should be as simple as possible quickly to stop the bleeding purposes. Can do a hysterectomy excision or subtotal resection or only rip the suture and bilateral tubal ligation, subject to the specific circumstances of large doses of effective antibiotics prevent infection before and after surgery.

⑧Uterine rupture, shock, and as far as possible local rescue to avoid because of transportation and increase the shock and bleeding. However, if restricted to local conditions must be transferred in a large number of transfusion blood transfusion, antishock conditions, as well as abdominal bandage after transhipment.

3.8.11　Prevention

Uterine rupture seriously endanger the mother and child life, and the vast majority of uterine rupture can be avoided. So prevention is extremely important. Strengthen family planning publicity and implementation of reduce multi maternal; change the concept of childbirth, to promote natural childbirth to reduce the rate of cesarean section; prenatal care to correct the malposition, estimated delivery may have difficulty, or dystocia history, or caesarean production history, early hospital childbirth, closely observe the progress of labor, according to obstetric indications and previous surgery after determining the mode of delivery. Master the strict application of oxytocin indications for use, dosage, should be hand guard; uterine scar, and uterine malformations maternal trial production, the production process should be closely observed and the relaxation of the indications for cesarean section; strict observation of the production process, for the first exposed high,

管、宫颈和阴道，如发现有损伤，应同时行这些脏器的修补术。

⑦个别被忽略的、产程长、感染严重的病例，为抢救产妇生命应尽量缩短手术时间，手术宜尽量简单、迅速达到止血目的。能否做全子宫切除或次全切除术或仅裂口缝合术加双侧输卵管结扎术，须视具体情况而定，术前后应用大剂量有效抗生素防治感染。

⑧子宫破裂已发生休克者，尽可能就地抢救，以避免因搬运而加重休克与出血。但如限于当地条件必须转院时，也应在大量输液输血抗休克条件下以及腹部包扎后再行转运。

3.8.11　预防

子宫破裂严重危及母儿生命，且绝大多数子宫破裂是可以避免的，故预防工作极其重要。加强计划生育宣传及实施，减少多产妇；转变分娩观念，提倡自然分娩，降低剖宫产率；加强产前检查，纠正胎位不正，估计分娩可能有困难者，或有难产史，或有剖宫产史者，应提早住院分娩，密切观察产程进展，根据产科指征及前次手术经过决定分娩方式。严格掌握应用缩宫素的指征、用法、用量，同时应有专人守护；对有子宫瘢痕、子宫畸形的产妇试产，要严密观察产程并放宽剖宫产指征；严密观察产程，对于先露高、有胎位异常的孕妇试产更应仔细观察；避免损伤性大的阴道助产及操作，如中高位产钳、宫口未开全

abnormal fetal position, pregnant women trial production should be carefully observed; avoid traumatic vaginal delivery and operation such as high forceps, the cervix does not open full-that is, midwifery, negligibility shoulder first exposed row Deflection of placenta accreta forcibly dig.

3.8.12　Uterine rupture repair

3.8.12.1　Indications

Uterine rupture repair is the surgical method for treatment of uterine rupture and is applied to the following situations:

1. The rupture is neat and easy to suture.

2. Rupture to surgery time is shorter, not more than 24 h.

3. No concurrent infection.

4. No damage of uterine artery.

5. No uterine malformations.

6. The desire to give birth again.

3.8.12.2　Preparations before surgery

1. Skin preparation, catheter placement.

2. The rapid establishment of intravenous access, and prepare blood transfusion anti-shock treatment. If necessary, placement of central venous pressure, combined urine monitoring, estimated blood loss. Maternal severe shock, should be transferred in a timely manner, to avoid delays or lost rescue opportunity.

3. Uterine rupture, whether it is the exploration of the part or full, are required to immediately line laparotomy. Vaginal operative delivery often makes the gap to expand, increasing the degree of uterine rupture, causing re-bleeding leading to shock, or caused by other intra-abdominal organ injury and repair difficulties.

4. The preoperative use of broad-spectrum antibiotics.

即助产、忽略性肩先露行内倒转术、胎盘植入时强行挖取等[1]。

3.8.12　子宫破裂修补术

3.8.12.1　适应证

子宫破裂修补术是用于治疗子宫破裂的手术方法,适用于以下情况:

1.破裂口整齐,易缝合。

2.破裂至手术时间较短,不超过 24 h。

3.无并发感染。

4.未损伤子宫动脉。

5.无子宫畸形。

6.渴望要求再生育者。

3.8.12.2　手术前的准备工作

1.备皮,安放导尿管。

2.迅速建立静脉通道,备血、输血抗休克治疗。必要时置放中心静脉压,联合尿量监测,估计失血量。严重休克的产妇,应及时转院,避免延误或失去抢救机会。

3.子宫破裂无论是部分的还是完全的,均需立即行剖腹探查。阴道手术分娩常使裂口扩大,加重子宫破裂的程度,引起再度出血而导致休克,或造成腹腔内其他脏器的损伤,而修补困难。

4.术前开始使用广谱抗生素。

3.8.12.3　Surgical procedures

Caesarean section in the fetus and hemostasis

Remove the midline vertical incision, and cut the abdominal wall into the abdominal cavity. Edge suction of blood in the abdominal cavity to the side of exploration, the break of the fetus and placenta from the uterus into the abdominal cavity should hold the tire quickly enough, remove the fetus and placenta, the Ministry of Palace direct injection of oxytocin or oxytocin by intravenous push forward 20 U contraction of the uterus to reduce bleeding. Oval clamp or Alice clamp live rupture hemostasis. If the fetus outside the womb, from the tear with scissors along the break extended to less vascular parts of the delivered fetus. Uterine margin of the oval clamp, careful hemostasis. Check the ureter, bladder, cervix and vagina with or without injury.

The lower uterine segment rampant break repair

Generally the lower edge of the bladder peritoneum of the lower edge of the free gap has been shrinking to the deeper parts of the bladder boundaries are not easily distinguishable carefully to find the edge of break up and down and filed with Alice clamp with curved forceps to lift the visceral peritoneum, check bladder injury. Gently push the bladder and along the edge a little free from the uterus break, so as not to hurt the bladder suture. Such as the first pruning scar for scar dehiscence after suture, the suture must be aligned. Embedding continuous suture of catgut line on the 2nd layer of the first layer, second layer line continuous mattress suture, tension sutures to ensure a good break closed. The best bladder anti-peritoneal fold incision embedded.

On both sides of the lower uterine segment break

Repair rampant with the following paragraph break, but be careful to not hurt the uterine vessels and ureters when the suture. Ureteral injury due to

3.8.12.3　手术步骤

剖腹取胎和止血

取下腹中线纵切口,切开腹壁进入腹腔。边吸腹腔内的血边探查,若胎儿和胎盘已从子宫破口进入腹腔,应迅速握住胎足,取出胎儿和胎盘,同时宫体部直接注射缩宫素或由静脉推进缩宫素20 U,使子宫收缩减少出血。用卵圆钳或艾利斯钳夹住破裂口止血。若胎儿一部分在子宫外,应从破口处用剪刀顺破口向血管少的部位延长,娩出胎儿。用卵圆钳夹子宫创缘,仔细止血。检查输尿管、膀胱、宫颈和阴道有无损伤。

子宫下段横行破口修补

游离裂口下缘的膀胱腹膜,一般下缘已缩至较深部位,与膀胱界限不易分辨,仔细找到破口上下缘并用艾利斯钳夹提起,用弯血管钳提起膀胱腹膜反折,检查有无膀胱损伤。并沿子宫破口下缘稍作游离轻轻推开膀胱,以免缝合时伤及膀胱。如为瘢痕裂开者需先修剪瘢痕后再缝合,缝合时一定要对齐。以2号肠线行全层连续缝合第一层,第二层行连续褥式包埋缝合,拉紧缝线,保证破口封闭良好。最好用膀胱反折腹膜将切口包埋。

子宫下段两侧破口

修补方法同下段横行破口,但要注意缝合时勿伤及子宫血管及输尿管。输尿管的损伤多因解

the anatomical relationship between unclear, and the clamp forceps, surgical mistake tie, or mistakenly cut due. If the above damage, should be detected immediately ureteral anastomosis. Such as suture, punctured blood vessel formation of hematoma, should be promptly cut serosa to clear blood clots, complete hemostasis.

Broad ligament hematoma

Incision the left broad ligament hematoma of uterine rupture in the side of the uterus, injury to the uterus of the great vessels or branch to form a huge hematoma in the broad ligament. Must first open the broad ligament before and after the leaves, free uterine artery ascending branch of its accompanying vein ligation to avoid clamp damage the ureter and bladder. Adnexectomy line when necessary. If the bleeding is still severe or hematoma continues to expand but can not find a significant bleeding viable internal iliac artery ligation.

Suspected infection

For uterine culture, metronidazole rinse the uterine cavity, abdominal cavity, place the drainage tube drainage in the posterior fornix or the lower abdomen.

3.9　Cardiac Disease in Pregnancy

Key words

1. heart disease in pregnancy
2. hemodynamic
3. cardiac output
4. hemoptysis
5. fatiguing syncope
6. cyanosis
7. clubbing of fingers
8. neck vein distention
9. systolic murmur
10. diastolic

剖关系不清,而被血管钳钳夹、手术误扎或被误切所致。如发生上述损伤,应及时发现,立即行输尿管吻合术。如缝合时刺破血管形成血肿,要及时剪开浆膜清除积血,彻底止血。

阔韧带血肿

切开左侧阔韧带血肿子宫破裂于子宫的侧面,伤及子宫大血管或分支,形成阔韧带内巨大血肿。需先打开阔韧带前后叶,游离子宫动脉上行支及其伴随的静脉进行结扎,避免钳夹损伤输尿管与膀胱。必要时行附件切除术。如果出血仍严重或血肿不断扩大而找不到明显的出血点,可行髂内动脉结扎术。

疑有感染

应作宫腔培养,后用灭滴灵冲洗宫腔、盆腹腔,放置引流管于后穹窿或下腹部进行引流。

3.9　妊娠合并心脏病

关键词

1. 妊娠合并心脏病
2. 血流动力学
3. 心输出量
4. 先天性心脏病
5. 劳累性晕厥
6. 发绀
7. 杵状指
8. 颈静脉怒张
9. 收缩期杂音
10. 舒张期的

11. arrhythmia

12. pulmonary hypertension

13. heart failure

14. electrocardiography

15. ventricular septal defects

16. peripartum Cardiomyopathy

3.9.1 Main content

3.9.1.1 Incidence

Heart disease complicates about 1% of pregnancies. Congenital heart lesions now constitute at least half of all cases of heart disease encountered during pregnancy.

3.9.1.2 Physiological considerations with heart disease in pregnancy

The marked hemodynamic changes stimulated by pregnancy have a profound effect on underlying heart disease in the pregnant women. The most important consideration is that cardiac output is increased by 30%-50% during pregnancy.

3.9.1.3 Prognosis

The likelihood of a favorable outcome for the mother with heart disease depends upon：

1. the functional cardiac capacity.

2. other complications that further increase cardiac load.

3. the quality of medical care provided.

3.9.2 Congenital heart disease in offspring

Many congenital heart lesions appear to be inherited as polygenic characteristics. Thus，it might be expected that some women with congenital lesions would give birth to similarly affected infants.

3.9.3 Diagnosis of heart disease

Many of the physiological changes of normal pregnancy tend to make the diagnosis of heart disease more difficult.

11. 心律不齐

12. 肺动脉高压

13. 心力衰竭

14. 心电图

15. 室间隔缺损

16. 围生期心肌病

3.9.1 主要内容

3.9.1.1 发病率

妊娠合并心脏病约占 1%。目前先天性心脏病至少占妊娠合并心脏病的一半。

3.9.1.2 孕期心脏病的生理性变化

妊娠引起的明显血流动力学改变对心脏病孕妇产生严重的影响。最重要的变化是妊娠期心输出量增加 30%～50%。

3.9.1.3 预后

妊娠合并心脏病孕妇良好的预后依赖于：

1. 心功能良好。

2. 是否有导致心脏负担进一步加重的其他并发症。

3. 所提供的医疗保健质量。

3.9.2 子代中的先天性心脏病

多数先天性心脏病为多基因遗传。因而，某些患先天性疾病的妇女可能生出患相似病变的婴儿。

3.9.3 心脏病的诊断

正常妊娠的生理性变化中有许多因素可使心脏病的诊断造成困难。

1. Symptoms：

(1) progrssive dyspnea or orthopnea.

(2) paroxysmal nocturnal dyspnea.

(3) hemoptysis.

(4) fatiguing syncope.

(5) chest pain related to fatigue or emotion.

2. Signs：

(1) cyanosis.

(2) clubbing of fingers.

(3) persistent neck vein distention.

(4) systolic murmur grade 3/6 or greater.

(5) diastolic murmur.

(6) cardiomegaly.

(7) persistent arrhythmia.

(8) persistent split-second sound.

(9) pulmonary hyertension.

3. Investigation：

(1) electrocardiography.

(2) chest X-ray cardiomegaly.

(3) echocardiography：the widespread use of echocardiography has allowed accurate diagnosis of most heart diseases during pregnancy.

3.9.4　Clinical grading

Grade Ⅰ：

Uncompromised-patients with cardiac disease and no limitation in physical activity.

Grade Ⅱ：

Slightly compromised-patients with cardiac disease and slightly limitation in physical activity.

Grade Ⅲ：

Markedly compromised-patients with cardiac disease and marked limitation in physical activity.

Grade Ⅳ：

Severely compromised-patients with cardiac disease and inability to perform any physical activity without discomfort.

1. 症状：

(1)进行性呼吸困难或端坐呼吸。

(2)阵发性夜间呼吸困难。

(3)咯血。

(4)劳累性晕厥。

(5)与劳累或情绪有关的胸痛。

2. 体征：

(1)发绀。

(2)杵状指。

(3)持续性颈静脉怒张。

(4)3/6级或以上的收缩期杂音。

(5)舒张期杂音。

(6)心脏扩大。

(7)持续性心律失常。

(8)持续性第二心音分裂。

(9)肺动脉高压征。

3. 辅助检查：

(1)心电图检查。

(2)胸部 X 线检查:心脏扩大。

(3)超声心动图检查:其广泛应用使妊娠期的绝大多数心脏疾患得以准确诊断。

3.9.4　临床分级

Ⅰ级：

心脏病患者情况好,体力活动不受限。

Ⅱ级：

心脏轻度受损,体力活动轻度受限。

Ⅲ级：

心脏明显受损,体力活动明显受限。

Ⅳ级：

心脏严重受损,不能进行任何体力活动,否则引起不适。

3.9.5 Management

Individualization is essential in assuring optimal outcome.

1. Management requires a team approach, involving obstetrician, cardiologist, anesthesiologist, and other specialists.

2. Four concepts affecting management:

(1) 50% increase in blood volume and cardiac output by the early third trimester.

(2) Further fluctuations in volume and cardiac output in the peripartum period.

(3) A decline in systemic vascular resistance, about 20% below normal value.

(4) Hypercoagulability is of special importance in women requiring anticoagulation with coumarin derivatives in the nonpregnant state.

3.9.5.1 Management of grade Ⅰ and Ⅱ

Women in grade Ⅰ and most in grade Ⅱ go through pregnancy without morbidity.

1. Infection has proved to be an important factor to induce cardiac failure, each women should receive instructions to avoid contact with persons who have respirtory infections.

2. Cigarette smoking is prohibited, because of its effects on heart as well as the propensity to cause upper respiratory infections.

3. Labor and delivery:

(1) Delivery should be accomplished vaginally unless there are obstetrical indications for cesarean delivery.

(2) Relief from pain and apprehension are especially important. Continuous epidural analgesia is recommended.

(3) During labor, the mother should be kept in a semirecumbent position with lateral tilt. Pulse rate above 100 per minute or respiratory rate above 24, particularly when associated with dyspnea, may

3.9.5 处理

为确保最佳效果需个体化对待。

1. 治疗需要一个梯队参与，包括产科医生、心脏病专家、麻醉科医生以及其他科的专家。

2. 影响处理的四个概念：

(1) 晚孕早期血容量和心输出量增加 50%。

(2) 围生期血容量和心输出量进一步波动。

(3) 循环系统血管阻力下降，低于正常值 20%。

(4) 高凝状态，在未孕时即需行双香豆素衍生物抗凝的妇女中尤为重要。

3.9.5.1 Ⅰ级和Ⅱ级的处理

患Ⅰ级和绝大多数Ⅱ级心脏病的妇女均可度过妊娠期而不发病。

1. 感染是引起心力衰竭的重要因素，应指导每位孕妇避免与有呼吸道感染的患者接触。

2. 禁止吸烟，因其有影响心脏和导致上呼吸道感染的倾向。

3. 临产和分娩：

(1) 除非有产科剖宫产指征，一般应经阴道分娩。

(2) 缓解疼痛及消除焦虑尤为重要。推荐硬膜外麻醉镇痛。

(3) 产程中产妇应保持半卧侧倾斜位。如脉搏＞100 次/min 或呼吸＞24 次/min，尤其伴有呼吸困难时提示将发生心室衰竭。

suggest impending ventricular failure.

(4) It is essential to remember that delivery itself will not necessarily improve the maternal condition and emergency operative delivery may be particularly hazardous.

（5）Intrapartum heart failure—The proper therapeutic approach will depend upon the specific hemodynamic status and underlying cardiac lesion.

3.9.5.2　Management of delivery period

Cardiac patients should be delivered vaginally unless obstetric indications for cesarean are present. The patient should be instructed to avoid pushing during the second stage of labor because the associated increase in intraabdminal pressure increase venous return and cardiac output and can lead to cardiac decompensation. The second stage of labor is assisted by performing an outlet forceps delivery or by the use of a vacuum extractor.

3.9.5.3　Puerperium

Postpartum hemorrhage, anemia, infection, and thromboembolism are much more serious complications of heart disease, possibly inducing postpartum heart failure in women with underlying disease. So it is important that meticulous care be continued into the puerperium.

3.9.5.4　Management of grade Ⅲ and Ⅳ

The important question in these women is whether pregnancy should be continued or not.

1. For early pregnancy pregnancy interruption should be considered. If the pregnancy is to be continued, prolonged hospitalization or bed rest will often be necessary.

2. Vaginal delivery is preferred in most cases, and cesarean delivery is limited to obstetri.

3. As for less severe disease, epidural analgesia for labor and delivery is usually recommended.

（4）应牢记分娩本身并不一定能改善母体状况，而急症手术分娩可能非常危险。

（5）产时心衰——治疗方法依赖于特定的血流动力学状况和心脏病变的情况。

3.9.5.2　分娩期处理

除非有剖宫产的产科指征，心脏病患者应阴道分娩。应指导患者在第二产程时不要屏气，因为屏气时增加腹内压，同时也增加静脉回流和心输出量，导致心脏代偿失调。第二产程时，应行出口产钳或负压助产。

3.9.5.3　产褥期

产后出血、贫血、感染和血栓栓塞是心脏病非常严重的并发症，常使有心脏病的产妇发生产后心力衰竭。因此产后护理很重要。

3.9.5.4　Ⅲ级和Ⅳ级的处理

重要的是能否继续妊娠。

1. 如果孕期尚早，应考虑终止妊娠。如继续妊娠常需长期住院治疗或卧床休息。

2. 对大多数病例理想的分娩方式是阴道分娩，剖宫产仅限有产科指征者。

3. 病情稍轻的产妇临产和分娩时推荐应用硬膜外麻醉。

3.9.6　Congenital heart disease

1. Septal defects：

（1）Atrial septal defects：Many of these cases are asymptomatic. Pregnancy is well tolerated unless pulmonary hypertension has developed.

（2）Ventricular septal defects：If the defect is less than 1.25 cm^2, pulmonary hypertension and heart failure do not develop.

2. Persisitent ductus arteriosus：Hypotension should be avoided whenever possible and treated vigorously if it develops. Prophylaxis for bacterial endocarditis should be given at delivery.

3. Cyanotic heart disease：The most commonly is the Fallot tetralogy.

（1）Effect on pregnacy：Maternal mortality approaches 10%. Miscarriage, FGR, preterm delivery, or fetal death can be caused.

（2）Labor and delivery：Vaginal delivery is preferred unless there is an obstetrical indication for cesarean delivery. Care must be taken to avoid sudden blood pressure decreases.

3.9.7　Peripartum cardiomyopathy

1. Used to describe peripartum heart failure with out readily apparent etiology.

2. Women who develop peripartum heart failure often have obstetrical complications that either contribute to or precipitate heart failure. For example, preeclampsia, acute anemia, and infection.

3. Women with cardiomyopathy present with sign and symptoms of congestive heart failure, including dyspnea, orthopnea, cough, palpitations, and chest pain.

4. The hallmark finding is usually impressive cardiomegaly.

5. Digoxin is given to treat heart failure unless complex arrhythmias is identified.

6. Angiotensin-converting enzyme inhibitors

3.9.6　先天性心脏病

1. 间隔缺损：

（1）房间隔缺损：大多无症状。如果不出现肺动脉高压则可很好地耐受妊娠。

（2）室间隔缺损：如果缺损不足 1.25 cm^2，不发生肺动脉高压和心衰。

2. 动脉导管未闭：无论何时都应避免低血压，一旦出现应及时治疗。分娩时应预防细菌性心内膜炎。

3. 青紫型心脏病：最常见的是法洛四联征。

（1）对妊娠的影响：母亲死亡率接近 10%。可导致流产、胎儿宫内生长受限、早产或胎儿死亡。

（2）临产和分娩：除非有产科剖宫产指征，否则最好经阴道分娩。必须小心避免血压突然下降。

3.9.7　围生期心肌病

1. 用于指无明显病因发生的围生期心力衰竭。

2. 发生围生期心衰的妇女通常有引起或加速心力衰竭的产科并发症，如先兆子痫、急性贫血、感染等。

3. 心肌病妇女伴有充血性心脏病的症状和体征，包括呼吸困难、端坐呼吸、咳嗽、心悸和胸痛。

4. 最具特征的发现为明显的心脏扩大。

5. 治疗心力衰竭，可使用洋地黄，除非证实有复杂的心律失常。

6. 降低后负荷，分娩前应避

should be avoided to reduce afterload if the women is undelivered.

7. Because there is a high incidence of associated pulmonary embolism, heparin is often recommended.

Test

Question: How to diagnose heart disease?

Reference answer:

1. Symptoms

(1) progrssive dyspnea or orthopnea.

(2) paroxysmal nocturnal dyspnea.

(3) hemoptysis.

(4) fatiguing syncope.

(5) chest pain related to fatigue or emotion.

2. Signs

(1) cyanosis.

(2) clubbing of fingers.

(3) persistent neck vein distention.

(4) systolic murmur grade 3/6 or greater.

(5) diastolic murmur.

(6) cardiomegaly.

(7) persistent arrhythmia.

(8) persistent split-second sound.

(9) pulmonary hyertension.

3. Investigation

(1) electrocardiography.

(2) chest X-ray cardiomegaly.

(3) echocardiography: the widespread use of echocardiography has allowed accurate diagnosis of most heart disease during pregnancy.

3.10　Intrahepatic Cholestasis of Pregnancy (ICP)

Key words

1. intrahepatic cholestasis
2. hyperbilirubinemia
3. bile acids

免应用血管紧张素转换酶抑制剂。

7. 因肺栓塞发生率高,常推荐应用肝素。

测试题

问题：如何诊断心脏病？

参考答案：

1.症状

(1)进行性呼吸困难或端坐呼吸。

(2)阵发性夜间呼吸困难。

(3)咯血。

(4)劳累性晕厥。

(5)与劳累或情绪有关的胸痛。

2.体征

(1)发绀。

(2)杵状指。

(3)持续性颈静脉怒张。

(4)3/6级或以上的收缩期杂音。

(5)舒张期杂音。

(6)心脏扩大。

(7)持续性心律失常。

(8)持续性第二心音分裂。

(9)肺动脉高压征。

3.辅助检查

(1)心电图检查。

(2)胸部X线检查:心脏扩大。

(3)超声心动图检查:其广泛应用使妊娠期的绝大多数心脏疾患得以准确诊断。

3.10　妊娠期肝内胆汁淤积症

关键词

1. 肝内胆汁淤积
2. 血胆红素增高
3. 胆汁酸

4. fetal distress

Intrahepatic cholestasis is characterized clinically by pruritus and icteras. The major histological lesion is intrahepatic cholestasis, centrilobular bile staining and no proliferation of inflammatory cells and mesenchymal cells.

3.10.1　Pathogenesis

The causes are unknown, possibly related to estrogen and genetic factors.

3.10.2　Clinical presentation

Most women with cholestasis develop pruritus in late pregnancy, although the syndrome occasionally occurs in the second trimester. There are no constitutional symptoms.

3.10.3　Laboratory testing

(1) Serum transacalnase activities: normal to moderately elevated, and seldomly exceed 250 IU/L.

(2) Hyperbilirubinemia: total plasma concentrations rarely exceed 4 to 5 mg/dl.

(3) Serum alkaline phosphatase: usually elevated than that in normal pregnancy.

(4) Bile acids: serum concentration of total bile acids may be elevated 10 to 100 folds.

3.10.4　Management

Pruritus associated with cholestasis is caused by elevated serum bile salts and may be quite troublesome.

(1) Antihistamines: orally administered antihistamines may provide some relief.

(2) Dexamethasonc: 12 mg daily for 7 days, results in prompt relief of pruritns. It is postulated that this is associated diminished estrogen synthesis as well as lowered serum tranasaminase level.

(3) Ursodeoxycholic acid: retrospective observations showed its efficacy.

4. 胎儿窘迫

其临床特征是瘙痒、黄疸，主要的组织学病变是肝内胆汁淤积，肝小叶中心染色而无炎性细胞或间质细胞增殖。

3.10.1　发病机制

病因不清楚，考虑其发病与雌激素及遗传等因素有关系。

3.10.2　临床表现

大多数妇女在妊娠晚期出现瘙痒，偶尔出现在中孕期。没有全身症状。

3.10.3　实验室检查

(1)血清转氨酶：正常或中度升高，很少超过 250 IU/L。

(2)血胆红素增高：浓度很少超过 4~5 mg/dl。

(3)血清碱性磷酸酶：与正常妊娠比升高。

(4)胆汁酸：胆酸的总含量可能会升高至 10~100 倍。

3.10.4　处理

胆汁淤积引起的瘙痒是由于血清胆盐升高，可能很不舒服。

(1)抗组胺药：口服抗组胺药可能会有所缓解。

(2)地塞米松：12 mg/d 共 7 天，瘙痒迅速缓解。推测可能与雌激素合成减少和血清肝酶的水平下降相关。

(3)熊脱氧胆酸：回顾性观察已证实其效果。

3.10.5 Effects on pregnancy

Preterm delivery, fetal distress and postpartum hemorrhage can be caused, and the incidence of pregnancy induced hypertension is increased.

3.11　Gestational Diabetes Mellitus

Key words

1. diabetes mellitus
2. gestational diabetes
3. diet
4. glucose monitoring
5. insulin
6. insulin dependent diabetics management, IDDM
7. diabetes ketotic acidosis, DKA

3.11.1　Diabetes

Perinatal complications and mortality associated with diabetes in pregnancy are 2-3 times higher than average.

However, optimal management generally results in a good outcome. Tight control of blood glucose is crucial for good outcome, so the optimum management of diabetes in pregnancy needs a team approach. Physicians/endocrinologists advise on alterations of insulin dosage and dedicated dieticians, specialist nurses, adviseres and obstetricians are also involved.

The following discussion will focus on management of diabetic women who become pregnant and will then address the issue of gestational diabetes. The first determination of glucose level of diabetic pregnant women should be performed under strict conditions.

The importance of advice prior to conception has already been stressed. It is imperative that the woman is confident in the management of her diabetes.

3.10.5　对妊娠的影响

可引起早产、胎儿窘迫、产后出血、增加妊娠高血压的发生。

3.11　妊娠合并糖尿病

关键词

1. 糖尿病
2. 妊娠期糖尿病
3. 饮食
4. 血糖监测
5. 胰岛素
6. 胰岛素依赖型糖尿病
7. 妊娠期糖尿病酮症酸中毒

3.11.1　糖尿病

妊娠期糖尿病造成围生期的并发症和死亡率比人均高 2～3 倍。

然而,如果采取最佳的处理方式通常会有一个很好的结果。获得良好结果的关键是严密控制血糖,孕期糖尿病的管理需要一个团队,内科医生指导胰岛素剂量,专门的营养师、专业护士、顾问、产科医生共同参与治疗。

下面将集中讨论糖尿病孕妇的管理和如何解决妊娠期糖尿病问题。第一次对孕期血糖的诊断要在一个非常严格的条件下进行。

孕前的咨询和建议的重要性之前已经强调,有必要使孕妇对自己糖尿病的处理有信心,在教

Before any improvements in education and dosage the woman must understand that there is a 2-3 fold increase in incidence of congenital malformation in diabetic cases but that this can be reduced by ensuring optimal blood glucose control. The risk of congenital malformation is related to the concentration of haemoglobin Aic, a marker of glucose control in the first trimester over a period of weeks. Other issues such as renal function, hypertension and assessment of laser treatment for retinopathy are also important.

During pregnancy, the diabetic woman should be reviewed every 2 weeks or even weekly depending upon the stage of the pregnancy and the control of blood sugar. Certain physiological changes occur during pregnancy and may affect carbohydrate metabolism.

1. Insulin concentration increases due to increased demand and the antagonistic action of placental hormones, *i. e.* human placental lactogen.

2. Blood glucose concentration does not change in normal pregnancy.

3. Preconception: Ensure optimal control of blood glucose. Investigate and treat any associated hypertension and renal or retinal disease.

4. First trimester: Strictly control blood glucose to avoid congenital realformations. Perform ophthalmology consultation.

5. Second and prenatal third trimester: Urinary tract and other infection, pre-term labour, preeclampsia, and unexplained stillbirth.

6. Delivery: Risk of dyslocia. Risk of shoulder dystocia.

7. Postpartum: Reduce insulin requirement and long term counsell.

8. Glycosuria is more likely to occur as there is a lower renal threshold for glucose.

In the first trimester, insulin requirements will increase with the pregnancy. This is thought to be

育和剂量改善之前,孕妇必须明白糖尿病会有 2～3 倍的概率发生先天性畸形,通过最佳的血糖控制可以减少先天性畸形的风险。先天性畸形的风险与糖化血红蛋白浓度 Aic 有关。血红蛋白 Aic 是早期妊娠血糖控制的一个标记,持续数周。同样重要的是其他问题,比如肾脏功能、高血压和需要激光治疗视网膜病变的评估。

妊娠糖尿病的妇女应该每周或每两周进行一次检查,这取决于怀孕的阶段和血糖的控制程度,某些生理变化发生在妊娠期间,可能会影响碳水化合物的代谢。

1. 胰岛素浓度增加是由于需求的增长和胎盘激素、催乳素的拮抗作用。

2. 正常妊娠时,血糖浓度不改变。

3. 妊娠前:确保最佳的血糖控制。调查和处理任何相关的高血压、肾脏或视网膜疾病。

4. 早期妊娠:严格控制血糖,防止先天性畸形、眼科会诊。

5. 中期和晚期妊娠:尿路及其他感染,早产和先兆子痫,不明原因的死产。

6. 分娩时难产风险。肩难产的风险。

7. 产褥期:减少胰岛素的需求,长期咨询。

8. 肾糖阈很低更可能发生糖尿病。

在早期妊娠,怀孕将使胰岛素的需求增加。这被认为是胎盘

due to the antagonistic action of hormones of placental origin against insulin. Much effort is therefore directed at controlling blood glucose tightly in the first trimester. The alterations in insulin dosage and the control are aimed to prevent the woman from a risk of hypoglycaemic attacks, and her tolerance to treatment will be much improved if she understands the objectives of the treatment.

Appropriate control of glucose concentrations will usually require bolus doses of short acting insulin with each meal and one or two doses of intermediate acting insulin. Home blood glucose monitoring systems is necessary. Any oral hypoglycaemic agents must be stopped prior to conception, and effects of insulin on fetus should be controlled.

Renal function should be checked at the time of the first visit. An ultrasound scan should be arranged to check viability and dates. This is especially important in the diabetic pregnancy as there is an increased risk of preterm delivery. Referral for retinal assessment should be arranged as retinopathy can deteriorate in pregnancy.

In the second trimester, the first concern is to ensure that issues and prenatal diagnosis have been fully discussed. Congenital malformafions that arise with greater frequency in diabetes include cardiac, CNS, skeletal and renal malformations, and very rare sacral agenesis, but these are more common in the diabetic population.

Serum screening for trisomy 21 cannot be relied upon in diabetes, therefore, nuchal fold scanning is preferred.

Once the pregnancy progresses beyond 20 weeks of gestation, attention is increasingly focused on risks of serious urinary tract infection, pre-term labour and hypertension-related problems, *e. g.*, pre-eclampsia.

Urinary tract infection requires prompt treatment in view of its association with preterm

来源的激素拮抗胰岛素的影响，因此妊娠前三个月严密控制血糖。胰岛素用量的变化和控制，目的是预防孕妇低血糖，如果患者能理解治疗的目标，那她对治疗的忍耐将大大提高。

适当控制血糖浓度通常需要每餐注射剂量短效胰岛素，和一个或多个剂量的中效胰岛素。家庭血糖监测系统是必要的。怀孕之前任何口服降血糖剂必须停止，需要优化控制胰岛素对胎儿不利影响。

一次看门诊的时候应该检查肾功能。超声扫描应安排检查的可行性和日期。特别重要的是妊娠糖尿病有增加早产的风险。推荐对视网膜评估，视网膜病变可能在怀孕期间恶化。

在第二妊娠期，最关心的是确保问题与产前诊断已经充分讨论。在糖尿病中先天性畸形出现的概率很大，包括心脏、中枢神经系统、骨骼和肾畸形以及非常罕见的骶骨发育不全，糖尿病人群却很常见。

血清筛查21三体不能依赖于糖尿病，因此颈项透明带扫描是首选。

一旦怀孕进展超过20周，需要关注严重尿路感染、早产和高血压相关的问题，如先兆子痫。尿路感染需要立即治疗，鉴于其与早产和糖尿病的风险不稳定。糖尿病控制不良偶尔会发生酮症酸中毒，这些需要密切管理有高

labour and the risk of glucose instability. Occasional ketotic episodes arise in poorly controlled diabetics. These require intensive management and pose a significant risk to the fetus. Preterm labour is also more common, which this may be related to over distension of the uterus from polyhydramnios. The incidence of pre-eclampsia is thought to be increased by two folds in the diabetic population. The diagnosis is often difficult in a population that have an increased incidence of hypertension and renal disease.

In the third trimester, the main problems are the risk of polyhydramnios and fetal macrosomia. These complications can be reduced by tighter control of blood glucose. Serial ultrasound assessment is usually arranged to allow early diagnosis.

There is an increased incidence of respiratory distress in babies born to diabetic mothers. Unfortunately there are also an increased incidence and sudden intrauterine death in the later third trimester. Such intrauterine deaths can be minimized by attempting to deliver early, i. e. 36-37 weeks.

The problem is that this is not appropriate for most fetuses and early delivery. These will be associated with high caesarean section rates and neonatal respiratory distress. Therefore, most patients are managed by awaiting spontaneous labour until approximately 39 weeks in the presence of good control and no complications. If there are significant concerns regarding glucose control or complications, delivery will be undertaken at 37-38 weeks.

Insulin is given via an infusion pump. Blood glucose is checked hourly, and the infusion rate is adjusted accordingly. Post partum, the insulin requirement will fall immediately to the pre-pregnancy level and insulin doses can be reduced accordingly.

Neonatal risks from maternal diabetes include:

风险的胎儿,早产也是较常见的,这可能与羊水早破有关。在糖尿病人群中先兆子痫发生率增加 2 倍。高血压和肾脏疾病的发病率增加在人群中往往难以诊断。

晚期妊娠的主要问题是羊水过多和巨大胎儿,严格地控制血糖可减少这些并发症。串行超声评估通常是安排允许早期诊断。

由于母亲患糖尿病使婴儿出生后发生呼吸窘迫的发病率在增加。不幸的也有发病率增加,在晚期妊娠可导致突然宫内死亡,这样在 36～37 周早产就可减少宫内死亡数。

问题是,这不适合大多数胎儿和早产儿,这些将与高剖宫产率、新生儿呼吸窘迫有关。因此,大多数患者的管理是等待自然分娩,直到约 39 周还良好控制,无并发症。如果有重要的血糖控制或并发症,分娩将在 37～38 周进行。

人工胰岛素通过输液泵给予。每小时检查一次血糖,并调整相应的输注速率。产后,对胰岛素的需求将立即下降到怀孕前的水平,从而胰岛素剂量可以减少。

母亲患糖尿病,新生儿的风险包括:

1. prematurity.

2. congenital malformation.

3. respiratory distress.

4. polycythaemia.

5. hypoglycaemia.

6. birth trauma, including brachial plexus injury.

3.11.2 Gestational diabetes

3.11.2.1 Screening for gestational diabetes

1. Fifty grams oral glucose load, administered between 24-28 weeks of gestation.

2. Non-fasting.

3. Venous plasma glucose measured 1 h later.

4. Plasma glucose ≥ 140 mg/dl indicates need for 3 hour GTT.

3.11.2.2 Diagnosis of gestational diabetes

1. One hundred grams oral glucose load, administered after overnight fast.

2. Test should be given after 3 days of unrestricted diet and activity.

3. Venous plasma glucose is measured after fasting for 0, 1, 2 and 3 h.

4. Two or more abnormal values = gestational diabetes.

3.11.2.3 Management of gestational diabetes

1. Diet：

(1)Ideal Body Weight (IBW)—100 lb/5 ft. Add 5 lb/inch for those ＞5 ft.

(2)kcal：36 kcal/kg or 15 kcal/lb of IBW＋100 kcal/trimester.

(3)Nutrients：40%-50% carbohydrates

    12%-20%   protein

    30%-35%   fat

2. Glucose monitoring（mg/dl）：

Desire dranges—Fasting 60-90

---

1. 早产。

2. 先天性畸形。

3. 呼吸窘迫。

4. 红细胞增多症。

5. 低血糖。

6. 出生创伤，包括臂丛神经损伤。

3.11.2 妊娠期糖尿病

3.11.2.1 妊娠期糖尿病筛查

1. 50 g 糖口服。在孕 24～28 周之间施行。

2. 不用禁食。

3. 1 h 后查静脉血糖。

4. 血糖≥140 mg/dl 水平需做 3 h 糖耐量试验。

3.11.2.2 妊娠期糖尿病的诊断

1. 经过一夜禁食后给予 100 g 葡萄糖口服。

2. 试验可在不严格限制饮食和活动后 3 天进行。

3. 在空腹、1 h、2 h 和 3 h 查静脉血糖。

4. 有二次或以上异常水平＝妊娠期糖尿病。

3.11.2.3 妊娠期糖尿病的处理

1. 饮食：

（1）理想体重（IBW）—5 英尺高的 100 lb，大于 5 英尺高的每英寸加 5 lb。

（2）千卡：36 kcal/kg，或 15 kcal/lb(IBW)，每孕期加 100 kcal。

（3）营养：40%～50%碳水化合物

    12%～20%   蛋白质

    30%～35%   脂肪

2. 血糖监测（mg/dl）：

理想的范围—空腹 60～90

2 hr after meal　100-140

Premeal　60-105

After meal　≤120

2:00 AM-4:00 AM　60

3. Insulin:

(1) usually used for continuous fasting glucose >105.

(2) anticipated eventual insulin requirements for gestational diabetic.

Week 6-18　0.7 U/kg

18-26　0.8 U/kg

26-36　0.9 U/kg

36-40　1.0 U/kg

* 1/2 these doses at the beginning.

(3) distribution:

AM 2/3: 2/3 NPH insulin, 1/3 regular insulin.

PM 1/3: 1/2 NPH insulin, 1/2 regular insulin.

(4) IDDM (Insulin dependent diabetics management) requires individualization.

3.11.3　Diabetes ketotic acidosis（DKA）during pregnancy

1. Laboratory assessment:

arterial blood gas, glucose, ketones, and electrolytes, once every 2 h.

2. Insulin:

Low dose: intravenous regular insulin.

Loading dose: 0.2-0.4 U/kg.

Maintenance dose: 2.0-10.0 U/kg.

3. Fluids:

(1) Isotonic NaCl.

(2) Total replacement in first 12 hr=4-6 L.

(3) 500-1 000 ml/h for 2-4 h.

(4) 250 ml/h until 80% is replaced.

4. Glucose:

Infuse 5% GNS when plasma glucose reaches

餐后 2h　100～140

餐前　60～105

餐后　≤120

晨 2～4 时　60

3. 胰岛素:

(1) 通常用于空腹血糖持续 >105。

(2) 孕期糖尿病胰岛素需要量的预测:

孕周6～18　0.7 U/kg

18～26　0.8 U/kg

26～36　0.9 U/kg

36～40　1.0 U/kg

* 开始用这些剂量的 1/2。

(3) 分布:

上午 2/3: 其中 2/3 中性鱼精蛋白胰岛素, 1/3 常规胰岛素。

下午 1/3: 其中 1/2 中性鱼精蛋白胰岛素, 1/2 常规胰岛素。

(4) 胰岛素依赖型糖尿病的处理需要个体化。

3.11.3　妊娠期糖尿病酮症酸中毒

1. 实验室辅助检查:

动脉血气、血糖、酮体、电解质, 每 2 h 一次。

2. 胰岛素:

低剂量:静脉内常规胰岛素;

负荷量:0.2～0.4 U/kg;

维持量:2.0～10.0 U/kg。

3. 液体:

(1) 等渗氯化钠。

(2) 初 12 h 内的总量=4～6 L。

(3) 500～1 000 ml/h,持续 2～4 h。

(4) 250 ml/h,直到补充 80%。

4. 血糖:

当血糖达 250 mg/dl 时开始

250 mg/dl.

5. Potassium：

(1)if initially normal or reduced，then add 40-60 mEq/L.

(2)if initially elevarted，then give 20-30 mEq/L once levels begin to decline.

6. Bicarbonate：

Add one amp（44 mEq）to 1 L of 0.45％ NS if pH is ＜7.10.

3.11.4　Management of Insulin dependent diabetics in pregnancy

1. Hemoglobin A should be determined during preconception and 1st trimester. Rate of malformations is 22％ for HbA＞8.5.

2. Fetal echocardiogram at 22 weeks.

3. Ultrasound at 18，22，26 and 38 weeks；consider amniocentesis at 38 weeks for maturity.

4. Consider cesarean if estimation of fetal weight（EFW）＞4 000 g（see section on shoulder dystocia）.

5. Blood sugar q 2 h in labor. If ＞120，start insulin drip（10 U in 1 000 ml）to keep BS 85-100 mg/dl.

6. If cesarean is selected，give AM insulin and perform AM C/S.

3.11.5　Case analysis and test

Medical Records：38-year-old to stop after 36 weeks，fetal disappeared on the 4th admission of the chief complaint. Usually menstrual cycle，last menstrual period September 8，2007，the expected date of June 15，2008. Menopause more than 40 days of the early response，natural relief for four weeks. Menopause 5 the beginning of a sense of fetal movement，four conscious fetal movement disappeared，found that "fetal death" by the B-mode ultrasound examination at a local hospital and transferred to our hospital induced labor. Nearly two

滴 5％葡萄糖氯化钠。

5. 钾：

（1）如果开始正常或降低，加 40～60 mEq/L。

（2）如果开始升高，一旦开始下降给予 20～30 mEq/L。

6. 碳酸氢钠：

如果 pH＜7.10，加 44 mEq 碳酸氢钠于 1 L 0.45％氯化钠中。

3.11.4　胰岛素依赖型糖尿病的孕期处理

1. 孕前和早孕期查血红蛋白 A。血红蛋白 A＞8.5 者畸形的发生率为 22％。

2. 22 周时做胎儿心脏超声心动图。

3. 在 18、22、26、38 周做超声检查，38 周时考虑检查羊水了解成熟程度。

4. 如果估计胎儿体重＞4 000 g，考虑剖宫产（见肩难产节）。

5. 分娩中 2 h 查一次血糖，如果 ＞120，开始胰岛素静滴（10 U 加入 1 000 ml）保持血糖在 85～100 mg/dl。

6. 如果选择剖宫产，则上午给予胰岛素，上午行剖宫产。

3.11.5　病例分析和习题

临床资料：经产妇，38 岁，以"停经 36 周，胎动消失 4 日"主诉入院。平素月经周期规律，末次月经 2007 年 9 月 8 日，预产期 2008 年 6 月 15 日。停经 40 余日出现早孕反应，持续 4 周自然缓解。停经 5 个月初感胎动，4 日前自觉胎动消失，在当地医院经 B 型超声检查发现"胎死宫内"，转来我院引产。患者近 2 个

months in patients with lower extremity edema, alleviate and gradually increased by rest, nearly a conscious increase in food intake, thirst, polydipsia. Nearly three days, headache, chest tightness, fatigue, ignoring the blurred and vaginal bleeding, vaginal fluid, two will be normal. Pregnancy recurring genital itching, kind of bean dregs leucorrhea, diagnosis and treatment were not. Denied a history of hypertension, nephritis, etc., to deny the history of infectious diseases such as tuberculosis and hepatitis, smoking and alcohol. Basal blood pressure 90/60 mmHg. His father suffered from diabetes for 5 years and died of diabetic nephropathy two months ago. Pregnant 4 production, abortion, natural childbirth 10 years ago, a female including infants, weight 4 100 g. The pregnancy and the last third trimester of pregnancy have polydipsia, polyphagia, polyuria symptoms, but blood sugar levels were not detected.

On admission examination: body temperature 36.8 ℃; pulse 102 times/min, blood pressure 160/100 mmHg, weight 91.8 kg. No anemia, normal heart and lung auscultation. Lower limbs with moderate edema. Obstetric examination: full-term pregnancy abdominal uterine length 38 cm, abdominal circumference 126 cm. Unheard and fetal heart rate. Supplementary examination: blood leukocyte $14.8 \times 10^9/L$, hemoglobin 132 g/L, hematocrit 0.38; urinary protein (＋＋), urine (＋＋), ketones (＋＋), specific gravity 1.030, no tube; total protein 57 g/L, albumin 30 g/L, transaminase normal; with normal renal function; fasting blood glucose twice 11.3 mmol/L, 13.2 mmol/L, arterial blood gas analysis: pH 7.44 and HCO_3^- 20 mmol/L, $PaCO_2$ 29.4 mmol/L, TCO_2 21.3 mmol/L. Blood clotting were normal; B-mode ultrasound examination: fetal head biparietal diameter of 8.0 cm, sheep level segment 8.0 cm, Yi plate Ⅱ level; fundus examination: A∶V＝1∶2.5, there is pressure trace characterization reflective enhanced artery, reflective dark cloud center of the macula; ECG: sinus tachycardia, heart rate 105 times/min.

月出现双下肢水肿,经休息后不缓解并逐渐加重,近1个月自觉进食量增加,口渴,多饮。近3日时有头痛、胸闷、乏力,无视物不清及阴道流血、阴道流液,二便正常。妊娠期反复出现外阴瘙痒,豆渣样白带增多,未予诊治。否认高血压、肾炎等病史,否认结核及肝炎等传染性疾病史,无烟酒嗜好。基础血压 90/60mmHg。其父患糖尿病 5 年,并于 2 个月前死于糖尿病肾病。孕 4 产 1,人工流产 2 次,10 年前曾自然分娩一女活婴,体重4 100 g。此次妊娠前和前次孕晚期均有多饮、多食、多尿症状,但未检测血糖水平。入院时查体:体温 36.8 ℃,脉搏 102 次/min,血压160/100 mmHg,体重 91.8 kg。无贫血貌,心肺听诊正常。双下肢中度水肿。产科检查:足月妊娠腹型,子宫长度 38 cm,腹围 126 cm。未闻及胎心。辅助检查:血白细胞 $14.8 \times 10^9/L$,血红蛋白 132 g/L,血细胞比容 0.38;尿蛋白 (＋＋),尿糖(＋＋),尿酮体(＋＋),尿比重 1.030,无管型;总蛋白 57 g/L,白蛋白 30 g/L,转氨酶正常值;肾功能正常;空腹血糖两次分别为 11.3 mmol/L、13.2 mmol/L,动脉血气分析:pH 7.44,HCO_3^- 20 mmol/L,$PaCO_2$ 29.4 mmol/L,TCO_2 21.3 mmol/L。凝血四项均正常;B 型超声检查:胎头双顶径 8.0 cm,羊水平段 8.0 cm,胎盘 Ⅱ 级;眼底检查:A∶V＝1∶2.5,有压迹征,动脉反光增强,黄斑中心反光暗浊;心电图:窦性心动过速,心率 105 次/min。

Test

Diabetes：

a. is associated with a decreased incidence of congenital abnormality.

b. is associated with postmaturity rather than prematurity，resulting in increased birth weights.

c. is associated with an increased incidence of respiratory distress in the neonate.

d. is associated with a reduced insulin requirement in pregnancy.

e. Maternal hypoglycaemia can occur in the puerperium.

Answers

a. False. The increased incidence is related to periconceptual control of the blood glucose concentration.

b. False. Prematurity is increased in diabetes. Birth weight is increased，though postmaturity is unlikely to arise as most diabetic women are delivered between 38 weeks and term. It is thought that birth weight is increased due to the effect of high insulin levels on the fetus.

c. True. This is more likely to arise due to prematurity， an increased incidence of hyaline membrane disease in infants of diabetic mothers，and a cardiomyopathy in the neonate.

d. False. There is a substantial rise in insulin requirement to overcome the antagonistic effect of placental hormones.

e. True. If insulin dosage is not reduced to levels approximating the requirement prior to pregnancy.

测试题

糖尿病：

a. 与先天性畸形的发病率下降相关。

b. 与过度成熟而不是早产相关联，从而增强出生体重。

c. 会增加新生儿呼吸窘迫的发病率。

d. 怀孕与胰岛素的需求减少有关。

e. 孕产妇低血糖可以发生在产褥期。

答案

a. 错误。发病率的增加和自我控制血糖浓度相关。

b. 错误。糖尿病中早产儿是增加的。出生体重增加，但不过度成熟，这是不可能出现的，就如大多数糖尿病妇女在 38 周和终止期限之间分娩。据认为，出生体重增加是由于胎儿高胰岛素水平。

c. 正确。早产儿，透明膜病变的糖尿病母亲的婴儿和心肌病的新生儿更容易增加发病率。

d. 错。胰岛素的要求大幅度增加，以填补胎盘激素的拮抗作用。

e. 正确。如果胰岛素用量不减少到怀孕前的水平。

3.12 Prenancy Associated with Sexually Transmitted Diseases

Key words

1. gonorrhea
2. syphilis
3. condyloma acuminata
4. sexually transmitted disease，STD
5. human papilloma virus，HPV
6. genital herpes
7. herpes simplex virus，HSV
8. chlamydia

3.12.1 Introduction

3.12.1.1 What is a sexually transmitted disease?

- STDs is also known as sexually transmitted infections(STI).
- Defined as the infections that can be transferred from one person to another through sexual contact.

3.12.1.2 Pregnance combined with STDs

The harm of pregnancy with sexually transmitted disease is that it can infect fetus or neonate through the vertical transmission，seriously affecting the health of the next generation.

3.12.1.3 Common STDs

- herpes
- condyloma acuminatum
- syphilis
- gonorrhea
- HIV/AIDS
- hepatitis B
- trichomoniasis

3.12 妊娠合并性传播疾病

关键词

1. 淋病
2. 梅毒
3. 尖锐湿疣
4. 性传播性疾病
5. 人乳头状病毒
6. 生殖器疱疹
7. 单纯疱疹病毒
8. 衣原体

3.12.1 介绍

3.12.1.1 什么是性传播疾病？

- STDs(性传播疾病)，简称性病或性传播感染(STI)。
- 是指可经性行为或类似性行为传播的一组传染病。

3.12.1.2 妊娠合并性传播疾病

妊娠合并性传播疾病的危害：在于可通过垂直传播感染胎儿或新生儿，严重影响下一代的健康。

3.12.1.3 常见性病的类型

- 生殖器疱疹
- 尖锐湿疣
- 梅毒
- 淋病
- 艾滋病
- 病毒性乙型肝炎
- 滴虫性阴道炎

3.12.2　Human immunodeficiency virus (HIV) infection

3.12.2.1　Etiology

Causative agents of the immunodeficiency syndrome are DNA retroviruses immunodeficiency viruses, HIV-1 and HIV-2. Their transmission is similar to that of hepatitis B virus. Sexual intercourse, especially among male homosexuals, is the major mode of transmission. The virus is also transmitted by blood or blood-contaminated products, and mothers may infect their infants.

3.12.2.2　Pathogenesis

The common denominator of clinical illness with HIV is profound immunosuppression. Thymus-derived (lymphocytes-T) lymphocytes defined phenotypically by the CD4 surface antigen are the principal targets. Viral DNA is integrated into cellular DNA to reduce celluar life by infection. The number of T cells drops insidiously and progressively, resulting eventually in profound immunosuppression.

3.12.2.3　Clinical manifestations

The incubation period from exposure to clinical disease is usually within 2-3 months, and the median time is about 10 years.

1. Symptoms:

In acute cases, the symptoms similar to those of many other viral infections and usually lasts for less than 10 days. Common symptoms include fever, night sweats, fatigue, rash, headache, lymphadenopathy, pharyngitis, myalgias, arthralgias, nausea, vomiting, and diarrhea.

2. $CD4^+$ count of less than $200/\mu l$ is also considered definitive for the diagnosis of HIV.

3. Serological testing:

The enzyme-linked immunoassay assay (ELISA) is usually used as a screening test for HIV

3.12.2　人免疫缺陷病毒(HIV)感染

3.12.2.1　病因

免疫缺陷综合征是由 DNA 逆转录病毒(称为人免疫缺陷病毒)HIV-1 和 HIV-2 引起的。其传播与乙型肝炎病毒相似,性交尤其在男性同性恋之间是其主要传播方式。也可通过血液或血制品传播,感染的母亲也可将其传给婴儿。

3.12.2.2　发病机制

HIV 的主要特征是严重的免疫抑制。胸腺来源的淋巴细胞(T-淋巴细胞)以 CD4 表面抗原的表现型为特征的是该病毒的主要靶细胞。病毒整合入淋巴细胞的 DNA,通过感染来缩短细胞的生存周期使患者的 T-淋巴细胞数急剧减少而最终导致严重的免疫抑制。

3.12.2.3　临床表现

从暴露至临床发病的潜伏期通常为 2～3 个月,中位数时间约为 10 年。

1. 症状:

急性发病类似于其他病毒感染症状,常常持续 10 天以内。常见症状包括:发热、盗汗、疲劳、皮疹、头痛、淋巴结病、咽炎、肌肉痛、关节痛、恶心、呕吐及腹泻。

2. $CD4^+$ 细胞计数少于 $200/\mu l$为确诊指标。

3. 血清学检测:

酶联免疫法(ELISA)常用以筛查 HIV 抗体的存在。

antibodies.

3.12.2.4　Maternal and fetus-infant infection

1. mother-to-infant transmission accounts for most HIV infection among children. Risk of prenatal transmission is about 25%.

2. Risk factors：

(1) CD4$^+$ count of less than 700/μl.

(2) preterm delivery (<34 weeks).

(3) membranes ruptured for more than 4 h.

(4) breast feeding increase postnatal HIV-1 transmission by 10%-20%.

3.12.2.5　Prevention of transmission

1. Blood and body fluid precautions should be used consistently in all patients：

(1) All health care workers who participate in invasive procedures must use appropriate barrier precautions to prevent skin and mucous-membrane contract with blood and other body fluids of all patients.

(2) If a glove is torn or there is a needle stick or other breakages, the glove should be removed and a new glove should be used as promptly as patient safety permits.

2. Prevention of vertical transmission：

Antiretroviral therapy and cesarean delivery.

3.12.2.6　Prenatal care

1. Monitor CD4 counts and viral load during each trimester if possible.

2. Check CD4 counts to determine need for pneunocystis carinii prophylaxis. Initiate prophylaxis when CD4<200/μl：

(1)trimethoprim：sulfamethoxazole (Septra DS) 800 mg/160 mg q day.

(2) iv pentamidine for severe disease in patients intolerant of TMP-SMX.

3. Antiviral regiment：

(1) Antepartum：100 mg zidovudine (ZDV),

3.12.2.4　母亲和胎儿——婴儿感染

1. 儿童中大多数 HIV 感染是由于母亲——婴儿垂直传播。产前传播的危险性约 25%。

2. 危险因素：

(1)CD4$^+$ 细胞计数小于 700/μl。

(2)早产(孕<34 周)。

(3)胎膜破裂大于 4 h。

(4)母乳喂养可使感染率增加 10%～20%。

3.12.2.5　传播的预防

1. 对所有病人的血及体液应进行防护：

(1)所有进行有创性操作的医务工作者均需使用合适的防护屏障,以免皮肤和黏膜与患者的血液和其他体液接触。

(2)如果手套破损或发现被针刺等损伤,应在病人安全允许的条件下,尽快更换新手套。

2. 垂直传播的预防：

抗逆转录病毒的治疗和剖宫产。

3.12.2.6　产前保健

1. 如果可能,每三个月检测一次 CD4 计数和病毒负荷。

2. 检查 CD4 计数决定是否需预防卡氏肺囊虫。当 CD4<200/μl,开始预防性治疗：

(1)甲氧苄氨嘧啶-新诺明：800 mg/160 mg/d。

(2)双戊烷：静滴,用于严重、不能耐受 TMP-SMX 的患者。

3.抗病毒方案：

(1)产前：叠氮胸苷(齐多夫

p. o., 5 times/day, starting at 14 weeks of gestation.

(2) Labor and delivery：ZDV i. v. loading dose 2 mg/kg over 1 h; then 1 mg/kg until delivery.

(3) Neonatal：ADV 2 mg/kg, p. o., q 6 hours for first 6 weeks of life since 8-12 hours postpartum.

3.12.2.7　Breast feeding

Breast feeding increase the risk of neonatal transmission and in general is not recommended in HIV-positive women.

3.13　Postpartum Haemorrhage

Key words

1. postpartum hemorrhage
2. uterine atony
3. retained placenta
4. placenta accrete
5. placenta increta
6. coagulation defects

3.13.1　Definition

Primary postpartum haemorrhage (PPH) is loss of blood estimated to be ＞500 ml, from the genital tract, within 24 h post delivery.
- Mild PPH means estimated blood loss of up to 1 000 ml.
- Severe PPH means any estimated blood loss over 1 000 ml.
- Secondary postpartum haemorrhage is abnormal loss of blood within 24 h-6 weeks post delivery.

3.13.2　Aetiology

The "Four Ts" mnemonic (Tone, Trauma,

定)：100 mg,口服,5 次/日,自孕 14 周开始。

(2)产时:叠氮胸苷:静滴,先给负荷剂量 2 mg/(kg·h);随后给予持续静滴 1 mg/kg 直至分娩。

(3)新生儿期:叠氮胸苷:2 mg/kg,口服,每 6 h 一次,从出生后 8～12 h 直至 6 周。

3.12.2.7　哺乳

哺乳会增加新生儿传播的危险,一般不推荐 HIV 阳性妇女母乳喂养。

3.13　产后出血

关键词

1. 产后出血
2. 子宫收缩乏力
3. 胎盘滞留
4. 胎盘粘连
5. 胎盘植入
6. 凝血功能障碍

3.13.1　定义

产后出血定义:胎儿娩出后 24 h 内失血超过 500 ml。

- 轻度产后出血定义:胎儿娩出后 24 h 内失血少于 1000 ml。
- 重度产后出血定义:胎儿娩出后 24 h 内失血超过 1000 ml。
- 继发性产后出血定义:胎儿娩出后 24 h 到 6 周内异常出血。

3.13.2　病因

4T 指子宫收缩乏力,胎盘因

Tissue, and Thrombin) can be used to detect specific causes. The most common cause of postpartum haemorrhage (PPH) is uterine atony. Atony and retained placenta are 80% of all cases; lacerations comprise the bulk of the other 20%. Cervical lacerations, uterine rupture, broad ligament haematoma and extra genital bleeding also need to be excluded.

3.13.3 Risk factors

Factors relating to the pregnancy:
- Antepartum haemorrhage in this pregnancy.
- Placenta praevia (15×risk).
- Multiple pregnancy (5×risk).
- Pre-eclampsia or pregnancy-induced hypertension (4×risk).
- Nulliparity (3×risk).
- Previous PPH (3×risk).
- Maternal obesity (2×risk).

Factors relating to delivery:
- Emergency Caesarean section (CS) (9×risk).
- Elective CS (4×risk)-especially if >3 repeat procedures.
- Retained placenta (5×risk).
- Mediolateral episiotomy (5×risk).
- Operative vaginal delivery (2×risk).
- Labour of >12 hours (2×risk).
- Pre-existing maternal haemorrhagic conditions.

3.13.4 Presentation

(1) Symptoms: continuous bleeding, which fails to stop after delivery of the placenta at the third stage.

(2) Signs: loss of >1000 ml may be accompanied by clinically apparent shock, ie tachycardia, hypotension.

(3) Investigations.

(4) Thorough examination of the lower genital tract. This may require theatre/anaesthesia.

(5) RBC, clotting screen, crossmatch.

素,软产道裂伤,凝血功能障碍。最常见为子宫收缩乏力和胎盘因素,占全部病例的80%,产道裂伤和其他因素占20%,所有需排除宫颈裂伤、子宫破裂、阔韧带血肿和其他生殖道出血的情况。

3.13.3 高危因素

与妊娠相关的因素包括:
- 本次妊娠产前出血
- 前置胎盘(15倍风险)。
- 多胎妊娠(15倍风险)。
- 产前子痫和高血压(4倍风险)。

- 初产妇(3倍风险)。
- 既往有产后出血史(3倍风险)。
- 孕妇肥胖(2倍风险)。

分娩因素:
- 急诊剖宫产。
- 阴道助产>3次剖宫产。
- 胎盘残留(5倍风险)。
- 会阴侧切(5倍风险)。
- 阴道手术助产(2倍风险)。
- 孕妇产程>12 h(2倍风险)。
- 孕妇有血液系统疾病。

3.13.4 临床表现

(1)阴道多量流血胎儿娩出后第三产程持续阴道出血。

(2)症状:当阴道出血>1000 ml临床上伴随脉搏细数、脉压缩小。

(3)检查。

(4)体格检查:彻底检查软产道,有时需在手术室麻醉下进行。

(5)红细胞凝血功能交叉配血做好输血准备。

(6) Hourly urine output.

(7) Continuous pulse/blood pressure or central venous pressure monitoring ECG, pulse oximetry.

3.13.5　Management

Ideally one of the emergency drills to be practised by the team on the labour ward.

- Call expert assistance.
- Secure IV access with 2×14-gauge cannulae.

- If the perceived blood loss is 500-1000 ml and there are no signs of clinical shock, basic measures, (crossmatch 2 units, RBC, clotting screen, IV access and monitoring clinical observations) should suffice.

- However, loss of greater than 1000 ml or any signs of shock should lead to full alert of the clinical team: experienced midwife, obstetric registrar (alert consultant), anaesthetic registrar (alert consultant), alert haematologist, alert transfusion service, call porters for transport of specimens and blood products.
- Oxygen should be given by mask at 8 litres per minute.
- Transfuse crossmatched blood (6 units initially) as soon as possible.
- Until then, infuse crystalloid or colloid.
- Use a warming device and a pressure cuff.
- Do not use dextrans.

- Give up to 1 litre of fresh frozen plasma (FFP) and 10 units of cryoprecipitate if clinically indicated. A new haemostatic agent-recombinant factor Ⅶ a-has had some clinical success, but its efficacy and safety is untested in clinical trials as yet.
- Monitor temperature and urine output (catheterise).
- Stop the bleeding.
- Ensure bladder empty and bimanually compress the

（6）测每小时尿量。

（7）持续监护脉搏血压和静脉压。

3.13.5　处理原则

最好是在产房由抢救小组抢救。

- 通知有经验的医生到场。
- 开通足够的静脉通道，使用 2 个 14 G 的套管针。
- 通过基本的测量，初步估计出血量在 500～1000 ml，没有休克的临床表现，一定要做好基本的测量，包括交叉配血 2 U、血常规、凝血功能、维持静脉通道和临床监护。
- 然而，若出血量超过 1000 ml 或有任何休克的表现，则需要全部的抢救人员到位，呼叫有经验的助产士、产科主任、麻醉师、血液科、检验科，还有特殊标本的转运和血液制品的准备。
- 每 8 L/min 的速度面罩给氧。

- 尽快输血配血（首次 6 个单位）。

- 到了这时，需要时补充晶体或胶体液。
- 使用温热设备并加压输入。
- 不使用右旋糖苷。
- 输新鲜冰冻血浆。有临床指征时输 10 单位冷沉淀。一种新的止血剂凝血因子血，有一定的临床成功率，但它的效果和安全性仍在临床试验阶段。
- 监测体温和尿量。
- 止血。
- 排空膀胱。

uterus ± rub up a contraction. A Sengstaken-Blakemore tube has been used to compress the uterus.

- Give IV syntocinon 10 units or IV ergometrine 500 micrograms.
- Try misoprostol 1 000 micrograms rectally.
- Exclude other causes than atony: Tissue (retained products of conception), Trauma (of the genital tract), Thrombin (abnormalities of coagulation).
- If pharmacological measures fail to control the haemorrhage, resort to surgery early:
- Bilateral ligation of the uterine arteries or bilateral ligation of the internal iliac (hypogastric) arteries.
- An alternative to ligation is embolisation with gelatin sponge. Uterine bracing suture, (the B-Lynch suture) to the anterior and posterior uterine walls has been shown to be effective and safe.

- Hysterectomy should be considered early, especially in cases of placenta accreta or uterine rupture.

3.13.6 Prevention

1. The active management of the third stage of labour; prophylactic oxytocics should be routinely used in the third stage of labour as they decrease the risk of postpartum haemorrhage (PPH) by 60%.

2. Good prenatalcare and education.

3.14 Postpartum Depression

Key words

1. postpartum depression
2. pharmacological
3. antidepressants
4. anxiolytic agents

- 双手按摩子宫,或用三腔管压迫子宫。
- 加强宫缩,缩宫素 10 单位静滴或静推。
- 米索前列腺醇直肠塞药。
- 排除其他原因的产后出血:胎盘因素,软产道裂伤,凝血功能障碍。
- 如果药物治疗失败,尽早采用手术治疗。
- 结扎盆腔血管:子宫动脉或双侧髂内动脉。
- 介入栓塞:行股动脉穿刺,插入导管至子宫动脉或髂内动脉,注入明胶海绵栓塞动脉。子宫前后壁的 B-Lynch 缝合也是有效和安全的方法。
- 若有胎盘植入或子宫破裂等情况需及时切除子宫。

3.13.6 预防

1. 正确处理产程。加强产后观察,产后 2 h 注意观察会阴有无血肿、生命体征、宫缩及阴道出血情况。产后常规注射催产素,有助于降低产后出血率。

2. 重视产前保健,加强孕前及孕期保健。

3.14 产后抑郁症

关键词

1. 产后抑郁症
2. 心理学家
3. 抗抑郁药
4. 抗焦虑药

3. 14. 1　Definition

Depression is considered postpartum if it begins within 3 to 6 months after childbirth, and similar to other depression that develops at any time.

3. 14. 2　Incidence

1. Depression disorders with an onset within 2 to 3 months of delivery develop in approximately 8 to 15 percent of postpartum women.

2. Women with a history of a depressive illness have a risk of postpartum depression of about 30 percent.

3. Adolescent women have a risk of postpartum depression of about 30 percent.

3. 14. 3　Criteria for diagnosis of depression

1. Major depression：

(1)At least five of the following symptoms for a 2 week period；one symptom must be either depressed mood or loss of interest or pleasure nearly every day：

①Depressed mood most of the day.

②Markedly diminished interest or pleasure in all，or almost all. Activities most of the day.

③Significant weight loss or weight gain when not dieting，or decrease or increase in appetite.

④Insomnia or hypersomnia.

⑤Psychomotor agitation or retardation.

⑥Fatigue or loss of energy.

⑦Feelings of worthlessness or excessive or inappropriate guilt.

⑧Diminished ability to think or concentrate.

⑨Recurrent thoughts of death，recurrent suicidal ideation without a specific plan or a suicidal attempt.

(2) The symptoms eallse clinically significant distress or impairment in social，occupational，or other important areas of functioning.

(3)Symptoms are not due to the direct effects of substance or general medical condition.

3. 14. 1　定义

产后抑郁症指产后 3～6 个月内开始的同其他任何时间发生的抑郁相似的抑郁症。

3. 14. 2　发病率

1. 将近 8％～15％的产后妇女在产后 2～3 个月发生抑郁症。

2. 有抑郁症病史的妇女，产后抑郁症的危险将近 30％。

3. 青春期妇女产后抑郁症的发病率约为 30％。

3. 14. 3　诊断标准

1. 严重产后抑郁：

(1)至少有以下五种症状持续两周；一种症状必须是情绪抑郁或几乎每天都无兴趣或不快乐。

①一天中大多数时间抑郁。

②一天中大多数时间对几乎所有活动明显缺乏兴趣和乐趣。

③当不节食，或减少或增加食欲会导致显著的体重增减。

④失眠或嗜睡。

⑤精神易激动或迟钝。

⑥疲乏或缺乏精力。

⑦无用感或过分或不恰当的内疚感。

⑧思考或精力集中能力减弱。

⑨总是有死的念头，反复出现的无计划的自杀观念或自杀的企图。

(2)症状导致临床明显的抑郁或社交、职业或其他重要方面的损害。

(3)症状不是由物质或一般医疗情况的直接影响所致。

（4）Symptoms are not within 2 months of the loss of alove one.

（5）In severe cases，may be accompanied by psychosis(bizarre or paranoid thought)．

2. Minor depression：Reqires 2 weeks'depressed mood and fewer than five symptoms.

3.14.4 Course

1. The natural course is one of gradual improvement over the 6 months after delivery.

2. In some cases the women may remain symptomatic for months to years.

3.14.5 Treatment

Supportive treatment alone is not sufficient for major postparttum depression. Pharmacological intervention and management in canjucfion with a psychiatrist is needed in most instances. Treatment options include antidepressants，anxiolytic agents，and eleetroconvulsive therapy.

3.15 Abnormal Labour

Key words

1. dystocia
2. cephalopelvic disproportion
3. persistent occiput-posteriou(POP) position
4. hands-and-knees positon
5. pelvic-rocking
6. delayed established(active) first stage
7. delayed second stage
8. a retained placenta
9. multiple births
10. breech presentation

3.15.1 Definition

■ Abnormal labor（Dystocia）is defined what have been categorized classically as abnormalities of the

（4）症状不是在两个月内失恋所致。

（5）在严重的病例也许会伴有精神病（古怪或类偏执的想法）。

2.轻微抑郁:有两周的抑郁情绪和少于五种症状。

3.14.4 病程

1.自然病程为产后 6 个月，是一个逐渐好转的过程。

2.有些病例症状会持续数月至数年。

3.14.5 治疗

仅用支持治疗对严重的产后抑郁症是不够的。大多数病例需要药物治疗和与心理学家联合治疗。治疗方法包括:抗抑郁药、抗焦虑药和电惊厥疗法。

3.15 异常分娩

关键词

1.难产
2.头盆不称
3.持续性枕后位
4.手膝支持俯卧位
5.骨盆晃动
6.第一产程活跃期延长
7.第二产程延长
8.胎盘滞留
9.多胎分娩
10.臀位

3.15.1 定义

■ 异常分娩（难产）通常经典的定义是:由于产力异常（子宫收缩

power (uterine contractions or maternal expulsive forces), the passenger (position, size, or presentation of the fetus), or the passage (pelvis or soft tissues).

力或母亲的屏气用力)、胎儿异常(胎位、胎儿大小和胎方位)、产道异常(骨盆和软产道),任何一个或一个以上因素出现异常,分娩就可能发生困难,称异常分娩(distocia),俗称"难产"。

- Because dystocia can rarely be diagnosed with certainty, the relatively imprecise term "failure to progress" has been used, which includes lack of progressive cervical dilation or lack of descent of the fetalhead or both. The term "cephalopelvic disproportion" describe a disparity between the size of the maternal pelvis and the fetal head that precludes vaginal delivery.

- 因为难产是一个比较难以确定的概念,常用其他相关的用语来描述难产,如"产程不进展",用来描述宫口扩张的延迟或胎儿下降延迟,或者说两种情况都存在。头盆不称用来描述阴道分娩中,胎头与母亲骨盆之间的不适应状态。

- The diagnosis of dystocia should not be made before an adequate trial of labor has been achieved.

- 对难产的诊断只有在经过了认真的试产后才能作出决定。

- As the distinction between "start of labour" and "false labour" can only be made after a period of carefully observation, the diagnosis of prolonged latent phase is usually better substituted by "false labour", and not dystocia.

- 因为临产的起点与假临产之间的分界不清,只能经过一段时间的仔细观察才能区分,所以对潜伏期延长的诊断,最好用假临产来代替,而不应当在这个时候诊断为难产。

3.15.2 Strateges to promote normal labour

In order to promote normal birth, a national practice guidelines on normal childbirth that address philosophy and practice expectations to provide evidence-based practices in all clinical settings should be developed, Promotion among childbirth educators and maternity care providers of knowledge about the birth process and evidence-based practices so that women and families can be informed about normal birth. Following strateges are recommended:

3.15.2 能够促进正常分娩的措施

为了促进正常分娩,应有一个国家层面的正常分娩指南,强调分娩的生理特征,保证在各级医疗保健部门能够实施有循证医学依据的服务方式。对正常分娩的健康教育人员和医疗服务人员进行有关正常分娩和循证医学的知识更新,以保证产妇和家人能够得到正确的信息。下列是有利于正常分娩应当提倡的措施:

- Waiting for spontaneous onset of labour until contradicted.

- Offer continuous support during labor from caregivers (nurses, midwives, or lay individuals) to

- 等待自然发动宫缩,除非有医学指征不允许这样做。

- 产程中所有服务人员(护士、助产士、其他非专业人员如导乐

women and their newborns.

- Encourage freedom of movement throughout labour for women in labour.
- Encourage of spontaneous pushing in the woman's preferred position during second stage of labour.

- Use of fetal surveillance by intermittent auscultation until indicated.

- Encourage of non-pharmacologic approaches to pain relief (such as tubs/showers, access to natural light, environmental designs/adaptations, quiet area).
- Offering pharmacologic measures as indicated according to order.
- No any routine interventions until indicated.

3.15.3　Strateges for prevention of dystocia

- Birthing as a natural process should be promoted by all health care professionals who provide antenatal care.
- Health care professionals should be committed to protecting, promoting, and supporting normal childbirth according to evidence-based practice.
- Normal birth should be accessible to all pregnant and birthing women and their families, so they should be able to make informed choices.
- There should be a valid reason (evidence-based practice) to intervene in the natural process when labour and birth are progressing normally.
- Risk assessment is a process continuing throughout pregnancy and birth. Referral of the woman to a higher level of care may be required when early signs of complications become apparent.
- Vaginal birth following a normal pregnancy is safer for mother and child than a Caesarean section.
- Caesarean section should be reserved for pregnancies in which there is threat to the health

师)都应当给予产妇连续性的支持照顾。

- 整个产程中鼓励产妇自由活动。
- 第二产程中支持鼓励产妇在自己感到舒适的体位按自己的意愿用力(自主的用力)。
- 应用间断性的胎心监护技术进行评估,除非有医学指征不允许这样做(需要持续监护)。
- 鼓励应用非药物镇痛方法减轻和缓解产痛,例如沐浴或盆浴,自然舒适的灯光、安静舒适的环境等。
- 对有指征都按医嘱应用药物镇痛。
- 除非有医学指征,不给予任何常规的干预措施。

3.15.3　难产的预防措施

- 所有从事孕产妇保健工作的人员都应提倡和促进正常分娩。
- 所有孕产妇保健人员都要遵守循证医学的实践方式,预防难产,促进和支持正常分娩。
- 对产妇及其家人提供正常分娩服务,使她们能够有选择分娩方式的权利。
- 当产程进展正常时,不应人为地干涉产程,除非有充分的循证医学的证据支持这样做。
- 对于分娩中危险因素的评估是连续动态的过程。及时发现产程中的异常情况,如果有必要,及时转诊到上级医院。
- 阴道分娩比剖宫产对母子更安全。
- 剖宫产只能用于当母子安全受到危险时的措施。对于没有产

of the mother and/or baby. A Caesarean section should not be offered to a pregnant woman when there is no obstetrical indication.

程指征的孕产妇不能做剖宫产术。

3.15.4　Persistent occiput-posteriou(POP) position

- Persistent occiput-posteriou(POP) position of the fetus is one of the most common complications encountered in obstetrics. For a fetus in an occiput-posteriou position to rotate to an occiput-anterior position, it must rotate 135 degrees(ROP to ROT to ROA or OA).
- Most cases this rotation is acccomplished before the fetus deliveried, it is reported that 70%-90% of OP will turn to OA when the fetus reached to the pelvic(in late phase of labour, usually when the cervical reached to the full dialation or later).
- some cases are not rotated to OA, and may be remained at OP position, labour progress may cease or the fetus may be born in a posterior position, that cases are recorded as the persistent occiput-posteriou position.

3.15.4　持续性枕后位

- 持续性枕后位是产科常见的并发症,如图 3-15-1 所示。枕后位的胎儿,需要经过 135°(如 ROP 到 ROT 到 ROA 或到正枕前 OA)。大多数情况下,在胎儿分娩前,能够完成旋转。
- 据报道,70%～90% 的枕后位当胎儿入盆后(在产程的后期,通常当宫口开全或开全后),转为枕前位分娩。
- 有些枕后位可能持续处于枕后位,产程进展迟缓,或者在枕后位分娩,这种情况称为持续性枕后位。

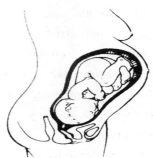

Figure 3-15-1　Occiput-posteriou position

图 3-15-1　枕后位

3.15.4.1　Maternal-fetal-neonatal risks

- The woman may suffer intense back pain in the labour process that is caused bythe fetal occiput compressing the sacral nerves.
- The woman had higher risk of severe perineal laceration.
- There is no increased risk of fetal mortality due to

3.15.4.1　枕后位对母子的危险性

- 因为胎儿枕骨压迫骶神经,产妇可能腰痛比较严重。
- 分娩时发生重度会阴裂伤的危险增加(如果以枕后位分娩)。
- 对于胎儿没有增加危险,除非

the occiput-posteriou position unless labour is protracted or an operative birth is performed.

3.15.4.2　Medical therapy

- Await spontaneous birth and offering supportive care as position changing on woman's will and nutrition support.
- Manual rotation to the anterior position and awaiting spontaneous birth.
- Forcep delviery at OP position.
- Forcep delvivery at OA postion (manual rotation or forcep assisted rotation.
- Fetus and mother conditions during labour should be observed closely and recorded.

3.15.4.3　Maternal posture changing in the facilitation of fetal position change

- Allow free of movement of the women during labour.

- Side-lying positon: the woman may be placed on one side and then asked to move to the other side as the fetus rotate.
- Knee-chest position or hands-and-knees positon provides a downward slant to the vaginal canal, directing the fetal head downward on descent, and is often effective in rotating the fetus.
- Pelvic-rocking: addition to position changing, as to maintaining a hands-and-knees position on the bed, the woman may do pelvic rocking to facilitate the rotation of fetus(Figure 3-15-2).
- In addition to these positons, the woman may want to sit on the toilet, walk around the room, stand beside the bed and lean forward with her hands on the bed and do the pelvicrock, rest in a whirlpool, or lie on her side in the bed. The woman's chioce should be respected and supportive care should be offered(Figure 3-15-3).

有产程延长或手术助产情况。

3.15.4.2　医疗措施

- 给予支持性照顾,协助产妇改变体位和饮食支持,等待自然分娩。
- 给予徒手协助旋转胎位到枕前,并等待自然分娩。
- 在枕后位应用产钳助娩。
- 在枕前位应用产钳助娩(徒手或用产钳转成枕前位后)。
- 产程中密切观察母亲和胎儿情况并做好记录。

3.15.4.3　母亲体位改变协助胎方位的改变

- 鼓励支持产妇在产程中保持自由活动。
- 侧卧:产妇可以先躺向一侧,再转向另一侧,以利于胎儿转动。

- 胸膝支持或手膝支撑的俯卧位时胎儿重力作用朝向产道,有利于胎头的下降和旋转。

- 骨盆的晃动:除了产妇体位的改变,如手膝支持俯卧位,产妇可能想晃动臀位来帮助胎头的转动,如图 3-15-2 所示。

- 除了上述的体位改变,产妇可能想坐到便器上、在房间内走动散步、靠床边站立、扶物前倾站立并晃动骨盆、或希望在浴盆里休息,或在床上侧卧。妇女的自身愿望应当得到尊重并给予支持,如图 3-15-3 所示。

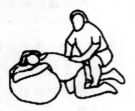

Figure 3-15-2　Hands-and-knees position and pelvic rocking

图 3-15-2　手膝支持俯卧位和骨盆晃动

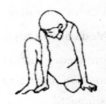

Figure 3-15-3　Woman position on choice

图 3-13-3　产妇自我选择的其他体位

3.15.4.4　Manual rotation of occiput-posteriou(pop) position

Manual rotation is an effective technique for reducing the cesarean delivery rate in patients with an occiput posterior or transverse position during labor. The risk of failure is higher when manual rotation is attempted before full dilatation , so manual rotation is recommended only when it is reached to full dilatation or later.

- The patient bladder emptied.
- The patient is placed in a dorsal recumbent (flat) position.
- When the uterus is relaxed (between the constractions), the operator gently places two fingers or, if possible, the entire hand (right hand for left occiput posterior [OP] and transverse [OT] positions and left hand for the right OP and OT positions) behind the fetal ear (right for left positions and left for right positions).
- During the uterine contraction, while the patient is pushing, the operator uses the pressure of the fingers to rotate the anterior fetal head, moving the occiput relative toward the anterior pelvic girdle.
- Fetal heart rate (FHR) is monitored continuously throughout these procedures.
- The maneuver can be performed again if the FHR is reassuring.

3.15.4.4　徒手旋转枕后位

在枕后位或横位产妇，徒手协助胎头旋转是一个有效的方法，能够降低剖宫产率。当宫口没有开全之前应用，失败概率增高，所以提倡在宫口开全或以后应用。方法如下：

- 产妇排空膀胱。
- 产妇取仰卧位（截石位）。
- 在两次宫缩之间，操作者轻轻置两手指（如果可能，用整个手掌）进入阴道置于胎儿耳后，左手用于左枕后、横，右手用于右枕后、横。
- 在子宫收缩并且产妇开始用力时，操作者用手指协助胎头向枕前位旋转，使枕骨朝向耻骨前方。
- 在操作过程中，要持续听诊监护胎心（发现异常要停止）。
- 如果胎心正常，该操作可重复进行。

3.15.5　Complicated labour: labour process

3.15.5.1　Delay in the established first stage

1. Definition

- Established(active) first stage of labour is a period of progressive cervical dilatation from 4 cm to full dilatation.
- A diagnosis of delay in the established first stage of labour needs to take into consideration all aspects of progress in labour and should include:
    → cervical dilatation of less than 2 cm in 4 hours for first labours.
    → cervical dilatation of less than 2 cm in 4 hours or a slowing in the progress of labour for second or subsequent labours.
    → descent and rotation of the fetal head.
    → changes in the strength, duration and frequency of uterine contractions.

2. Management of delay in the established first stage

- Where delay in the established first stage is suspected the following should be considered:
    → parity.
    → cervical dilatation and rate of change.
    → uterine contractions.
    → station and position of presenting part.
    → the woman's emotional state.
    → referral to the appropriate healthcare professional.
- Women should be offered support, hydration, and appropriate and effective pain relief.
- All women with suspected delay in the established first stage of labour should be advised to have a vaginal examination 2 hours later, and if progress is less than 1 cm a diagnosis of delay is made.
- In women confirmed delay in the established first stage of labour with intact membranes, amniotomy should be advised to the woman, and she should be advised to have a repeat vaginal examination 2 hours later whether her membranes are ruptured or intact.

3.15.5　产程异常

3.15.5.1　第一产程活跃期延长

1. 定义

- 第一产程活跃期是指自宫口开大 4 cm 到宫口开全的一段时间。
- 第一产程活跃期的诊断,需要考虑下列影响产程进展的可能因素:
    → 在初产妇,宫口在 4 h 内开大小于 2 cm。
    → 在经产妇,宫口在 4 h 内开大小于 2 cm。

    → 胎头下降和胎头旋转。
    → 子宫收缩的强度、持续时间、频率等是否正常。

2. 第一产程活跃期延长的处理

- 当怀疑有第一产程活跃期延长时,要关注以下情况:
    → 产妇的孕次、产次。
    → 宫口开大的程度和变化。
    → 子宫收缩。
    → 胎位及胎先露位置。
    → 产妇的精神心理状态。
    → 报告给相应的产科专家。
- 给予产妇支持关怀、饮食支持、有效的分娩镇痛措施。
- 对怀疑有活跃期延长的产妇,2 h 后要再次阴道检查,如果宫口扩张小于 1 cm,可以确诊。

- 确诊为活跃期延长的产妇,如果胎膜仍然完整,建议人工破膜。告之产妇 2 h 后要再次阴道检查(不管进行了人工破膜,还是未行破膜,均要再次检查)。

- Amniotomy alone for suspected delay in the established first stage of labour is not an indication to commence continuous EFM.
- When delay in the established first stage of labour is confirmed, the use of oxytocin should be considered. A full assessment, including an abdominal palpation and vaginal examination should be performed before making a decision about the use of oxytocin.
- Women should be informed that oxytocin will increase the frequency and strength of their contractions and that its use will mean their baby should be monitored continuously.
- Where oxytocin is used, the time between increments of the dose should be no more frequent than every 30 minutes.
- The woman should be advised to have a vaginal examination 4 hours after commencing oxytocin in established labour.
- If there is less than 2 cm progress after 4 hours of oxytocin, further obstetric review is required to consider caesarean section. If there is 2 cm or more progress, vaginalexaminations should be advised 4-hourly.
- Where a diagnosis of delay in the established first stage of labour is made, continuous EFM should be offered.
- Continuous EFM should be used when oxytocin is administered for augmentation.

3.15.5.2 Complicated labour: second stage

1. Definition and management
- Birth would be expected to take place within 3 hours of the start of the active second stage(from fulldilatation of the cervical and women start pushing spoutneously in most nulliparous women, and within 2 hours in most parous women.
- In nulliparous women, if after 1 hour of active second stage progress is inadequate, delay is

- 在单纯行人工破膜处理的产妇,不需要进行持续性的胎心监护。
- 当确诊为活跃期延长,应报告上级医生,考虑是否应用缩宫素。在决定是否需要应用缩宫素之前,要进行全面完整的评估检查。

- 应用缩宫素前,要告之产妇,缩宫素将使宫缩加强,在应用期间要持续监护胎儿情况(持续性的胎心监护)。
- 应用缩宫素期间,增加剂量的间隔时间不能短于 30 min。

- 应用缩宫素后 4 h,要进行 1 次阴道检查。

- 如果在应用缩宫素 4 h 后检查,宫口扩张小于 2 cm/4 h,要进一步评估,考虑剖宫产;如果宫口扩张大于 2 cm,4 h 后再次阴道检查。
- 确诊为活跃期延长的孕产妇要进行持续性胎心监护。

- 应用缩宫素的孕产妇要进行持续性胎心监护。

3.15.5.2 异常产程:第二产程

1. 第二产程异常的定义与处理原则
- 在大部分初产妇,第二产程的活跃期(自宫口开全并产妇自主用力开始)开始后,一般在 3 h 内结束分娩。在经产妇一般 2 h 内结束分娩。
- 在初产妇,如果第二产程活跃期开始后 1 h 未见明显的进展,怀

suspected. Following vaginal examination, amniotomy should be offered if the membranes are intact.

- A diagnosis of delay in the active second stage should be made when it has lasted 2 hours in nulliparous women and women should be referred to a healthcare professional trained to undertake an operative vaginal birth if birth is not imminent.

- A diagnosis of delay in the active second stage should be made when it has lasted 1hour in parous women and women should be referred to a healthcare professional trained to undertake an operative vaginalbirth if birth is not imminent.

- Where there is delay in the second stage of labour, or if the woman is excessively distressed, support and sensitive encouragement and the woman's need for analgesia are particularly important.

- Women with confirmed delay in the second stage should be assessed by an obstetrician but oxytocin should not be started.

- Following initial obstetric assessment for women with delay in the second stage of labour, ongoing obstetric review should be maintained every 15-30 minutes.

2. Delayed second stage and instrumental birth

- Instrumental birth should be considered if there is concern about fetal wellbeing, or for prolonged second stage.

- Instrumental birth is an operative procedure that should be undertaken with tested effective anaesthesia.

- If a woman declines anaesthesia, a pudendal block combined with local anaesthetic to the perineum can be used during instrumental birth.

- Caesarean section should be advised if vaginal birth is not possible.

3.15.5.3　Complicated labour: third stage

The third stage of labour is diagnosed as prolonged if not completed within 30 minutes of the

疑有第二产程活跃期延长。需要进行阴道检查,如果胎膜未破裂,要进行人工破膜。

- 在初产妇,如果第二产程活跃期超过 2 h 而不会立即分娩,需要报告给上级医院并考虑手术助产。

- 在经产妇,如果第二产程活跃期超过 1 h 而分娩仍旧不能立即完成,要报告上级医院并考虑手术助产。

- 当产妇出现第二产程延长,或产妇产程中出现极度紧张焦虑时,要给予支持鼓励和关怀,给予恰当的镇静麻醉措施以减轻疼痛。

- 确诊为第二产程延长的产妇,要报告上级医生会诊检查,但并不立即使用缩宫素。

- 在给予最初的检查评估后,每 15～30 min 要再次评估产程进展情况。

2.第二产程延长手术助产

- 第二产程延长或者胎儿情况出现异常时,要考虑进行手术助产。

- 手术助产是一个手术操作,要进行有效的麻醉镇痛。

- 如果产妇拒绝行椎管麻醉或静脉麻醉,可进行局部的神经阻滞麻醉。

- 如果不能进行手术助产,要准备行剖宫产术。

3.15.5.3　产程异常:第三产程

第三产程延长定义为自胎儿娩出到胎盘娩出超过 30 min(主

birth of the baby with active management and 60 minutes with physiological management.

Treatment of women with a retained placenta

- Intravenous access should always be secured in women with a retained placenta.

- Intravenous infusion of oxytocin should not be used to assist the delivery of the placenta.

- For women with a retained placenta oxytocin injection into the umbilical vein with 20 IU of oxytocin in 20 ml of saline is recommended, followed by proximal clamping of the cord.

- If the placenta is still retained 30 minutes after oxytocin injection, or sooner if there is concern about the woman's condition, women should be offered an assessment of the need to remove the placenta.

- Women should be informed that this assessment can be painful and they should be advised to have analgesia or even anaesthesia for this assessment. If a woman reports pain during the assessment, the healthcare professional must immediately stop the examination and address this need.

- If manual removal of the placenta is required, this must be carried out under effective regional anaesthesia (or general anaesthesia when necessary).

3.15.6 Complicated labour: Prolapsed cord

The cord is visible outside the vagina or can be felt in the vagina below the presenting part before the birth of the baby.

3.15.6.1 If at home or in community unit

- Instruct assistant (family, staff) to position the woman's buttocks higher than the shoulder.

- Refer urgently to hospital.

动的第三产程管理)、超过 1 h（生理性第三产程管理）。

胎盘滞留的处理

- 胎盘滞留的产妇,处理前首先要建立静脉通道。

- 不要应用静脉注射缩宫素来试图帮助娩出胎盘。

- 给予 20 IU 缩宫素混合 20 ml 生理盐水脐静脉内注射,并在远端(胎儿侧)钳夹脐带。

- 脐静脉注射缩宫素后,如果 30 min 后胎盘仍未娩出,或者产妇的情况出现变化,要告知产妇可能需要手工取出胎盘。要告知产妇取胎盘可能会带来疼痛,她需要进行麻醉。

- 如果产妇在取胎盘过程中有疼痛,要立即停止操作并进行相应处理,给予恰当的镇痛。

3.15.6 产程异常:脐带脱垂

如果在胎儿娩出前脐带出现于阴道外,或能够在阴道内触摸到脐带低于胎儿先露部,称为脐带脱垂。

3.15.6.1 如果孕产妇在家中或在社区医院

- 指导产妇(家属或服务人员),让产妇取臀部抬高位(高过肩部,趴位)。

- 迅速转送到医院。

3.15.6.2　If early labour

- Push the head or presenting part out of the Pelvis and hold it above the brim/pelvis with your hand onthe abdomen until caesarean section is performed.
- If transfer not possible, allow labour to continue.

3.15.6.3　If late labour

- Call for additional help if possible (for mother and baby).
- Prepare for Newborn resuscitation.
- Ask the woman to assume an upright or squatting position to help progress.
- Expedite delivery by encouraging woman to push with contraction.
- Explain to the parents that baby may not be well, probably dead.

3.15.7　Breech presentation

- On external examination fetal head felt in fundus.

- Soft body part (leg or buttocks) felt on vaginal examination.
- Legs or buttocks presenting at perineum.

3.15.7.1　If early labour

- Refer urgently to hospital.

3.15.7.2　If late labour

- Call for additional help.
- Confirm full dilatation of the cervix by vaginal examination.
- Ensure empty bladder.
- Prepare for newborn resuscitation.

3.15.7.3　Deliver the baby

- Assist the woman into a position that will allow the baby to hang down during delivery, for example, propped up with buttocks at edge of bed or onto her hands and knees (all fours position).

3.15.6.2　如果产妇处于分娩的早期

- 上推胎头或胎儿先露部分退出骨盆,并在腹部耻骨之上握住先露部分保持这一位置,直到剖宫产开始。
- 如果不能迅速转运,让产程继续进行。

3.15.6.3　在分娩晚期

- 寻求帮助。

- 准备新生儿复苏。
- 协助产妇取直立体位或蹲位,加快分娩。
- 鼓励产妇用力协助胎儿快速娩出。
- 告之产妇或家属胎儿的情况可能不好,有可能会发生死亡。

3.15.7　臀位

- 腹部检查时,发现胎儿头部位于宫底部。
- 有阴道检查时触及胎儿腿部或臀部。
- 在阴道外见到臀部或腿先露。

3.15.7.1　如果在分娩早期

- 迅速转到上级医院。

3.15.7.2　如果在分娩晚期

- 寻求帮助。
- 阴道检查评估宫口是否开全。

- 排空膀胱。
- 准备新生儿复苏。

3.15.7.3　娩出胎儿

- 协助产妇在合适的位置,能够让胎儿娩出后有悬空的空间,例如让产妇趴在床上,臀部移到床的边缘,或者手膝支持的

- When buttocks are distending, make an episiotomy.
- Allow buttocks, trunk and shoulders to deliver spontaneously during contractions.
- After delivery of the shoulders allow the baby to hang until next contraction.

3.15.7.4 If the head does not deliver after several contractions

- Place the baby astride your left forearm with limbs hanging on each side.
- Place the middle and index fingers of the left hand over the malar cheek bones on either side to apply gentle downwards pressure to aid flexion of head.
- Keeping the left hand as described, place the index and ring fingers of the right hand over the baby's shoulders and the middle finger on the baby's head to gently aid flexion until the hairline is visible.
- When the hairline is visible, raise the baby in upward and forward direction towards the mother's abdomen until the nose and mouth are free. The assistant gives supra pubic pressure during the period to maintain flexion.

3.15.7.5 If trapped arms or shoulders

- Feel the baby's chest for arms.

- If not felt: Hold the baby gently with hands around each thigh and thumbs on sacrum.

- Gently guiding the baby down, turn the baby, keeping the back uppermost until the shoulder which was posterior (below) is now anterior (at the top) and the arm is released.
- Then turn the baby back, again keeping the back uppermost to deliver the other arm.
- Then proceed with delivery of head as described above.

俯卧位(四肢着床位)。

- 在臀部即将娩出时,做会阴切开。
- 让臀部、躯干、肩部在宫缩时自然娩出。
- 在肩部娩出后,让胎儿自然地悬空,等待下一次宫缩。

3.15.7.4 如果经过几次宫缩胎头仍未自然娩出

- 让胎儿骑跨在操作者的左手前臂,四肢分别位于前臂的两侧。
- 左手的中指和食指置于胎儿的上颌骨两边稍加力牵引,协助胎头俯屈。
- 左手牵引的同时,右手中指置于胎头枕骨,食指与无名指分别置于两侧肩部,协助左手一起轻轻下拉胎头,直到发际可见。
- 当发际显现后,协助胎头上抬朝向母亲的腹部,依次娩出面部、嘴。另一个协作者在腹部给予耻骨上的加压,协助胎头取俯屈位利于娩出。

3.15.7.5 如果肩或上肢不能娩出

- 操作者手在胎儿胸部寻找胎儿的手臂。
- 如果不能触及手臂(上肢上举),操作者双手分别轻轻握住胎儿的双大腿,拇指置于胎儿的骶骨。
- 轻轻向下牵拉胎儿,并旋转,胎背向上,直到胎儿后肩转到前肩,手臂随之娩出。

- 同法旋转娩出另一侧上肢。

- 按上述方法继续娩出胎头。

3.15.7.6 If trapped head and baby is dead

- Tie a 1 kg weight to the baby's feet and await full dilatation.
- Then proceed with delivery of head as described above.

※ NEVER pull on the breech.

※ DO NOT allow the woman to push until the cervix is fully dilated. Pushing too soon may cause the head to be trapped.

3.15.8 Multiple births

3.15.8.1 Prepare for delivery

- Prepare delivery room and equipment for birth of 2 or more babies. Include：

  →more warm cloths.
  →two sets of cord ties and razor blades.
  →resuscitation equipment for 2 babies.
  →arrange for a helper to assist you with the births and care of the babies.

3.15.8.2 Second stage of labour

- Deliver the first baby following the usual procedure. Resuscitate if necessary. Label her/him Twin 1.

- Ask helper to attend to the first baby.
- Palpate uterus immediately to determine the lie of the second baby. If transverse or oblique lie, gently turn the baby by abdominal manipulation to head or breech presentation.
- Check the presentation by vaginal examination. Check the fetal heart rate.
- Await the return of strong contractions and spontaneous rupture of the second bag of membranes, usually within 1 hour of birth of first baby, but may be longer.
- Stay with the woman and continue monitoring her and the fetal heart rate intensively.

3.15.7.6 如果胎头不能娩出,胎儿已经死亡

- 在胎儿的足部给予 1 kg 的重量作牵引,等待宫口开全。
- 宫口开全后,按上述方法娩出胎儿。

※不要在臀部牵拉。

※在宫口开全之前不要让产妇用力。用力过早容易造成胎头的娩出困难。

3.15.8 多胎分娩

3.15.8.1 分娩准备

- 做好产房准备和仪器用物准备,准备 2 份或更多的婴儿用品,包括以下:
  →更多一份衣物。
  →双份的脐带结扎用品和刀片。
  →双份的新生儿窒息复苏用品。
  →寻求协助人员的帮助。

3.15.8.2 第二产程处理

- 按常规娩出第一个胎儿。如果有必要给予复苏处理。给予标注双胎第一个新生儿。
- 让协助者照顾第一个新生儿。
- 立即进行腹部检查,触诊第二个胎儿的胎位,如果是横位或斜产式,给予手法复位至头位或臀位(并给予协助固定)。
- 行阴道检查确诊胎位。听诊评估胎心。
- 等待宫缩加强,等待第二个胎儿的胎膜自然破裂。通常在第1个胎儿娩出 1 h 内,但有时候也会等待更长时间。
- 陪伴产妇,持续地监护胎心和评估母亲情况。

- Remove wet cloths from underneath her. If feeling chilled, cover her.
- When the membranes rupture, perform vaginal examination to check for prolapsed cord. If present, see Prolapsed cord.
- When strong contractions restart, ask the mother to bear down when she feels ready.
- Deliver the second baby. Resuscitate if necessary. Label her/him Twin 2.

- After cutting the cord, ask the helper to attend to the second baby.
- Palpate the uterus for a third baby. If a third baby is felt, proceed as described above. If no third baby is felt, go to third stage of labour.

※ Do not attempt to deliver the placenta until all the babies are born.

※ Do not give the mother oxytocin until after the birth of all babies.

3.15.8.3　Third stage of labour

- Give oxytocin 10 IU IM after making sure there is not another baby.
- When the uterus is well contracted, deliver the placenta and membranes by controlled cord traction, applying traction to all cords together.
- Before and after delivery of the placenta and membranes, observe closely for vaginal bleeding because this woman is at greater risk of postpartum haemorrhage. If bleeding, see.
- Examine the placenta and membranes for completeness. There may be one large placenta with 2 umbilical cords, or a separate placenta with an umbilical cord for each baby.

3.15.8.4　Immediate postpartum care

- Monitor intensively as risk of bleeding is increased.
- Provide immediate Postpartum care.

- 更换湿透的衣物,如果产妇感到冷,给予保暖衣物。
- 当胎膜破裂后,行阴道检查,触诊有无脐带脱垂。

- 当宫缩开始加强,让产妇在宫缩时用力,如果她感到能够用力。
- 娩出第二个胎儿,如有需要给予复苏处理。标注为双胎之第二个新生儿。
- 断脐后,让协助者照顾第二个新生儿。
- 进行腹部触诊,有无第三个胎儿,如果有,按上述处理(保持胎位为头位或臀位)。

  如果没有第三个胎儿,按第三产程处理。

※不要试图娩胎盘,直至全部胎儿娩出。

※不要给予母亲缩宫素,直到所有胎儿都娩出。

3.15.8.3　第三产程处理

- 在确定没有胎儿在子宫内后,给予母亲 10 IU 缩宫素注射。
- 当子宫收缩良好时,轻轻牵拉全部的脐带,按常规娩出胎盘。

- 多胎分娩的产妇产后出血的危险性增加,在胎盘娩出前和娩出后,都要严密观察产后出血情况。
- 仔细检查胎盘和胎膜是否完整。可能是一个胎盘上有两根脐带,或两个胎盘上分别有两根脐带。

3.15.8.4　产后护理

- 严密观察产后出血情况。
- 给予产后常规的护理照顾。

→ Keep mother in health centre for longer observation.

→ Plan to measure haemoglobin postpartum if possible.

→ Give special support for care and feeding of babies.

3.15.8.5 Delayed interval delivery of the twin, DIDT

After immature delivery of the first infant in women with multifetal pregnancies, attempts have been made to delay the delivery of remaining twins, triplets, and higher-order multiples to improve perinatal outcome, provided there is no contraindications to the mother and fetus, and the contraction of the uterus vanished.

Contraindications to delayed delivery

- non reassuring status of the remaining fetus(es).
- intrauterine infection.
- severe blood loss, or prerupture of the placenta.
- rapid delivery of the remaining fetuses.
- severe abnormal of the second or third baby.
- pretupture of the membrane of the second baby.

3.15.9 Vaginal birth after previous cesarean delivery

- Vaginal birth after previous cesarean delivery (VBAC) is safe and effective for mother and fetus if recommended guidelines are in place and appreciated.
- Physicians should provide patients balanced information on what is known and what areas are controversial.
- Facilities should have a general VBAC policy that is agreed on by the obstetrics and gynecology department, with a built-in monitoring and evaluation system.
- The cesarean delivery rate can be lowered by judicious use of VBAC; however, one must never forget the potential for a uterine rupture, especially in patients who have had an induction or augmentation of labor.

→ 注意:产妇需要在产科中心进行更长时间的观察。

→ 准备测量产后血色素水平。

→ 给予新生儿特殊照料和开始哺乳。

3.15.8.5 延迟双胎第二胎分娩时间

延迟双胎第二胎分娩时间 (delayed interval delivery of the twin, DIDT)是指在第一胎儿流产或早产后,子宫收缩逐渐消退,无分娩的其他指征,为提高尚未娩出的第二胎儿的生存机会,将第二胎儿保留在子宫内继续维持妊娠数天或数周后出生。

延迟双胎第二胎分娩时间的禁忌证

- 胎儿情况不确定。
- 绒毛膜羊膜炎。
- 有阴道出血,胎盘早剥。
- 宫口开大,早产临产。
- 胎儿有严重畸形。
- 另一胎也发生胎膜早破。

3.15.9 剖宫产术后阴道分娩

- 剖宫产后阴道分娩对于母亲和胎儿是安全有效的分娩方式,如果能够规范实施实践指南。
- 医生要向孕妇提供信息权衡利害关系,包括哪些确定的信息和有争议的问题。
- 医疗机构应当有全体妇产科人员通过的剖宫产后顺产的实践指导,有健全的评估监测和评估系统。
- 正确应用剖宫产后阴道分娩能够有效降低剖宫产率,但同时也应当注意,子宫破裂的危险性是存在的,尤其是在那些引产和加强宫缩的病例。

3.15.9.1　Indications for VBAC candidate

ACOG Selection Criteria for Attempting VBAC(2)

- One or two previous low transverse cesaream deliveries.
- Climically adequate pelvis.

- No other uterine scars or previous rupture.

- Physician readily available throughout labor, capable of monitoring labor, and performing an emergency cesarean delivery.
- Availability of anesthesia and personnel for emergency cesarean delivery.

3.15.9.2　Contraindications for VBAC

ACOG Contraindications for Attemping VBAC(2)

- Previous classical or T-shaped incision or other transfundal uterine surgery.
- Contracted pelvis.
- Medical or obstetric complication that precludes vaginal delivery.
- Inability to perform immediate emergency cesarean delivery because of unavailable surgeon, anesthesia, sufficient staff, or facility.

3.15.9.3　Management during labour

- Once trials of labor after previous cesarean delivery (TOLAC): TOLAC has begun, continuous electronic fetal monitoring is necessary.
- Signs and symptoms of uterine rupture may include:
  - →fetal bradycardia.
  - →increased uterine contractions.
  - →vaginal bleeding.
  - →loss of fetal station.
  - →new onset of intense uterine pain.

3.15.9.1　试产的条件

美国妇产科学会剖宫产后顺产试产标准

- 前次剖宫产术式为子宫下段横切口。
- 此次妊娠具有阴道分娩条件，无相对头盆不称。
- 无再次子宫损伤史，如子宫穿孔、子宫肌瘤剔除等子宫有瘢痕。
- 产程中有产科医生能够持续地观察和监护分娩过程，能够实施紧急剖宫产手术。
- 具有较好的医疗监护设备及随时抢救的条件，麻醉师和其他紧急手术的人员到位。

3.15.9.2　试产的禁忌证

美国妇产科学会剖宫产后顺产试产标准

- 前次古典式或 T 形状的子宫切口，或其他经过宫底部的子宫手术。
- 骨盆狭窄。
- 有产科并发症或其他情况不能阴道分娩。
- 医院没有进行急症剖宫产的条件，如缺少产科医生、麻醉师、人员不足或其他条件限制。

3.15.9.3　产程管理

- 剖宫产后阴道分娩，开始试产（产程开始）后，要进行持续性胎心监护。
- 观察子宫破裂的症象，包括：
  - →胎心变慢。
  - →子宫收缩增强。
  - →阴道出血。
  - →胎位不能触及。
  - →子宫其他部位出现异常的剧烈的疼痛。

- Augmentation or induction of labor with oxytocin increases the risk of uterine rupture though the risk is still low (1%-2. 4%).

※ The ACOG Committee on Obstetric Practice recommends that misoprostol not be used for induction of labor in women with prior Caesareans or major uterine surgery.

3. 15. 10　Basic neonatal resuscitation

3. 15. 10. 1　Basic principle

- All relevant healthcare professionals caring for women during birth should attend a course in neonatal resuscitation at least annually, which is consistent with the algorithm adopted in the 'Newborn life support course' developed by the Resuscitation Council (UK).
- Basic resuscitation of newborn babies should be initiated with air.
- Oxygen should be available for babies who do not respond once adequate ventilation has been established.
- Emergency referral pathways for both the woman and the baby should be developed and implemented for all birth settings.

3. 15. 10. 2　Monitoring and treatment of women with meconium-stained liquor

- Continuous EFM should be advised for women with significant meconium-stained liquor, which is defined as either dark green or black amniotic fluid that is thick or tenacious, or any meconium-stained amniotic fluid containing lumps of meconium.
- Amnioinfusion should not be used for the treatment of women with meconium-stained liquor.

- 注意:应用缩宫素引产或加强宫缩会增加子宫破裂的危险,尽管发生率并不高(1%~2.4%)。

※ 美国妇产科医师协会指出,米索不能用于剖宫产后阴道分娩的引产,因为增加子宫破裂的危险。

3. 15. 10　新生儿基础生命救护

3. 15. 10. 1　基本要求

- 所有从事孕产妇健康服务的人员都要进行新生儿抢救的培训至少每年 1 次,培训内容与程序需与国家统计标准保持一致。

- 新生儿复苏最初要应用空气进行复苏。
- 如果在建立了有效的通气后,新生儿仍未恢复反应,要给予氧气。
- 所有的孕产妇服务机构都要建立有关孕妇与新生儿抢救转诊的临床路径指南。

3. 15. 10. 2　羊水污染时的监护与处理

- 如果羊水深绿或黑色黏稠状,或有块样胎便,要给予持续性的胎心监护。
- 在羊水污染的产妇中,不提倡应用羊膜腔灌注作为治疗方法。
- 羊水污染产妇的新生儿复苏准备。
- 羊水污染的产妇分娩时,要有经过新生儿复苏培训的人员在场。

3.15.10.3　Resuscitation of babies with meconium-stained liquor

- If significant meconium-stained liquor is identified, healthcare professionals trained in FBS should be available in labour and healthcare professionals trained in advanced neonatal life support should be readily available for the birth.

- Suctioning of the nasopharynx and oropharynx prior to birth of the shoulders and trunk should not be carried out.

- The upper airways should only be suctioned if the baby has thick or tenacious meconium present in the oropharynx.

- If the baby has depressed vital signs, laryngoscopy and suction under direct vision should be carried out by a healthcare professional trained in advanced neonatal life support.

- If there has been significant meconium staining and the baby is in good condition, the baby should be closely observed for signs of respiratory distress. These observations should be performed at 1 and 2 hours of age and then 2-hourly until 12 hours of age.

Case analysis

Case 1

Mao, age 28, admission at 8th of may in 2012 by "pregancy 40+4 weeks, lower abdomical pain for 7 hours". Normal pregnancy procedure, single fetus in vertical presentationi. BPD 99 mm, FL 73 mm, AFI 139 mm, placenta 2 classes. Viginal examinaition: cervical dialation 0.5 cm, S-3, 80% affacement, intact membrane.

2012-5-8 22:00 Viginal examinaiton: cervical dialation 2 cm. Large fontanelle is at 1 clock. Normal fetus heart beat, intact membrane. Indicate her move around, she feels lighter pain when in sitting position.

3.15.10.3　羊水污染的新生儿复苏

- 当胎头娩出后,立即开始吸引清理咽喉部,在胎肩和躯干未娩出前进行。

- 气管内吸引只用于有明显的口咽部胎粪污染情况下(不作常规吸引)。

- 如果新生儿呼吸不好,要由经过培训的专业人员进行气管插管和气管内吸引。

- 如果有明显的胎粪污染但新生儿情况良好,要密切观察新生儿的呼吸情况。至少每1小时1次,连续2次,然后每2小时1次至少到产后12 h。

病例分析

病例1

毛××,28岁,以"停经40+4周,下腹痛7小时"为主诉于2012年5月8日8:30入院。孕期检查正常。B超显示:单胎头位,BPD 99 mm,FL 73 mm,AFI 139 mm,胎盘2级。阴查宫颈容受80%,宫口0.5 cm,S-3,未破膜。

2012年5月8日22:00自诉开始规律腹痛,夜间睡眠不佳。

2012年5月9日8:50阴查:宫口容纳2指松,大囟在1~2点之间,前羊膜囊突。胎心基线正常,变异反应好。指导自由

10:25 Urine once. Contraction is becoming stronger. Free movement, sit, walk or stand up. Ditect heart beat of fetus in 30 mins intervals.

13:00 Viginal examination: cervical dialation is 4 cm, S-0, intacet membrane, small fontanelle is at 7 clock, the woman feels tension and want to do cesearen section due to the severe pain, encourage her and offer masage on the back.

14:00 Viginal examination: cervical dialation is 6 cm. S-0. No cervical swelling. Encourage walking aroud.

15:00 Auto rupture of membrane, viginal examination: cervical dialation is 7 cm, S+1, large fontanelle is at 12 clock, severe pain, asking for ceserean section, offer encouragement, lie on left side for rest.

17:00 Viginal examination: cervical 9 cm, S+2. Large fontanelle is at 12 clock.

17:15 Full dialation of the cervical, S+3. Large fontanelle is at 12 clock. Starting pushing in supine position.

17:35 No obvious descent of head, getting the woman off the bed and changing to squattiong positon, pushing for 20 mins.

17:50 Visible head of fetus, small fontanelle is at 1 clock(LOA).

18:01 Baby is deliveried normally. One loop of umbilical cord aroud the neck. Weight is 3650 g, Apgar score is 10 at 1 to 5 mins.

Questions

1. Explain the function of women positioin changing during the labour.

2. What is persistent "Occiput posterior position", how to care for twomen with "OPP"?

体位,下产床自主坐位,诉:坐位时疼痛较躺卧减轻。

10:25 自解小便一次。小便后宫缩渐频,自由体位,或站或坐,或走。间断 30 min 听取胎心。

13:00 阴查:宫口开大 4 cm,S-0,前羊膜囊存。小囟 7 点。宫缩渐强,产妇诉:想剖宫产,予以心理指导,宫缩时在其腰骶部指压按摩。

14:00 阴查:宫口开大 6 cm,S-0,宫颈无水肿。继续自由体位。

15:00 阴查:宫口开大 7 cm,胎膜自破,S+1,正枕后位,自诉宫缩痛难忍要求剖宫产,继续鼓励心理指导。指导左侧卧位。

17:00 阴查:宫口开大 9 cm,S+2,正枕后位。

17:15 宫口开全,S+3,正枕后位。仰卧位用力。

17:35 宫口开全,20 min 左右先露继续下降不理想,躺产床上用力效果不佳,指导下床蹲位用力 10 min。

17:50 再次上产床,拨露够大,胎位 LOA。

18:01 以 LOA 顺产一女婴,脐带绕颈一周,评 10 分,重 3650 g。

试分析:

1. 产妇的体位变化在分娩中有何作用?

2. 持续性枕后位的诊断要点是什么?如何护理枕后位产妇促进顺产?

Case 2

A patient who progressed normally during the first stage of labour until a cervical dilatation of 7 cm reaches full dilatation of the cervix after a further 5 hours. At the last examination 3/5 of the fetal head is still palpable above the pelvic brim while 3 + moulding is found on vaginal examination. The patient is prepared for the second stage of labour and is asked to bear down with contractions.

1. What complications would you expect when you consider the patient's progress during the first stage of labour?

2. What would be the most likely cause of a prolonged second stage in this patient?

3. Do you agree with the decision to allow the patient to bear down because she is fully dilated?

4. How should this patient be managed further if she is at a clinic?

5. What arrangements must be made to make the transfer of this patient as safe as possible?

Test

1. A doctore is performing a vaginal assessment on a pregnant woman in labour, and notes the presence of the umbilical cord protruding from the vagina. Which of the following would be the initial action of the dorctor?　　　　　　　(　)

   A. place the woman in the hip-up position

   B. push the cord back into the vagina

   C. call another staff by telephone

   D. offer sedation medicine to the mother

   E. pull the baby out immediately

2. Which of the following signs indicated that the woman may be in the second stage of the labour process?　　　　　　　(　)

   A. The woman begins to expel clear vaginal liquid

   B. The contractions are regular and painfull

   C. The membranes have ruptured

病例 2

一产妇,第一产程进展良好,宫口开大 7 cm 后 5 h 宫口开全,检查发现 3/5 的胎头仍然能够在腹部触及,阴道检查发现胎头 3 度的高变形。产妇准备进入第二产程,试图让产妇用力。

1. 产妇发生了什么样的并发症?产程进展是否正常?

2. 影响产妇产程进展最可能的原因是什么?

3. 你同意让产妇用力吗,因为宫口已经开全?

4. 如果是在基层的社区医院,如何管理这个产妇?

5. 如果产妇要转到上级医院,应当如何处理?

    D.　The cervical is completely dilated

    E.　The head of the fetus are at ＋3 position

3. Ragarding occipito posterior positions, which of the following is the proper answers?　　（　　）

    A.　the anterior fontanelle is in the posterior aspect of the pelvis

    B.　minority of this conditions will rotate to anterior prior to full dilatation

    C.　somecases will be deliveried by caesarean section

    D.　it can not be deliveried by ventouse

    E.　none of those cases are normal deliveried

4. Which of the following conditions are of high risk of uterine rupture?　　（　　）

    A.　had a history of hypertension

    B.　hypotonic contractions

    C.　preterm delivery

    D.　history of ceasarean section

    E.　prelabour repture of membrances this time

5. For woman suspected delayed in established labour, which of the interventions should be done in priotity?　　（　　）

    A.　to have a vaginal examination half hours later for a suspected delayed in labour

    B.　to put the woman in bed rest on her back

    C.　continuous EFM should be offered to women with suspected delayed in labour after amniotomy

    D.　oxtocin should be offered routinely

    E.　appropriate and effective pain relief should be offered

Reference answer

Case 1

    1. Free of movement and beinig allowed to adapt to the most comfortable postion whaterver the woman may like is the basic principle of normal labour care, it could shourten the labour process, resulting in less pain for women during labour, and

病例 1

    1. 产妇在产程中能够自由活动,并根据自身的感觉,选择自己感到最舒适的体位,是产程中的支持性照顾基本原则,能够缩短产程,减轻产痛,并预防胎儿宫内

less abnormal fetus unassure nse conditions.

2. Persistent opposite postion is difinded when the fetus head remained at occipit posterior position when at late labour process(the full dialation of the cercical or later).

Most cases of OP can rotate to OA during labour, to facilite the rotate, maternal position changing is essencial factors, and women should be given the choice to changing what ever position she prefer and side-lying and turn to another side, keens down, hands and knees postion, standing forward with supporting, pelvic rockinig, etc, may be efficient in the rotation of fetus.

Case 2

1. A prolonged estabilished first stage (active first stage of labour) of labour as the patient's progress in labour was slower than expected between 7 cm and full dilatation.

2. Cephalopelvic disproportion as indicated by an unengaged fetal head and 3+moulding.

3. No. As the patient has cephalopelvic disproportion, a caesarean section must be performed.

4. She must be referred to a hospital with facilities to perform a caesarean section.

5. The patient must lie on her side and an intravenous infusion must be started. If there are no contra-indications, the contractions must be stopped with intravenous hexoprenaline (Ipradol) or oral nifedipine (Adalat). If there is any concern about the condition of the fetus, the patient must be given face mask oxygen.

Test

1. A 2. D 3. C 4. D 5. D 6. E

窘迫缺氧。

2. 持续性枕后位是指在产程的晚期(宫口开全后或更晚),胎头仍然持续在枕后位的状态。

大部分的枕后位能够转成枕前位顺利分娩。为了促进胎儿自然转位,母亲体位的改变是最重要的因素。产妇可以在侧卧位并改变方向,跪,手膝支持俯卧,向前持物站立,晃动骨盆等,是可能有效的方法。

病例 2

1. 第一产程的活跃期延长,因为产妇从宫口开大 7 cm 到开全的时间超过了正常的活跃期时间。

2. 产妇产程异常的最可能原因是头盆不称,因为胎头有严重的变形和不能入盆。

3. 不同意让产妇用力。因为产妇有严重的头盆不称,可能要行剖宫产结束分娩。

4. 如果是在基层的社区医院,要及时转送到上级医院。

5. 如果要转运产妇,产妇应侧卧位,建立静脉通道,给予曲马多(Ipradol)或 nifedipine (Adalat)口服以减弱宫缩的强度,除非有其他并发症适合用药。如果有胎儿情况异常,应给予产妇面罩吸氧。

3. 16　Multiple Pregnancy

Key words

1. twin pregnancy
2. monoamnionic twin pregnancy
3. diamnionic twin pregnancy
4. monochorionic twin pregnancy

Incidence：twins 3：200 pregnancies；triplets 1：10 000.

Predisposing factors：Previous twins；FH of twins（dizygotic only）；increasing maternal age （< 20yrs 6. 4：1 000，> 25yrs 16. 8：1 000）；induced ovulation and IVF （1% of all UK pregnancies of which 25% are twin）；race origin （1：150 pregnancies for Japanese，1：36 in Nigerian Igbo women）. The worldwide rate for monozygotic （monochorionic） twins is constant at 3-5：1 000.

Early prepnancy：Uterus too large for dates；hyperemesis. Later there may be polyhydramnios. The signs are that > 2 poles may be felt；there is a multiplicity of fetal parts；2 fetal heart rates may be heard（reliable if heart rates differ by > 10 beats/min）. Ultrasound confirms diagnosis （and at 10-14 weeks can distinguish monochorionic from dichorionic twins）.

3. 16. 1　Complications during pregnancy

Polyhydramnios and pre-eclampsia is commoner （10% in singleton pregnancies； 30% in twins）. Anaemia is commoner （iron and folate requirements are increased）. APH incidence increases （6% for twins VS 4. 7% for singletons） due to both abruption and placenta praevia （large placenta）. Fetal complications. Perinatal mortality for twins is 36. 7：1 000 （8：1 000 if single；73：1 000 for triplets）.

3. 16　多胎妊娠

关键词

1. 双胎妊娠
2. 单羊膜囊双胎
3. 双羊膜囊双胎
4. 单绒毛膜双胎

发病率：双胎 3：200；三胎 1：10 000。

诱发因素：既往双胎史；双胎家族史（仅为双卵双胎）；女性年龄增长（<20 岁，6. 4：1 000；> 25 岁 16. 8：1 000）；促排卵和试管婴儿（英国 1% 的妊娠中 25% 是双胞胎）；种族起源（日本的妊娠 1：150，在尼日利亚的伊博女人 1：36），全球发生率（单绒毛膜双胎）双胞胎是 3～5：1 000。

早期妊娠特点：子宫较孕周增大，早孕反应剧烈，后期可能有羊水过多。B 超见 2 个孕囊，多个胚芽，听到 2 个胎心音，（两者相差 >10 次/min），B 超在 11～14 周可以区分单绒毛膜双胎和双绒毛膜双胎。

3. 16. 1　妊娠期的并发症

羊水过多和先兆子痫是常见并发症（占单胎的 10%，双胎的 30%），由于铁和叶酸的缺乏，贫血较常见。产前出血发病率增加（6%，单胎是 4. 7%），因为胎盘面积增大，前置胎盘和胎盘早剥发生率增加。

胎儿并发症：双胎围产期死亡率为 36. 7：1 000（单胎为 8：

The main problem is prematurity. Mean gestation for twins is 37 weeks, for triplets 33 weeks. Growth restricted babies are more common (growth the same as singletons up to 24 weeks but may be slower thereafter). Malformation rates are increased 2-4 times, especially in monozygotic twins. Severe disability rate 1.5% for singletons, 3.4% for twins. Ultrasound is the main diagnostic test. Selective fetocide (eg with intracardiac potassium chloride) is best used before 20 weeks in the rare instances where it is indicated. With monozygotic twins, placental vascular anastomoses may result in disparate twin size and one being born plethoric (so jaundiced later), the other anaemic (ie twin-twin transfusion). If one fetus dies in utero it may become a fetus papyraceous which may be aborted later or delivered prematurely. Complications of labour PPH is more common (4%-6% in singletons 10% in twins). Malpresentation is common (cephalic/cephalic 40%, cephalic/breech 40%, breech/breech 10%, cephalic/transverse (Tv) 5%, breech/Tv 4%, Tv/Tv 1%). Rupturing of vasa praevia, increased rates of cord prolapse (0.6% singleton, 2.3% twins), premature separation of the placenta and cord entanglement (especially monozygous) may all present difficulties at labour. Despite modern technology some twins remain undiagnosed, staff are unprepared, and syntometrine may be used inappropriately, so delaying delivery of the second twin. Epidural anaesthesia is helpful for versions.

3.16.2　Management

- Ensure adequate rest(need not entail admission).

- Use ultrasound for diagnosis and monthly checks on fetal growth.

- Give additional iron and folate to the mother during pregnancy.

1 000,三胎为 73∶1000)。

主要问题为早产,平均孕龄双胎是 37 周,三胎是 33 周。胎儿生长受限更常见(双胎 24 周前生长速度与单胎速度相同,24 周后较单胎减慢)。畸形率增加2～4 倍,尤其是在单卵双胎中。重度残疾率单胎为 1.5%,双胎为 3.4%。超声是诊断的主要方法。选择性减胎术(在胎心内注射氯化钾)最好在 20 周之前使用,适用于双胎之一异常,手术指征充分者。对于单卵双胎,胎盘血管吻合可致双胎大小不同,其中一胎血容量增加(今后出现黄疸),另一个胎儿贫血(比如双胎输血综合征),如双胎之一死亡形成纸样儿被吸收或早产分娩。分娩并发症 PPH 更常见,单胎为 4%,双胎为 10%。胎位异常较为常见(40%头/头,40%头/臀,10%臀位/臀位,5%头/横,4%臀/横,1%横/横)。前置血管破裂,脐带脱垂,胎盘早剥,脐带缠绕等均给分娩带来困难。运用现代科技,仍有部分双胎诊断不清,工作人员无准备,宫缩剂不适当地被使用,造成第二胎延迟分娩,在胎位不正时可改硬外麻行外倒转术。

3.16.2　孕期处理

- 确保充足的休息(未必需要住院)。
- 每月用 B 超监测胎儿的生长。
- 怀孕期间的母亲提供额外的铁和叶酸。

- More antenatal visits，eg weekly from 30 weeks (risk of eclampsia).
- Tell the mother how to identify preterm labour, and what to do. Monitoring cervical length and fFN.

Consider induction at 40weeks. Have an IVI running in labour and an anaesthetist available at delivery. Pediatricians (preferably one for each baby) should be present at delivery for resuscitation should this be necessary (second twins have a higher risk of asphyxia). Monozygous or dizygous? Monozygous twins are always same-sex and in 75% membrane consists of 2 amnions and1 chorion (if in doubt send for histology).

IVF babies，and psychological consequence of triplets

With 2 million IVF babies born worldwide since 1978 it is apparent that there are increased problems for pregnancy and offspring, not merely just those of multiple pregnancy. These are：

- Multiple birth：affects 1 in 4 IVF pregnancies. Monozygotic twins are also commoner. The rate of triplets was 5× pre-IVF rates by 1998 but are now only twice, as only 2 eggs are implanted into women <40 years old.

Older mother effects：so more pre-eclampsia, pregnancy induced hypertension, caesarean section delivery, and diabetes in the mothers(all of which have implications for offspring).

- Donor egg problems：pregnancy induced hypertension is 7. 1 times more common if nulliparous women receive donated eggs than for standard IVF.
- Genetic defects：Beckwith-Wiedeman syndromeis 6 times commoner in IVF babies and there is concern that intracytoplasmic sperm injection (ICSI) techniques could encourage chromosomal abnormalities or cystic fibrosis in offspring of men with azoospermia or oligospermia, so screening of these men for cystic fibrosis carrier status and chromosomal abnormalities before

- 更多的产前检查，如从 30 周（子痫的风险）开始每周检查。
- 告诉母亲如何识别早产，以及做什么。监测宫颈长度和阴道分泌物 fFN(胎儿纤维连接蛋白)。

考虑 40 周前分娩。分娩时有麻醉师与儿科医生(最好一个孩子一个医生)在场。做好新生儿窒息复苏的准备。双胎中的第二个具有较高的窒息风险。是单绒毛膜单胎还是双绒毛膜双胎？单绒毛膜双胎都是性别相同的，其中的 75% 为两层羊膜，一层绒毛膜。

试管婴儿和三胞胎的心理后果

自 1978 年以来全世界有 200 万试管婴儿出生，很明显，有关妊娠和子代的问题也随之增加。不仅仅是多胎妊娠的问题，还有多次"生育"占 IVF 的 1/4，单绒毛膜双胎也更加常见，至 1998 年 IVF 中的三胎妊娠率增加了五倍，但现在只有 2 倍，因为现在<40 岁的妇女只植入 2 个受精卵。

高龄产妇效应：高龄孕妇更易出现子痫前期、妊娠期高血压、剖宫产、糖尿病等。(所有这些都影响到了后代。)

捐卵的问题：捐卵的初孕妇妊娠期高血压率是正常 IVF 的 7.1 倍。

遗传缺陷：Beckwith-Wiedeman 综合征 IVF 胎儿发病率是正常人的 6 倍。现在认为单精子注射技术(ICSI)可能会增加无精或少精男性子代的染色体异常或囊性纤维瘤的发病率。所以推荐对这些男性在 ICSI 前进行囊性纤维

performing ICSI is recommended.

　　• Low birthweight is 1. 75 times commoner for singleton IVF babies compared to naturally conceived babies （and very low birthweight 2. 7-3 times commoner）. Part of this is due to prematurity, part to growth restriction.

Interestingly low birthweight is particularly correlated to the number of gestation sacs at earliest scan, even if a baby ends up as a singleton. IVF twins are less commonly low birthweight compared to naturally conceived twins.

　　• Prematurily is twice as common in IVF singleton babies compared to those naturally conceived, 3 times more common for prematurity<32 weeks. Again it is commoner if there was originally >1 gestation sac. Current practice is to implant only 2 embryos in mothers <40 yrs; though 3 may be implanted if she is>40 yrs.

3. 17　Genetic Counseling, Prenatal Screening and Prenatal Diagnosis

Key words

1. genetic counseling
2. prenatal diagnosis
3. Down's syndrome
4. nuchal translucency
5. thalassemia

The first half of pregnancy can become a time of constant "exams" to see if the baby can be allowed to graduate to the second half of pregnancy. Those at high and, increasingly, those at low risk of having an abnormal baby are offered prenatal diagnosis to allow better treatment of the expected defect, or （more often）if they would wish to terminate any abnormal fetus.

瘤的筛查。

　　单胎 IVF 胎儿发病率是自然受孕的 1. 75 倍（极低体重儿是自然受孕的 2. 7 到 1. 3 倍）,部分由于早产,部分由于发育受限,有趣的是,低体重与最早的 B 超所见孕囊的数目相关。即使最后妊娠结局为单胎依然如此。试管婴儿的妊娠双胎较自然受孕双胎发生概率低。

　　早产 IVF 单胎是自然妊娠单胎的两倍,小于 32 周的早产发生率为自然受孕的 3 倍。同样,如果早期孕囊数大于 1,发病率增高。英国目前的做法是在小于 40 岁的女性身上只放两个,大于 40 岁的可以放 3 个。

3. 17　遗传咨询、产前筛查 与产前诊断

关键词

1. 遗传咨询
2. 产前诊断
3. 唐氏综合征
4. 颈项透明带
5. 地中海贫血

　　妊娠的前半阶段是产前咨询的时期,我们要检查胎儿可否进入后半阶段,那些高危的有异常风险的胎儿将接受产前诊断,以便对出现的问题做更好的治疗,或者更通常地她们想终止妊娠放弃异常的胎儿。

High-risk pregnancies

1. Maternal age＞35.

2. First or second trimester serum screen is positive.

3. Previous abnormal baby or one of the parents has abnormal chromosome.

4. Unknown reason for still birth and abnormal fetus.

5. Severn single gene carrier in one of the parents.

6. Abnormal ultrasound finding.

7. Exposure to high dose of radio-rays, virus or harmful medicine.

8. Other conditions.

Ultrasound at 11-14 weeks is useful for dating pregnancy and for nuchal translucency screening. Further anomaly scan is at ～ 18weeks. Skilled operators can detect many external and internal structural anomalies. Ultrasound is best at detecting externally impinging structural abnormalities, eg anencephaly/spina bifida. Internal structural abnormality detection rate, eg for heart disease and diaphragmatic hernia, remains＜50％. Fetuses with false ＋ ve suggestion of abnormality are mostly associated with "soft signs" on ultrasound, eg nuchal thickening (eg trisomy 21), choroid plexus cysts (trisomies 18 and 21), and echogenic bowel(trisomy 2l and cystic fibrosis). Use of "soft signs" may increase false＋ves 12-fold.

α-Fetoprotein(AFP)is a glycoprotein synthesized by the fetal liver and GI tract Fetal levels fall after 13 weeks, but maternal (transplacental) serum AFP continues to rise to 30 weeks. Maternal AFP is measured at 17 weeks. In 10％ with a high AFP there is a fetal malformation, eg an open neural tube

高危风险包括

1. 孕妇年龄达 35 岁或以上。

2. 孕早、中期血清筛查阳性的孕妇。早期异常婴儿或遗传家庭史。

3. 夫妇一方为染色体病患者,或曾妊娠、生育过染色体病患儿的孕妇。

4. 有不明原因自然流产史、畸胎史、死胎或死产史的孕妇。

5. 怀有严重单基因遗传病高风险胎儿的孕妇。

6. 有异常胎儿超声波检查结果者。

7. 孕早期曾患过严重的病毒感染,或接受较大剂量放射线,服用过可能致畸药物。

8. 其他情况。

11～14 周超声检查确定胎儿孕龄和颈项透明带厚度 nuchal Translucency(NT)检查,进一步的胎儿解剖学 B 超在 18 周,开始由熟练的超声医生检查,可以检查出很多外在和内在的结构畸形。B 超最适合检查胎儿的外部结构异常,比如无脑儿、脊柱裂。内部结构的异常检出率,比如心脏病、膈疝约小于 50％,检查为假阳性的胎儿大多数为超声软指标,比如 NT 增宽(21 三体),脉络丛囊肿(18 及 21 三体),肠管强回声(21 三体和囊状纤维瘤),运用软指标可以增加假阳性率 12 倍。

α-甲胎蛋白(AFP) 是由胎儿肝脏和消化道产生的糖蛋白,其在胎儿内的水平 13 周后下降,但孕妇(通过胎盘的)血清 AFP 持续增高直到孕 30 周,孕妇 AFP 在孕 17 周可以检测到。AFP 增

defect (but closed defects are missed), exomphalos, posterior urethral valves, nephrosis, GI obstruction, teratomas. Turner's syndrome (or normal twins). In ～30% of those with no malformation, there is an adverse outcome, eg placenta abruption and third trimester deaths. Closely monitoring is necessary. In 40with a low AFP have a chromosomal abnormality (eg Down's). AFP is lower in diabetic mothers. As this test is non-specific on its own, it is of use for preliminary screening; those with abnormal values may be offered further tests.

Amniocentesis is done under continuous ultrasound control. Fetal loss rate is 0.5%-1% at ～16 weeks' gestation. Amniotic fluid AFP is measured (a more accurate screen for neural tube defects than maternal serum), and cells in the fluid are cultured for karyotyping (+enzyme and gene probe analysis). Cell culture takes 3wks, so an abnormal pregnancy must be terminated at a late stage.

Chorionic villus biopsy：At 10$^+$ weeks, placenta is sampled by transcervical or transabdominal approach under continuous ultrasound control. Karyotyping takes 2 weeks, enzyme and gene probe analysis 3 days, so termination for abnormality is earlier, safer, and less distressing than after amniocentesis. Fetal loss rate is ～4%. Use up to 20weeks (cordocentesis preferable thereafter) It does not detect neural tube defects and is not recommended in dichorionic multiple pregnancy.

Fetoscopy is carried out with ultrasound guidance to find external malformations, do fetal blood samples, or biopsy. Fetal loss rate is ～4%.

High resolution ultrasound and fetal nuchal translucency (NT)

• Early scans(at 11-14 weeks) may detect 59% of those with structural abnormality and 78%of those with chromosome abnormality. It is best at detecting CNS defects, neck abnormalities, GL, and renal defects：less good for spina bifida, heart and limb

高者 10％伴有胎儿畸形，比如神经管缺陷（不包括闭合的缺陷）、腹壁裂、尿道下裂、肾病、消化道梗阻、畸胎瘤、特纳综合征（或正常双胎），约 30％不伴有胎儿畸形，但有不良妊娠结局，比如胎盘早剥和晚孕死胎，需要密切监护胎儿。在糖尿病孕妇中 AFP 下降，因为 AFP 是一个非特异指标，所以用以初始的筛查，当有异常时，须作进一步的检查。

羊膜腔穿刺术，是在 B 超监护下进行，16 周时胎儿流产率0.5％～1％。羊水 AFP 在神经管畸形时增高。羊水细胞经过培养后进行核型分析，细胞培养需要三周时间，所以异常的妊娠在晚些时候需要终止。

绒毛活检（CVS），在孕 10$^+$周在持续 B 超引导下经阴道或腹部取绒毛，核型分析需两个星期时间，基因分析需 3 天，所以相对于羊水检查胎儿畸形的终止妊娠时间更早、更安全，心理压力更小，胎儿的丢失率约 4％，大于 20周后可考虑脐带穿刺，CVS 不能诊断神经管缺陷，不建议用于双绒膜双胎。

胎儿镜，是在超声引导下检查胎儿外在的畸形，采用胎儿血标本或胎儿活检，胎儿丢失率约 4％。

高分辨率超声及胎儿颈项透明层检查

高分辨率超声，早期 11～14周检查可以检查出 59％的结构畸形，78％的染色体异常，它最佳用于检测神经管缺陷、颈部异常、泌尿系缺陷，其次为检测中枢神

defects. With a combination of early and later scans up to 81% of malformations may be diagnosed.

• Fluid accumulation in the neck at 11-44 weeks' gestation(increased fetal nuchal translucency, FNT) may reflect fetal heart failure; and be seen in serious anomaly of the heart and great arteries.

• There is a strong association between chromosomal abnormality and FNT. In one study, 84% of karyotypically proven trisomy 21 fetuses had a nuchal translucency >3 mm at 10-13 weeks' gestation (as did 4.5% of chromosomally normal fetuses).

• The greater the extent of FNT, the greater the risk of abnormality.

• It is useful for screening twins as early detection is best, for if selective fetocide is to be used risk of miscarriage is 3-fold higher if done after 16 weeks. Monochorionic twins have a higher false+ve rate for nuchal translucency thickness than dichorionic twins or singletons.

In the 25% of monochorionic twins with FNT discordance of >20%, more than 30% had early fetal death or severe twin-twin transfusion syndrome (10% if less disordance).

• Note that the degree of neck flexion during the ultrasound examination May influence nuchal measurements.

• Other "soft marker" for Down's syndrome are fetal nasal bone appearance, the Doppler velocity wave form in the ductus venosus and tricuspid regurgitation.

Case analysis

Question：

What's the treatment for the following patients?

×××, female, 30 years old, G1P0, 17 weeks pregnant. Down 1∶190, past history, no genetic history. Physical examination and previous history were normal.

×××, female, 29 years old, children with thalassemia

经系统缺陷、脊柱裂、心脏和四肢缺陷,早孕和中孕联合可以诊断出 81% 的畸形。

11～14 周 NT 增宽见于:胎儿心衰,严重的胎儿心脏及大血管畸形。

胎儿 NT 增宽与染色体畸形密切相关,84% 的核型分析证实为 21 三体的胎儿在 10～13 周 NT 大于 3 mm,而正常胎儿仅有 4.5% NT >3 mm。

NT 增厚程度越高,胎儿畸形程度越高。

NT 对于双胎妊娠的早期诊断是最好的方法,因为它可以进一步做选择性减胎术,而 16 周后的减胎流产率增加 3 倍。单绒毛膜双胎 NT 增宽的比例较双绒毛膜双胎和单胎增加。

25% 的单绒毛膜双胎之间 NT 差异 >20%,其中 30% 出现双胎之一死亡和双胎出血综合征。(在差异较小的双胎中 TTTS 发生率为 10%)

注意胎儿颈部俯屈的程度将影响 NT 的测量。其他的 21 三体软指标包括胎儿鼻骨的存在,静脉导管的血流和三尖瓣的反流等。

案例分析

问题：

下列病人如何处理?

×××,女,30 岁,G1P0,孕 17 周。唐氏 1∶190,既往史正常,无遗传史。体检及既往史均正常。

×××,女,29 岁,有一地贫

who died at 19 weeks of pregnancy and ventricular arrhythmias, the couples are thalassemia carriers. Physical examination and previous history were normal.

患儿夭折，孕 19 周，室性心律不齐，该夫妇双方均为地贫携带者。体检及既往史均正常。

Answer：

1. Do aminocentesis for fetal karatyping.

2. Do aminocentesis for fetal gene analyzing of thalassemia.

答案：

1. 产前诊断查羊水染色体。

2. 产前诊断查羊水地贫基因。

附：产前筛查流程图

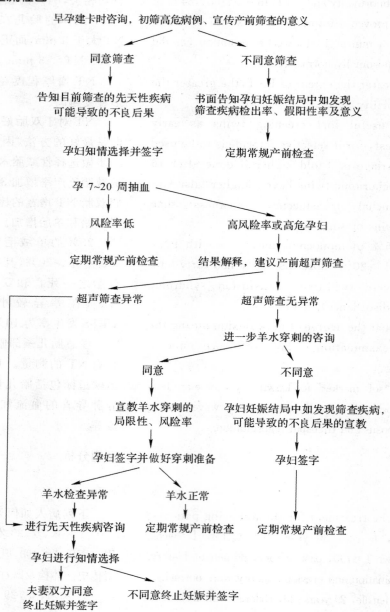

Chapter 4　Gynaecology

第 4 章　妇科

4.1　Hiatory-taking in Gynaecology

4.1　妇科病史采集

Key words

1. last menstrual period，LMP
2. leucorrhea
3. ruritus vulvae

关键词

1. 末次月经日期
2. 白带
3. 外阴瘙痒

To adequately evaluate the gynaecologic patient，it is important to establish a rapport during the history taking. The patient needs to tell her story to an interested listener who does not allow body language or facial expressions to imply disinterest or boredom. One should avoid cutting off the patient's story, because doing so may obscure important clues or other problems that may have contributed to the reasons for the visit.

The following outline varies from the routine medical history because，in evaluating the gynaecologic patient，the problem often can be clarified if the history is obtained in the following order.

在妇科病史采集中，为充分评估患者的情况，需要与其建立信任关系。患者所面对的倾听者应该耐心，不应表现出任何漠不关心或厌烦的肢体语言和面部表情。医生不应打断患者的叙述，以免遗漏有助于解决就诊患者疾病的重要线索。

以下列出的病史采集要点与常规内科病史采集有所不同。因为在评估妇科病人时，如果病史按以下顺序获得，问题常常可分类。

4.1.1　Demographic details

Name，age，date of birth，occupation.

4.1.1　个人资料

姓名、年龄、出生日期、职业。

4.1.2　Presenting complaint

Ask the patient to tell you in her own words what she perceives the main symptom or symptoms to be. Document each in order of severity.

4.1.2　当前主述

让患者用自己的语言表述其对主要症状的感觉。按症状的严重性依次记录。

4.1.3　History of presenting complaint

More detailed questioning will depend on the

4.1.3　现病史

根据患者主述的性质展开，

nature of the presenting complaint as the following：

1. The exact nature of the symptom.

2. The onset.

(1) When and how it began (*e. g.* suddenly, gradually—over how long?)

(2) If longstanding, why is the patient seeking help now?

3. Periodicity and frequency.

(1) Is the symptom constant or intermittent?

(2) If intermittent, how long does it last each time?

(3) What is the exact manner in which it comes and goes?

(4) How does it relate to the menstrual cycle?

4. Change over time.

5. Exacerbating and relieving factors.

6. Associated symptoms.

7. The degree of functional disability caused.

4. 1. 4 Menstrual history

1. Age of menarche (first menstrual period). Normally about 12 years but can be early as 9 or as late as 16.

2. Date of last menstrual period (LMP).

3. Duration and regularity of periods (cycle).

(1) Normal menstruation lasts 4-7 days.

(2) Average length of menstrual cycle is 28 days (*i. e.* the time between first day of one period and the first day of the following period) but can vary between 21 and 42 days in normal women.

4. Menstrual flow：whether light, normal, or heavy.

5. Menstrual pain：whether occurs prior to or at the start of bleeding.

6. Irregular bleeding：*e. g.* intermenstrual blood-loss, post-coital bleeding, etc.

7. Associated symptoms：bowel or bladder dysfunction, pain.

按以下步骤详细询问现病史：

1. 症状的准确性质。

2. 症状的起始过程。

(1) 何时及如何起病（如突然，逐渐，多久）?

(2) 如起病已久，为何现在才来就诊?

3. 周期性和频率。

(1) 症状是持续性还是间歇性?

(2) 如为间歇性，每次持续多久?

(3) 发作和缓解的模式如何?

(4) 与月经周期的相关性?

4. 随时间的改变。

5. 加重和缓解因素。

6. 相关症状。

7. 导致功能障碍的程度。

4. 1. 4 月经史

1. 月经初潮年龄。通常为12 岁，也可为 9～16 岁之间。

2. 末次月经日期(LMP)。

3. 月经周期的持续时间和规则性。

(1) 正常经期持续 4～7 天。

(2) 正常月经周期平均为 28天（即上一周期第一天到下一周期第一天的间隔），也可为 21～42 天。

4. 月经量：是否少，正常或多。

5. 月经期疼痛：是否发生在出血前或出血时。

6. 不规则出血：如月经间期出血、性交后出血等。

7. 相关症状：肠道或膀胱功能障碍，疼痛。

8. Hormonal contraception or HRT.

9. Age at menopause (if this has occurred).

4.1.5　Past gynaecological history

Record all details of：

1. Previous cervical smears，including date of last smear，any abnormal smear results，and treatments received.

2. Previous gynaecological problems and treatments including surgery and pelvic inflammatory disease.

3. It is also essential to ask sexually active women of reproductive age about contraception，including methods used，duration of use and acceptance，current method，as well as future plans.

4.1.6　Past obstetric history

1. Gravidity and parity.

2. Document the specifics of each pregnancy：

(1) Current age of the child and age of mother when pregnant.

(2) Birth weight.

(3) Complications of pregnancy，labour，and puerperium.

(4) Miscarriages and terminations. Note gestation time and complications.

4.1.7　Past medical history

Pay particular attention to any history of chronic lung or heart disease and make note of all previous surgical procedures.

4.1.8　Drug history

Ask about all mediction/drugs taken（prescribed，over the counter and illicit drugs）. Record dose，frequency，as well as any known drug allergies.

Make particular note to ask about the oral contraceptive pill（OCP）and hormone replacement therapy（HRT）if not done so already.

8. 激素避孕或激素替代治疗。

9. 绝经年龄（如已绝经）。

4.1.5　妇科既往史

记录以下细节：

1. 既往宫颈涂片情况，包括日期，任何异常结果和接受的治疗。

2. 既往妇科问题和处理，包括手术和盆腔炎性疾病。

3. 对于生育年龄的性活跃妇女，有必要询问避孕情况，包括方法、持续时间和接受程度，现用方法和未来计划。

4.1.6　产科既往史

1. 妊娠次数和产次。

2. 记录每次妊娠的细节。

(1) 子女年龄和妊娠时的年龄。

(2) 子女出生体重。

(3) 妊娠、分娩和产褥期并发症。

(4) 流产和终止妊娠。记录妊娠时间和并发症。

4.1.7　内科既往史

尤其注意慢性肺病或心脏病病史，并记录所有既往手术史。

4.1.8　药物史

询问所有使用药物（处方药、非处方药和违禁药品）。记录剂量、服药频率和已知药物过敏情况。

详细询问口服避孕药（OCP）和激素替代治疗（HRT）情况。

4.1.9　Family history

Note especially any history of genital tract cancer, breast cancer and diabetes.

4.2　Gynaecological Examination

The gynaecological examination should include a full abdominal examination before proceeding to the pelvic, speculum, and bimanual examinations.

Explain to the patient that you would like to examine their genitalia and reproductive organs and reassure them that the procedure will be quick and gentle.

You should have a chaperone present, particularly if you are a male.

As always, ensure that the room is warm and well lit, preferably with a moveable light source and that you will not be disturbed.

The examination should follow an orderly routine. The authors' suggestion is shown below. It is standard practice to start with the cardiovascular and respiratory systems—this not only gives a measure of the general health of the patient but establishes a "physical rapport" before you examine more delicate or embarrassing areas.

Table 4-2-1　Framework for the gynaecological examination

1. General inspection.
2. Cardiorespiratory examination.
3. Abdominal examination.
4. Pelvic examination:
(1)External genitalia—inspection.
(2)External genitalia—palpation.
(3)Speculum examination.
(4)Bimanual examination("PV" examination).

4.1.9　家族史

尤其注意家族成员中生殖器肿瘤、乳腺癌和糖尿病史。

4.2　妇科检查

完整的腹部检查为妇科体格检查的组成部分,应在盆腔检查、窥检和双合诊之前进行。

检查之前,向患者说明需要检查内外生殖器官,并且整个过程会快速而轻柔,以便征得患者的同意和配合。

男医师对患者进行妇科检查时,应有一名女伴在场。

检查室应保持温暖和光线充足,最好具备可移动的光源,并且确保不被打扰。

检查应该遵循一定顺序,编者推荐如下:常规操作是先从心血管和呼吸系统检查开始,这样既可以了解患者的一般健康情况,又能建立一种"生理默契",以减轻之后检查隐私、尴尬部位时患者的紧张心理。

表 4-2-1　妇科检查的基本框架

1. 全身一般检查。
2. 心血管和呼吸系统检查。
3. 腹部检查。
4. 盆腔检查:
(1)外生殖器——视诊。
(2)外生殖器——触诊。
(3)窥器检查。
(4)双合诊("PV"检查)。

4.2.1　General inspection and other systems

Always begin with a general examination of the patient including temperature, hydration, coloration, nutritional status, lymph nodes, and blood pressure. Note especially:

- Distribution of facial and body hair, as hirsutism may be a presenting symptom of various endocrine disorders.
- Height and weight.
- Examine the cardiovascular and respiratory systems in turn.

4.2.2　Abdominal examination

A full abdominal examination should be performed. Look especially in the periumbilical region where transverse incisions from caesarean sections and most gynaecological operations are found.

4.2.3　Pelvic examination

The patient should be allowed to undress in privacy and, if necessary, to empty her bladder first.

4.2.3.1　Set up and positioning

Before starting the examination, always explain to the patient what will be involved. Ensure the abdomen is covered. Ensure good lighting and remember to wear disposable gloves.

Ask the patient to lie on her back on an examination couch with both knees bent up and let her knees fall apart—either with her heels together in the middle or separated.

The lithotomy position, in which both thighs are abducted and feet suspended from lithotomy stirrups is usually adopted when performing vaginal surgery.

4.2.1　全身各系统检查

检查从一般情况开始,包括体温、是否脱水、皮肤着色、营养状况、浅表淋巴结以及血压等。着重记录:

- 面部及身体毛发的分布,如多毛症,可为多种内分泌紊乱疾病的症状。
- 身高和体重。
- 依次检查心血管系统和呼吸系统。

4.2.2　腹部检查

腹部检查应该全面完整,尤其要注意脐周区域,可见剖宫产和多数妇科手术的切口。

4.2.3　盆腔检查

盆腔检查前,让患者除去多余衣物,必要时排空膀胱,注意保护患者隐私。

4.2.3.1　准备工作和体位

检查前需告知患者进行盆腔检查的内容,确保遮盖腹部和充足照明,检查者注意佩戴一次性手套。

要求患者仰卧在检查床上,双膝弯曲,保持分开,双足可放在中间或分开。

妇科患者取截石位,双腿放置于腿架上,使大腿外展,足部悬垂,将臀部移到床边,能充分暴露会阴部,常用于阴道手术。

4.2.3.2　Examination of the external genitalia

1. Inspection

Uncover the mons to expose the external genitalia making note of the pattern of hair distribution.

Apply a lubricating gel to the examining finger.

Separate the labia from above with the forefinger and thumb of your left hand.

Inspect the clitoris, urethral meatus, and vaginal opening.

Look especially for any:

(1)Discharge.

(2)Redness.

(3)Ulceration.

(4)Atrophy.

(5)Old scars.

Ask the patient to cough or strain down and look at the vaginal walls for any prolapse.

2. Palpation

Palpate the length of labia majora between the index finger and thumb.

(1)The tissue should feel pliant and fleshy.

Palpate for Bartholin's gland with the index finger of the right hand just inside the introitus and the thumb on the outer aspect of the labium majora.

(2)Batholin's glands are only palpable if the duct becomes obstructed resulting in a painless cystic mass or an acute Bartholin's abscess. The latter is seen as a hot, red, tender swelling in the posterolateral labia majora.

4.2.3.3　Speculum examination

Speculum examination is carried out to see further inside the vagina and to visualize the cervix. It also allows the examiner to take a cervical smear or swabs.

There are different types of vaginal specula (Figure 4-2-1) but the commonest is the Cusco's or bivalve speculum. Many departments and clinical

4.2.3.2　外生殖器检查

1. 视诊

暴露阴阜,观察外阴发育及阴毛分布情况。

将润滑剂涂到用于检查的右手手指上。

用左手的拇指和食指分开阴唇。

检查阴蒂、尿道口和阴道口。

特别注意是否有:

(1)分泌物;

(2)发红;

(3)溃疡;

(4)萎缩;

(5)陈旧疤痕。

要求患者咳嗽或向下用力,观察阴道壁是否有脱垂。

2. 触诊

用食指和大拇指触摸测量大阴唇长度。

(1)正常组织柔软、丰满。

将右手食指伸入阴道口,拇指置于大阴唇外侧,仔细触诊巴氏腺。

(2)只有在腺管阻塞导致无痛囊肿或急性巴氏腺脓肿时,巴氏腺才能被触及。急性巴氏腺脓肿表现为位于大阴唇后外侧的发红发热、触痛明显的肿大物。

4.2.3.3　窥器检查

为进一步检查阴道内部和宫颈,需要进行窥器检查。同时可以进行宫颈涂片或拭子。

阴道窥器的种类不一,最常用的是 Cusco 窥器,又称鸭嘴或双叶窥器(图 4-2-1)。现在临床

areas now used plastic/disposable specula. There do not have a thumb-screw but a ratchet to open/close the blades. It is important that you familiarize yourself with the operation of the speculum before examining a patient so that you can concentrate on the findings.

上常用一次性塑料窥器,用棘齿代替了传统 Cusco 窥器的脚螺丝来开合叶片。在给患者检查前,熟悉窥器的使用非常重要,可以使检查者专注于临床所见。

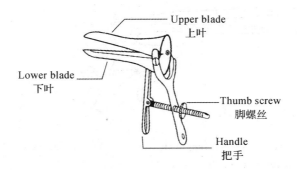

Figure 4-2-1　Cusco speculum
图 4-2-1　Cusco 窥器

Inserting the speculum

1. Explain to the patient that you are about to insert the speculum into the vagina and provide reassurance that this should not be painful.

2. Warm the speculum under running water and lubricate it with a water-based lubricant.

3. Using the left hand, open the lips of the labia minora to obtain a good view of the introitus.

4. Hold the speculum in the right hand with the main body of the speculum in the palm (Figure 4-2-2) and the closed blades projecting between index and middle fingers.

5. Gently insert the speculum into the vagina held with your wrist turned such that the blades are in line with the opening between the labia.

6. The speculum should be angled downwards and backwards due to the angle of the vagina.

7. Maintain a posterior angulation and rotate the speculum through 90° to position handles anteriorly. When it cannot be advanced further, maintain a downward pressure and press on the thumb piece to

插入窥器

1. 告知患者你准备插入窥器,整个过程一般不会感觉痛苦。

2. 用流水加温窥器,叶片上涂蘸水性润滑剂。

3. 用左手分开小阴唇,暴露阴道口。

4. 右手持窥器,将其主体部分握于手掌(图 4-2-2),用食指和中指夹住突出并合上的叶片。

5. 手握窥器,转动腕部,使叶片方向与阴唇之间开口方向一致,然后轻柔地将窥器插入阴道。

6. 窥器应该根据阴道的走向,以向下、向后的角度向阴道内推进。

7. 保持向后的角度,旋转窥器 90°使窥器的把手朝前。当感觉窥器前进到底并遇到阻力时,保持一种向下的压力,同时指压

hinge the blades open exposing the cervix and vaginal walls.

8. Once the optimum position is achieved, tighten the thumbscrew.

窥器的拇指片,利用铰合打开双叶,便可以暴露宫颈和阴道壁。

8.确定窥器的最佳位置后拧紧脚螺丝。

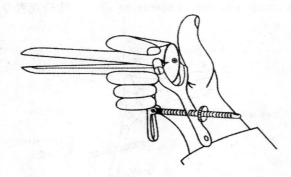

Figure 4-2-2　Hold the speculum in the right hand such that the handles lie in the palm and blades project between the index and middle fingers

图 4-2-2　右手持窥器,将其把手握于手掌,用食指和中指夹住突出并合上的叶片

Findings

Inspect the cervix which is usually pink, smooth and regular.

1. Look for the external os (central opening) which is round in the nulliparous female and slit-shaped after childbirth.

2. Look for cervical erosions which appear as strawberry-red areas spreading circumferentially around the os and represent extension of the endocervical epithelium onto the surface of the cervix.

3. Identify any ulceration or growths which may suggest cancer.

4. Cervicitis may give a mucopurulent discharge associated with a red, inflamed cervix which bleeds on contact. Take swabs for culture.

Removing the speculum

This should be conducted with as much care as insertion. You should still be examining the vaginal walls as the speculum is withdrawn.

1. Undo the thumbscrew and withdraw the speculum.

临床所见

检查宫颈,正常呈粉红、光滑和规则。

1.观察宫颈外口,未产妇为圆形,经产妇为裂纹形状。

2.观察宫颈糜烂情况,其表现为宫颈外口周围的草莓红色区域,外观潮湿而不光滑,是宫颈管上皮延伸至宫颈表面所致。

3.注意辨别宫颈局部的溃疡或增生,可能提示癌症的存在。

4.宫颈炎可能表现为黏液脓性分泌物并伴有宫颈发红发炎,有触血。需取分泌物拭子做培养。

移除窥器

和插入窥器一样,移除窥器也要小心轻柔。退出窥器时,仍需检查阴道壁。

1.旋开脚螺丝,再退出窥器。

2. The blades should be held open until their ends are visible distal to the cervix to avoid causing pain.

3. Rotate the open blades in an anticlockwise direction to ensure that the anterior and posterior walls of the vagina can be inspected.

4. Near the introitus, allow the blades to close taking care not to pinch the labia or hairs.

4.2.3.4　Bimanual examination

Digital examination helps identify the pelvic organs. Ideally the bladder should be emptied, if not already done so. This examination is often known as per vaginam or simply "PV".

Getting started

Explain again to the patient that you are about to perform an internal examination of the vagina, uterus, tubes, and ovaries and obtain verbal consent.

The patient should be well positioned. Expose the introitus by separating the labia with the thumb and forefinger of the gloved left hand.

Gently introduce the lubricated index and middle fingers of the right hand into the vagina.

1. Insert your fingers with the palm facing laterally and then rotate 90° so that the palm faces upwards.

2. The thumb should be abducted and the ring and little finger flexed into the palm (Figure 4-2-3).

2.在看到窥器叶片末端远离宫颈前,双叶应保持张开,以免引起疼痛。

3.逆时针方向旋转张开的叶片,确保阴道前、后壁也能检查到。

4.当窥器退至阴道口附近时,合上双叶,注意不要掐住阴唇或阴毛。

4.2.3.4　双合诊检查

指检有助于了解盆腔器官的一般情况。此时患者最好保持膀胱空虚,否则应该先排空膀胱。双合诊又称经阴道检查,简称PV。

准备工作

再次告知患者你准备进行阴道内检查,了解阴道、子宫、输卵管和子宫的情况,并获得患者口头同意。

患者取截石位,检查者戴手套用左手分开阴唇,暴露阴道口。

检查者右手食指和中指蘸润滑剂,轻柔地插入阴道。

1.手掌朝侧面,手指插入,再旋转90°使手掌面朝上。

2.拇指外展,环指和小指自然向掌面弯曲(图 4-2-3)。

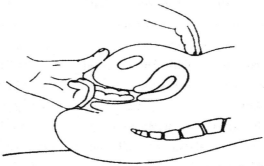

Figure 4-2-3　Bimanual examination of the uterus

图 4-2-3　双合诊检查子宫

Vagina, cervix and fornices

Feel the walls of the vagina which are slightly rugose, supple and moist.

Locate the cervix—usually pointing downwards in the upper vagina.

1. The normal cervix has a similar consistency to the cartilage in the tip of the nose.

2. Assess the mobility of the cervix by moving it from side to side and note any tenderness (excitation) which suggests infection.

Gently palpate the fornices either side of the cervix.

Uterus

Place your left hand on the lower anterior abdominal wall about 4 cm above the symphysis pubis.

Move the fingers of your right "internal" hand to push the cervix upwards and simultaneously press the fingertips of your left "external" hand towards the internal fingers.

1. You should be able to capture the uterus between your 2 hands.

2. Note the following features of the uterine body:

(1)Size: a uniformly enlarged uterus may represent pregnancy, fibroid or endometrial tumour.

(2)Shape: multiple fibroids tend to give the uterus a lobulated feel.

(3)Position.

(4)Surface characteristics.

(5)Any tenderness.

(6)Remember that an anteverted uterus is easily palpable bimanually but a retroverted uterus may not be.

Assess a retroverted uterus with the internal fingers positioned in the posterior fornix.

Ovaries and fallopian tubes

Position the internal fingers in each lateral fornix (finger pulps facing the anterior abdominal wall) and place your external fingers over each iliac fossa in turn.

1. Press the external hand inwards and

阴道,宫颈和阴道穹窿

正常阴道壁为多皱褶、柔软和潮湿的。

宫颈通常位于阴道上部,指向下。

1. 正常宫颈触诊与鼻尖软骨硬度相似。

2. 用指尖上下左右推动宫颈,评估宫颈的活动度,并注意有无触痛(刺激),提示感染的存在。

在宫颈的侧方,轻柔触诊阴道穹窿。

子宫

将左手置于患者下腹前壁,耻骨联合上方约 4 cm 处。

用置于阴道内的右手手指向上推起宫颈,同时位于腹部的左手手指向下按压腹壁,两手相互配合。

1. 两手相互迎合,可以扪清子宫情况。

2. 注意子宫体的以下特征:

(1)大小:均匀增大的子宫可见于妊娠、子宫肌瘤或子宫内膜癌。

(2)形状:多发子宫肌瘤触诊为分叶状。

(3)位置。

(4)表面特征。

(5)有无压痛。

(6)前倾位的子宫容易触及,而后倾位的子宫可能无法触及。

将阴道内手指置于后穹窿有助于后倾位子宫的触诊。

卵巢和输卵管

将阴道内手指置于侧穹窿(指腹朝向前腹壁),另一只手置于髂窝,依次检查双侧附件。

1. 置于腹部的手指向内向下

downwards and the internal fingers upwards and laterally.

2. Feel the adnexal structures (ovaries and fallopian tubes), assessing size, shape, mobility and tenderness.

(1)Ovaries are firm, ovoid and often palpable. If there is unilateral or bilateral ovarian enlargement, consider benign cysts (smooth and compressible) and malignant ovarian tumours.

(2)Normal fallopian tubes are impalpable.

(3)There may be marked tenderness of the lateral fornices and cervix in acute infection of the fallopian tubes (salpingitis).

Masses

It is often not possible to differentiate adnexal from uterine masses. However, there are some general rules:

1. Uterine masses may be felt to move with the cervix when the uterus is shifted upwards while adnexal masses will not.

2. If suspecting an adnexal mass, there should be a line of separation between the uterus and the mass, and the mass should be felt distinctly from the uterus.

3. Whilst the consistency of the mass may help to distinguish its origin in certain cases, an ultrasound may be necessary.

Finishing the examination

Withdraw your fingers from the vagina, and inspect the glove for blood or discharge.

Re-drape the genital area and allow the patient to re-dress in privacy, offer them assistance if needed.

4.2.3.5　Taking a cervical smear

Theory

Many countries have screening programs to detect pre-malignant conditions of the cervix. Women between the ages of 20 and 65 years receive an

按压,同时阴道内手指向上向外推。

2.触诊附件结构(卵巢和输卵管),评估大小、形状、活动度及有无压痛。

(1)卵巢为实性卵圆体,常可扪及。如扪到单侧或双侧增大的卵巢,应考虑卵巢良性或恶性肿瘤,前者触诊光滑并可压缩。

(2)正常输卵管无法触及。

(3)急性输卵管感染(输卵管炎)时可有侧穹窿和宫颈的明显触痛。

包块

通常附件区包块和子宫包块较难鉴别。以下是一些鉴别要点:

1.推动宫颈时,子宫包块会随着子宫的向前移动而被触摸到,附件区包块则不会。

2.疑为附件区包块时,触诊感觉其应与子宫分离,有较明显的分隔线。

3.同时,在某些病例中,包块的硬度也有助于判断其来源,必要时可以做超声检查。

结束检查

退出阴道内的手指,并检查手套上有无血迹和分泌物。

遮盖会阴部,让患者穿上衣物,注意保护隐私,必要时给予帮助。

4.2.3.5　宫颈涂片

原理

很多国家对 20 到 65 岁的妇女提供每 3 年一次的宫颈癌前病变筛查。其原理是取少许宫颈鳞

invitation to attend for screening every 3 years. A sample of cells from the squamo-columnar junction are obtained and a cytological examination performed to look for evidence of cervical intraepithelial neoplasia (CIN). This stage of the condition can be easily and successfully treated.

In order to minimize the number of inadequate samples, liquid based cytology (LBC), usually thinprep cytologic test (TCT), is used.

Equipments

1. Specula of different sizes.

2. Disposable gloves.

3. Request form.

4. Sampling device—plastic broom (Cervix-Brush).

5. Liquid-based cytology vial—preservative for sample.

6. Patient information leaflet.

Before you start

1. Ensure the woman understands purpose of examination.

2. Discuss how and when she will receive the results.

3. Provide a patient information leaflet.

4. Document the date of last menstrual period.

5. Document the use of hormonal treatment (*e. g.* contraception, HRT).

6. Record the details of last smear and previous abnormal results.

7. Ask about irregular bleeding (*e. g.* post-coital or post-menopausal).

8. Where appropriate, offer screening for Chlamydia infection (under 25 years, symptomatic).

Procedure

1. Prepare woman as for vaginal examination remembering to make her comfortable and allow privacy.

2. Write the patient's identification details on LBC vial.

柱状上皮进行细胞学检查,检测有无宫颈上皮内瘤变(CIN),此阶段容易成功治愈。

为了减少所需样品量,一般进行液基细胞学(LBC)检查,通常是薄层液基细胞学检测(TCT)技术。

检查用品

1. 不同型号的阴道窥器。

2. 一次性手套。

3. 申请表。

4. 采样器——塑料刷(宫颈刷)。

5. 液基细胞瓶——保存样品。

6. 患者信息单。

准备开始

1. 向患者说明检查目的。

2. 告知患者检查结果的领取事宜。

3. 发放患者信息单。

4. 记录末次月经日期。

5. 记录激素使用史(如避孕药物、激素替代治疗)。

6. 记录最后一次涂片情况和以往异常结果。

7. 询问阴道不规则出血情况(如性交后或绝经后出血)。

8. 25岁以下有症状者,可进行衣原体感染筛查。

步骤

1. 按阴道检查要求进行准备,保证患者舒适和保护隐私。

2. 在LBC瓶上写上患者个人信息。

3. Insert speculum to identify and visualize cervix, record any abnormal features of the cervix.

4. Insert the plastic broom so that the central bristles of the brush are in the endocervical canal and the outer bristles in contact with the ectocervix (Figure 4-2-4).

3. 插入窥器，观察并记录宫颈情况。

4. 插入宫颈刷，使中央刷毛深入宫颈管内，周围刷毛接触宫颈阴道部（图 4-2-4）。

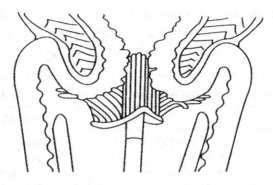

Figure 4-2-4　Representation of how to use a cervix-brush.
Note that the longer, central bristles are within the cervical canal whist the outer bristles are in contact with the ectocervix

图 4-2-4　宫颈刷使用示意图
注意长的中央刷毛深入宫颈管内，同时周围刷毛接触宫颈阴道部

5. Using pencil pressure, rotate the brush 5 times in a clockwise direction.

6. Rinse the brush thoroughly in the preservative (ThinPrep) or break off brush into the preservative.

7. Place in transport packaging with completed request form.

8. Remove the speculum and allow the patient to re-dress in privacy.

5. 稍加压力，顺时针转动宫颈刷 5 次。

6. 将宫颈刷完全浸入薄层液基保存液漂洗，折断刷头留在保存液中。

7. 将申请表和液基细胞瓶一起送检。

8. 取出窥器，让患者穿上衣物，注意保护隐私。

4.3　Infections

4.3　炎症

Key words

1. Bartholin's cyst
2. atrophic vaginitis
3. bacterial vaginosis
4. pelvic inflammatory disease

关键词

1. 巴氏腺囊肿
2. 萎缩性阴道炎
3. 细菌性阴道病
4. 盆腔炎性疾病

4.3.1　Vulval infections

4.3.1.1　Learning objectives

You should know：

1. How to recognize and treat genital warts.

2. The pathophysiology of Bartholin's swellings.

3. The implications of painless vulval ulceration.

4. The implications of a genital herpes simplex infection. Infections of the vulva may present as swellings，ulceration or infestations（Table 4-3-1）.

Table 4-3-1　Presentations of vulval infections

Vulval swellings	
Infective	*Non-infective*
● Warts	● Tumor
● Vulval abscess	● Sebaceous cyst
● Bartholin's abscess	● Lipoma
● Molluscum contagiosum	● Hernia
Vulval ulcers	
Infective	*Non-infective*
● Herpes simplex	● Vulval carcinoma
● Primary or secondary syphilis	● Basal cell carcinoma
● Chancroid	● Trauma
● Granuloma inguinale	
● Lymphogranuloma venereum	
Vulval infestations	
● Lice	
● Scabies	

4.3.1.2　Vulval swellings

1. Genital warts

Etiology

Genital warts are caused by infection with the human papillomavirus（HPV）. HPV types 16 and 18 are associated with an increased risk of preinvasive and invasive neoplasia of the cervix.

Transmission

Genital warts are usually transmitted by sexual contact，and have an incubation period of up to 8 months. The warm moist skin folds of the vulva are ideal conditions for the virus.

4.3.1　外阴炎症

4.3.1.1　学习目标

你应该了解：

1. 如何识别和处理生殖器疣。

2. 巴氏腺肿胀的病理生理。

3. 无痛性外阴溃疡的可能疾病。

4. 生殖道单纯疱疹感染的可能疾病。外阴感染性疾病可表现为肿胀、溃疡或侵染（如表4-3-1）。

表 4-3-1　外阴炎的表现

外阴肿胀	
感染性	非感染性
● 疣	● 肿瘤
● 外阴脓肿	● 皮脂囊肿
● 巴氏腺脓肿	● 脂肪瘤
● 触染性软疣	● 疝
外阴溃疡	
感染性	非感染性
● 单纯疱疹	● 外阴癌
● 原发或继发性梅毒	● 基细胞癌
● 软下疳	● 外伤
● 腹股沟肉芽肿	
● 性病性淋巴肉芽肿	
外阴侵染	
● 虱	
● 疥疮	

4.3.1.2　外阴肿胀

1. 生殖器疣

病因

生殖器疣是感染人乳头瘤病毒（HPV）引起的。HPV 16 和 18 型可增加侵袭前和侵袭性宫颈瘤变的风险。

传播途径

生殖器疣通常由性接触传播，潜伏期可达 8 个月。外阴温暖潮湿的皮肤皱襞是病毒理想的生存环境。

Clinical manifestations

The clinical appearance is of multiple small papillary excrescences which are most common on the vulval and perineal skin. Warty lesions may also be found in the vagina and on the cervix.

Warts are generally painless, but they may cause skin irritation and are usually a cosmetic concern to the patient. The particular strains of papillomavirus responsible for genital warts differ from those causing common skin warts.

Examination

Women with genital warts should be offered a cervical smear and colposcopic examination of the cervix because of the association with cervical intraepithelial neoplasia. Screening should be undertaken for other sexually transmitted diseases (STDs) such as gonorrhea, trichomonas and Chlamydia. During pregnancy genital warts often enlarge markedly. There is a small risk of neonatal infection at delivery which may result in laryngeal papillomas.

Treatment

Treatment is best carried out at a genitourinary clinic which has facilities for STD screening and contact tracing. Caustic agents such as podophyllin or trichloracetic acid are applied twice weekly to the lesions, taking care to avoid contact with the surrounding skin. Excision, diathermy or laser is reserved for large or resistant warts.

Treatment of warts does not lead to eradication of the virus from the genital tract, and characteristic warty cytological changes may persist on cervical smears. Genital warts may recur, particularly in the immune-compromised patient.

2. Vulval abscess

The vulval skin is prone to cellulitis and abscess formation. This commonly starts with staphylococcal infection at the base of a hair follicle or in a sebaceous gland. The clinical course is of increasing pain and

临床表现

最常见的临床症状为外阴及其周围皮肤上多个小乳头状突起的赘生物。阴道和宫颈上也可发现疣状病变。

疣一般为无痛性,但可引起皮肤刺激,影响外观。引起生殖道疣的乳头瘤病毒类型与引起一般皮肤疣的不同。

查体

因为与宫颈上皮内瘤变有关,患生殖器疣的女性应行宫颈刮片和阴道镜检查。应做包括淋病、滴虫和衣原体在内的其他性传播疾病的筛查。妊娠期间,生殖器疣常明显扩大。有一定概率可使新生儿产时感染,导致新生儿喉乳头状瘤。

处理

患者最好到生殖泌尿专业诊所治疗,可以进行性传播疾病筛查和接触追踪。使用腐蚀性试剂如足叶草碱或三氯乙酸涂抹患处,每周两次,小心防止接触周围皮肤。大范围或顽固性疣考虑用切割、透热或激光治疗。

治疗疣不能完全清除生殖道的病毒,宫颈刮片可以持续发现特征性疣状细胞学改变。生殖器疣可能复发,尤其是在免疫力低下的患者。

2.外阴脓肿

外阴皮肤容易发生蜂窝织炎和脓肿形成。起源于毛囊基底或皮脂腺葡萄球菌感染。临床过程为逐渐加重的疼痛和肿胀,之后

swelling followed by a discharge of pus. Early treatment with antibiotics may avert this but once a fluctuant swelling has developed incision and drainage is required.

3. Bartholin's cyst and abscess

The duct of the Bartholin's gland which opens out on the posteromedial aspect of the labium majus is prone to obstruction. Secretions then build up and dilate the duct to form a Bartholin's cyst, which may reach the size of an egg. These are usually painless but if the cyst becomes infected an extremely painful abscess develops. This will require drainage, and pus should be sent for culture and sensitivity. Bartholin's cysts are treated by marsupialization, which involves eversion and suturing the cyst wall, so allowing it to drain.

4. Molluscum contagiosum

Molluscum contagiosum is a contagious virus with causes small pearly white skin papules, which may occur on the vulval and perineal skin. Treatment is by piercing the lesion with phenol on the end of an orange stick.

5. Vulval ulceration

Vulval ulceration is commonly due to infection and rarely due to malignancy. Acutely painful ulcers are usually due to genital herpes, whereas the syphilitic chancre is painless.

6. Herpes simplex

Etiology

Genital herpes simplex virus infection (herpes simplex virus [HSV] type 1 or 2) is common STD. The primary attack occurs following sexual contact with an infected person, after an incubation period of 7 days.

Clinical manifestations

Acutely painful vulval ulceration, occasionally preceded by prodromal tingling, is the most prominent feature. Systemic symptoms such as headache and photophobia are not uncommon. The

有脓性分泌物排出。早期使用抗生素治疗可以防止加重,一旦形成有波动感的肿胀,则需要切开引流。

3. 巴氏腺囊肿和脓肿

巴氏腺导管开口于大阴唇中后部,容易堵塞。如分泌物积聚会使导管扩张,形成巴氏腺囊肿,可达到鸡蛋大小。一般为无痛性,但如囊肿感染,可形成疼痛明显的脓肿。因此需要引流,脓液做培养和药敏试验。巴氏腺囊肿可行造口术,外翻缝合囊肿壁以利引流。

4. 触染性软疣

触染性软疣是一种接触传染的病毒,可以导致外阴及其周围皮肤上珍珠白色的小丘疹。治疗方法为用尖棒蘸苯酚刺破疣体。

5. 外阴溃疡

外阴溃疡主要由感染引起,偶尔可因恶性病变导致。急性疼痛的溃疡一般有生殖器疱疹引起,而梅毒硬下疳是无痛性的。

6. 单纯疱疹

病因

生殖器单纯疱疹感染(HSV 1 或 2 型)是一种常见的性传播疾病。首次发病在与患者性接触后,潜伏期为 7 天。

临床表现

最主要特征为急性疼痛性外阴溃疡,少数发生溃疡前有麻刺感。全身症状有头痛,畏光等并不少见。开始的小囊泡经过 14

vesicles process over 14 days to weeping infectious ulcers，which then crust over and finally heal like a cold sore. The cervix is usually infected and may be covered in vesicle. The inguinal lymph nodes may be enlarged and tender.

Diagnosis

The diagnosis is confirmed by culture of vesicle fluid.

Outcome

After a primary infection the herpes virus is carried for life in the dorsal root ganglia. Recurrent attacks of genital herpes often follow, which may be triggered by stress, illness or sexual intercourse. These attacks are rarely as severe as the primary attack, and may even pass unnoticed, which allows infection to be easily transmitted to other sexual partners. Recurrent attacks of painful ulceration together with the knowledge that the virus is carried for life frequently leads to long-term psychosexual difficulties amongst sufferers.

Complications

1. Urinary retention.
2. Secondary bacterial infection.
3. Neonatal infection.

Treatment

Cure is not possible as the viral genome becomes integrated into the host neuronal cell deoxyribonucleic acid（DNA），and antiviral agents can only act when the virus is replicating. During acute attacks, pain relief is by simple analgesics and warm salt bathing. Acyclovir is given orally 200 mg five times daily for 5 days in conjunction with acyclovir ointment, which speeds healing of the ulcers and reduces the duration of infectivity. Famciclovir and valaciclovir are newer antiviral agents having improved bioavailability and longer half-lives, thus allowing less frequent administration.

Long-term antiviral therapy can be used to

天发展为有传染性的渗出性溃疡，之后结痂，最后像冷疱样愈合。宫颈通常受累，满布小囊泡。腹股沟淋巴结可有肿大和压痛。

诊断

通过囊液培养可以确诊。

结局

初次感染疱疹病毒后，病毒终生存在于背根神经节，之后压力、生病或性交等可触发生殖器疱疹反复发作。这些发作没有首次发病严重，甚至不被患者发现，所以很容易传给其他性伴侣。反复疼痛性溃疡发作以及得知终生携带病毒会导致患者长期的性心理障碍。

并发症

1. 尿潴留。
2. 继发细菌感染。
3. 新生儿感染。

处理

因为病毒基因组整合到宿主神经细胞的 DNA 中，而抗病毒药物仅在病毒复制时才能发挥作用，所以该病不可能完全治愈。在急性期，使用普通镇痛药和热盐水浸浴可缓解疼痛。口服阿昔洛韦 200 mg，5 次/天，共 5 天，同时局部使用阿昔洛韦软膏，可加速溃疡的愈合并缩短传染期。泛昔洛韦和伐昔洛韦是较新抗病毒药物，具有更高的生物利用度和更长的半衰期，可以减少用药次数。

长期抗病毒治疗可以降低复

reduce the frequency of acute attacks in those patients suffering from recurrent infections.

7. Syphilis

The primary chancre of syphilis is painless, and this may present as a highly infectious vulval ulcer. The incubation period is 9-90 days, by which time the spirochete has disseminated throughout the body. The characteristic lesion of secondary syphilis is condylomata lata, which appear as moist flat infective erosions on the vulva, vagina or cervix. Treatment is a 10-day course of procaine penicillin. All patients should be referred to a genitourinary clinic for full STD screening, treatment, contact tracing and follow-up.

Serological testing for syphilis is part of routine antenatal screening, because of the risk of transmission to the fetus. This practice has enabled the virtual elimination of congenital syphilis.

8. Vulval infections

Lice

A particular type of louse called Pediculosis pubis may be found clinging to pubic hairs, using its three sets of legs. Clinical features are intense pruritus and sky blue spots at the bite sites. Both sexual partners should be treated with 1% gamma benzene hexachloride powder.

Scabies

Scabies is caused by s small slow-moving mite called *Sarcoptes scabei* which is transmitted by prolonged close physical contact. The female burrows under the skin and lays eggs, which causes unbearable itching. A favorite site is in the finger clefts.

Diagnosis is made by deroofing the burrow and extracting the mite for identification under a microscope. Treatment is with 25% benzyl benzoate solution.

发患者急性发作的频率。

7. 梅毒

梅毒初期的硬下疳是无痛性的,而此时的外阴溃疡具有高度传染性。潜伏期为9~90天,期间梅毒螺旋体播散到全身。二期梅毒特征性病变为扁平湿疣,表现为外阴、阴道或宫颈上潮湿扁平的感染性糜烂。治疗方法是使用普鲁卡因青霉素,疗程10天。患者应到生殖泌尿专科诊所进行全套STD筛查、治疗、接触追踪和随诊。

梅毒存在垂直传播给胎儿的风险,因此梅毒血清学检测是常规产前筛查的一部分,这样可以真正消除先天性梅毒。

8. 外阴侵染

虱

虱的一种特殊类型叫做阴虱,它用三对足黏附在阴毛上。临床特点是剧烈瘙痒和被咬部位天蓝色斑点。性伴侣双方都应使用1%丙种六氯苯粉末治疗。

疥疮

疥疮是由一种叫做疥螨的移动缓慢的小恙虫导致的,长期身体密切接触可被传染。雌性藏于皮下隧道中产卵,导致无法忍受的瘙痒。最易侵犯的部位是手指缝。刮破皮肤隧道,挑取疥虫在显微镜下鉴定即可诊断。治疗用25%苯甲酸苄酯溶液。

4.3.2　Vaginal infections

4.3.2.1　Learning objectives

You should：

1. Understand how the vagina maintains an acidic environment.

2. Know how to manage the common symptom of vaginal discharge.

3. Be aware that chlamydia infection may be asymptomatic.

4. Understand how alterations in vaginal pH may occur.

The healthy vagina is colonized by the *Lactobacillus*, which prevents infection by other micro-organisms. The *Lactobacillus* metabolizes glycogen, which is produced by the squamous epithelial cells under the influence of estrogen, to lactic acid. This maintains a vaginal pH of 4.5. Any conditions which reduce the vaginal acidity or eradicate the *Lactobacillus* will predispose to infection.

4.3.2.2　Vaginal discharge

1. Definition

The healthy vagina produces a variable amount of physiological vaginal discharge. This is called leucorrhea.

2. Physiology

It is yellowish/white in color and does not cause any irritation or offensive smell. It contains a mixture of secretions from endometrial and cervical glands, exfoliated vaginal cells, bacterial flora and white blood cells.

It has a cyclical variation in common with cervical mucus, so women may notice their discharge increases at mid-cycle or prior to menstruation. Vaginal discharge may increase in pregnancy and in women who are using the combined oral contraceptive pill, both of which cause benign

4.3.2　阴道炎症

4.3.2.1　学习目标

你应该：

1. 理解阴道如何维持酸性环境。

2. 了解怎样处理一般阴道分泌物症状。

3. 注意衣原体感染可能为无症状性。

4. 理解阴道 pH 值怎样改变。

正常女性阴道有乳酸菌群居,可抑制其他微生物引起的感染。乳酸菌将雌激素影响下阴道鳞状上皮细胞产生的糖原代谢成乳酸,从而维持阴道 pH 值为 4.5。任何破坏阴道酸性环境或杀灭乳酸菌的情况都可以使阴道易于感染。

4.3.2.2　阴道分泌物

1. 定义

正常阴道可产生量多少不一的生理性阴道分泌物,叫做白带。

2. 生理

白带的颜色为淡黄色或白色,不产生刺激或臭味,是子宫内膜和宫颈腺体、脱落阴道上皮细胞、细菌群落和白细胞的混合物。

因为正常宫颈黏液存在周期性改变,所以女性自身会发现在月经周期中期或月经来潮之前分泌物增多。妊娠期妇女和使用复方口服避孕药的女性的阴道分泌物增多,因为激素可导致宫颈内

hyperplasia of the endocervical glands. This appearance may be recognized on visualizing the cervix as a bright red vascular area. It is termed cervical ectopy.

Excessive vaginal discharge is a common gynecological complaint, which should always be investigated. Careful examination of the vulva for signs of inflammation and discharge should be followed by vaginal speculum examination to enable swabs to be taken for microbiological identification of any infective organism, and to visualize the cervix to look for carcinoma.

3. Pathological cause of vaginal discharge

(1)Common infectious causes

①*Candida albicans*

②*Trichomonas vaginalis*

③*Gardnerella vaginalis*

④*Chlamydia trachomatis*

(2)Other infectious causes

①Beta-hemolytic *Streptococcus*

②*Neisseria gonorrhea*

③Herpes simplex virus

④Human papillomavirus

(3)Other pathological causes

①Chemical vaginitis

②Foreign body

③Chronic cervicitis

④Cervical polyps

⑤Cervical tumors

⑥Urinary or faecal fistulae

⑦Childhood vulvovaginitis

4. Candidiasis

Etiology

Candidiasis is the most common cause of infective vaginal discharge. *Candida albicans* is a yeast which thrives in moist skin folds. It is frequently found in asymptomatic women and it can often be isolated from the bowel. It is not usually sexually transmitted but may be carried by the

腺体良性增生。视诊可见宫颈呈鲜红色血管区域,称为宫颈柱状上皮异位。

阴道分泌物过多是妇科常见主述,应该查找原因。仔细检查外阴有无炎症迹象,行阴道窥检取分泌物拭子做感染性微生物学鉴定,并观察宫颈有无肿瘤。

3.阴道分泌物的病理原因

(1)常见感染性因素

①白色念珠菌

②阴道毛滴虫

③阴道加德那菌

④沙眼衣原体

(2)其他感染性因素

①B 组溶血性链球菌

②淋病奈瑟菌

③单纯疱疹病毒

④儿童期外阴阴道炎

(3)其他病理因素

①化学性阴道炎

②异物

③慢性宫颈炎

④宫颈息肉

⑤宫颈肿瘤

⑥尿瘘或粪瘘

⑦幼儿外阴阴道炎

4.念珠菌病

病因

念珠菌是感染性阴道分泌物最常见的病因。白色念珠菌是一种容易生长在潮湿皮肤皱褶的真菌。常见于无症状的女性,常可从肠道中分离出来。不常通过性传播,但可由未环切包皮的男性

uncircumcised male.

Diagnosis

The usual symptoms are vulval pruritus and vaginal soreness. Predisposing factors are diabetes, poor hygiene, nylon underwear and use of broad spectrum antibiotics.

The diagnosis is made on the clinical grounds of finding a thick white cheesy discharge together with the culture of the organism from a swab.

Treatment

Treatment is with clotrimazole vaginal pessaries, together with clotrimazole cream if vulvitis is present, or with oral fluconazole.

Recurrent infection is a common problem. This is thought to occur as a result of reinfection from a persistent bowel reservoir of organisms. Treatment is then with long-term courses of antifungal drugs. Advice should be given to wear loose cotton underwear and skirts to prevent excessive perspiration, and any predisposing factors such as diabetes should be identified and remedied.

5. Trichomonas

Diagnosis

This causes a yellowish-green vaginal discharge, and a characteristic "strawberry cervix" due to the prominent appearance of blood vessels. Trichomonas may also be carried asymptomatically in the vagina. It can be sexually transmitted so both partners should be screened for other sexually transmitted diseases.

Diagnosis can be made by dark ground microscopic examination of a sample from the posterior vaginal fornix. The protozoa can be seen swimming around by whipping movements of their flagellae.

Treatment

Treatment is with metronidazole. This should be given to both partners, with the advice to avoid alcohol during treatment. The dose is 400 mg 8-

携带。

诊断

常见症状为外阴瘙痒和阴道疼痛。易患病的因素包括糖尿病,卫生情况不佳,穿着尼龙内裤以及使用广谱抗生素。

临床上发现白色浓稠干酪样分泌物,加上阴道拭子培养出念珠菌,即可诊断该病。

治疗

治疗用克霉唑阴道栓剂,如有外阴炎加用克霉唑乳膏,或口服氟康唑。

反复感染是一个常见的问题,原因被认为是对持续存在的肠道菌群的再感染。治疗方法为长疗程使用抗真菌药物。应建议患者穿宽松棉质内裤和裙子,以防止过度出汗,并且还应积极诊断和治疗糖尿病等易患病因素。

5. 毛滴虫

诊断

毛滴虫可引起黄绿色阴道分泌物,以及血管突出造成的特征性"草莓状宫颈"。毛滴虫也可以无症状地存在于阴道中。因其可通过性传播,伴侣双方均应行其他性传播疾病的筛查。

用暗视野显微镜检查取自阴道后穹窿的样本,发现毛滴虫通过摆动鞭毛游弋即可诊断此病。

治疗

使用甲硝唑治疗,伴侣双方应同时治疗,期间避免饮酒。用法为每 8 h 一次,每次 400 mg,

hourly for 5 days, or 2 g as a single dose.

6. Bacterial vaginosis

Bacterial vaginosis is a common vaginal infection among women of reproductive age. It is caused by the anaerobic bacterium *Gardnerella vaginalis*. It causes a grey discharge and a fishy odor, although many women are asymptomatic. Microscopic examination of the discharge reveals typical "clue cells", which are vaginal epithelial cells exhibiting surface dimpling from attached bacteria. Treatment is with metronidazole.

Untreated vaginal infection with gardnerella increases the risk of ascending infection resulting in pelvic inflammatory disease. In pregnancy, gardnerella infection is associated with both premature rupture of the membranes and chorioamnionitis.

7. Chlamydia

Chlamydia is an important cause of pelvic inflammatory disease. Screening has identified the organism in 8% of women attending for termination of pregnancy, and it is frequently found in association with other sexually transmitted diseases.

In common with gonorrhea, infection in the female may be asymptomatic. Cervical infection with chlamydia presents with vaginal discharge secondary to cervicitis. The organism is difficult to isolate by culture, but the diagnosis can be made by fluorescent monoclonal antibody or polymerase chain reaction testing. Women giving a history of a recent change in sexual partner together with a vaginal discharge should be referred to a genitourinary clinic for full genital microbiological screening, contact tracing and follow-up.

Treatment is with a tetracycline such as doxycycline 100 mg 12-hourly for 14 days, or a single 1 g dose of azithromycin. Successful control of infection depends on investigation and treatment of the sexual partner.

共 5 天或单次给药 2 g。

6. 细菌性阴道病

细菌性阴道病是生育年龄妇女常见的一种阴道感染。病原体为厌氧的阴道加德那菌，可引起灰白色，有鱼腥味的分泌物，尽管很多妇女没有症状。分泌物显微镜检可发现典型的"线索细胞"，即附着细菌表面凹凸不平的阴道上皮细胞。治疗用甲硝唑。

加德那菌阴道感染如不治疗，会增加上行感染风险，导致盆腔炎性疾病。在妊娠期，加德那菌感染与胎膜早破和绒毛膜羊膜炎有关。

7. 衣原体

衣原体是盆腔炎性疾病的重要致病因素。在 8% 终止妊娠的妇女中检测到该病原体，该病通常与其他性传播疾病共同存在。

和淋球菌一样，女性感染衣原体可能为无症状性。宫颈感染衣原体表现为继发于宫颈炎的阴道分泌物。衣原体难以通过培养的方法分离，但能用荧光单克隆抗体或多聚酶链式反应检测确诊。对于近期更换性伴侣并出现阴道分泌物的女性，应到生殖泌尿专科诊所进行全套生殖道微生物学筛查，接触追踪和随诊。

治疗用四环素类抗生素，如多西环素每 12 h 一次，每次 100 mg，共 14 天，或单次给予 1 g 阿奇霉素。性伴侣要同时检查和治疗，才能确保有效控制感染。

8. Vulvovaginitis

Vulvovaginitis presents with an offensive vaginal discharge, and is seen in all age groups.

Childhood vulvovaginitis usually occurs due to under-estrogenisation of the vagina. Estrogen cream and attention to hygiene are indicated.

In women of reproductive age the common causes of vaginal discharge are infections with thrush, gardnerella and trichomonas. Rarer causes include a chemical vaginitis from an allergic reaction to detergents, douches, bath salts or deodorants. A foreign body in the vagina such as a forgotten tampon is an unusual cause, which may result in the toxic shock syndrome. This is a severe systemic infection with circulatory collapse due to release of staphylococcal toxins.

Vaginal discharge in post-menopausal women is usually due to bacterial vaginitis. The long-term effect of low estrogen levels results in the vaginal skin becoming thin and easily traumatized, and lacking in glycogen. Colonisation with the *Lactobacillus* thus decreases and the pH rises, allowing pathogenic bacteria to infect the vagina. The possibility of a carcinoma should be remembered in this age group, particularly if the discharge is blood-stained.

4.4 Infections of the Cervix

Key words

1. gonorrhea
2. chronic cervicitis

4.4.1 Learning objectives

You should:

- Know how to investigate suspected cervical infection.

8. 外阴阴道炎

外阴阴道炎表现为阴道分泌物有异味,所有年龄阶段的女性均可发生。

儿童型外阴阴道炎一般由去雌激素化引起。可用雌激素乳膏,并注意卫生。

生育期女性阴道分泌物最主要的致病因素包括念珠菌病、加德那菌和毛滴虫。其他少见的病因包括洗涤剂、灌洗剂、浴盐或除臭剂过敏所致的化学性阴道炎。阴道内异物,罕见的如被遗漏的棉塞,可导致中毒性休克综合征。这是一种由葡萄酒菌毒素引起的伴有循环衰竭的严重系统感染。

绝经后女性的阴道分泌物通常由细菌性阴道炎引起。低雌激素水平的长期作用导致阴道壁变薄,容易受创伤,缺乏糖原,使寄居的乳酸杆菌减少,pH 值增高,导致致病菌感染阴道。在这个年龄阶段还应该考虑肿瘤的可能性,尤其当分泌物为血性时。

4.4 宫颈感染

关键词

1. 淋病
2. 慢性宫颈炎

4.4.1 学习目标

你应该:

- 理解如何对可疑宫颈感染进行检查。

Acute infection of the cervix may be chlamydial, gonococcal or herpetic in origin. It may present with vaginal discharge, but is also commonly asymptomatic. The cervix usually looks red and many bleed easily on contact. Cervical swabs, colposcopy and cervical biopsy are all helpful in diagnosis.

4.4.2　Gonorrhea

Gonorrhea is sexually transmitted infection caused by the Gram-negative diplococcus *Neisseria gonorrhea*. The incubation period is 2-5 days. It infects the mucous membranes of the cervix, urethra, anus, rectum and oropharynx. It may present with generalized malaise, vaginal discharge and dysuria, but some cases are asymptomatic. Untreated infection can persist as a chronic cervicitis or progress to a more severe and generalized illness. The potential sequelae of gonorrhea infection include infertility, chronic pain and menstrual dysfunction.

If gonorrhea infection is suspected, swabs should be taken from the urethra, cervix and rectum, put onto Stuart's transport medium, and screening undertaken for other STDs.

4.4.2.1　Complications of gonorrhea

1. Pelvic inflammatory disease
2. Bartholin's abscess
3. Joint pains
4. Skin rash
5. Endocarditis

4.4.2.2　Treatment

A single dose of a long-acting penicillin is given by intramuscular injection. In cases of penicillin allergy, spectinomycin is effective. Tetracycline is often given in addition to eradicate possible chlamydial infection. Follow-up with repeat swabs is essential to confirm eradication, as some strains of the gonococcus have acquired penicillin resistance.

宫颈急性感染可能来自衣原体、淋球菌或疱疹，可表现为阴道分泌物，但也可以无症状。宫颈通常发红并流血。宫颈刮片、阴道镜以及宫颈活检均有助于诊断。

4.4.2　淋病

淋病是一种通过性传播感染革兰染色阴性双球菌属的淋病奈瑟菌引起。潜伏期为2～5天，可感染宫颈、尿道、肛门、直肠和口咽的黏膜。临床上可表现为全身乏力，有阴道分泌物，排尿困难，某些病例也可以无症状。如感染不治疗，可延续成慢性宫颈炎或加重发展成全身性疾病。淋病可能的后遗症包括不孕症、慢性盆腔痛和月经紊乱。

如怀疑淋球菌感染，应行尿道、宫颈和直肠拭子，接种到Stuart's转移培养基，并做其他性传播疾病筛查。

4.4.2.1　淋病的并发症

1. 盆腔炎性疾病
2. 巴氏腺脓肿
3. 关节疼痛
4. 皮疹
5. 心内膜炎

4.4.2.2　治疗

单次肌内注射长效青霉素。对青霉素过敏者，大观霉素有效。为消除可能伴随的衣原体感染，通常合用四环素。因某些淋球菌菌株可获得青霉素抗性，所以需多次复查拭子以确保治愈。

4.4.3　Chronic cervicitis

Chronic cervicitis causes a chronic persistent vaginal discharge. Cervical and vaginal swabs should be taken to exclude infection. In chronic cervicitis there is often no specific infection isolated. The cervix just appears enlarged and has copious mucous secretion from the glands. Obstruction of the gland openings results in mucous retention cysts, called Nabothian follicles. The naked eye appearance is of an enlarged irregular cervix with cystic lesions. Together with a firm irregularity on digital examination this can lead to a clinical suspicion of cancer. If there is doubt about the clinical appearance of the cervix a cervical smear and urgent referral for colposcopy is indicated. Provided specific infections and neoplasia have been excluded, destruction of the inflamed columnar epithelium by cauterization or cryotherapy may produce a cure.

4.5　Acute Pelvic Inflammatory Disease

Key words

1. endometritis
2. salpingitis
3. tub, ovarian abscess, TOA

4.5.1　Learning objectives

You should:

1. Understand the implications of pelvic inflammatory disease.

2. Know how to manage suspected pelvic inflammatory disease.

3. Be able to construct a differential diagnosis from the symptoms and signs in a case of suspected pelvic inflammatory disease.

Pelvic inflammatory disease refers to infection involving the upper genital tract. It usually results

4.4.3　慢性宫颈炎

慢性宫颈炎引起慢性持续性阴道分泌物。应行宫颈和阴道拭子排除感染。慢性宫颈炎病例中,通常分离不出特殊病原菌,而只是宫颈看起来肥大,腺体分泌大量黏液,如腺体开口堵塞可导致黏液潴留囊状,称为纳氏滤泡。宫颈肉眼看上去为增大不规则的囊状病变,如指诊感觉坚硬不规则,则临床怀疑宫颈癌。如临床视诊有所怀疑,应行宫颈涂片和紧急阴道镜检查。如排除特殊感染和瘤变,可用烧灼或冷冻疗法破坏发炎的柱状上皮,获得治愈。

4.5　急性盆腔炎

关键词

1. 子宫内膜炎
2. 输卵管炎
3. 输卵管卵巢脓肿

4.5.1　学习目标

你应该:

1. 理解盆腔炎性疾病的表现。

2. 了解如何处理可疑的盆腔炎。

3. 能够从可疑盆腔炎的症状和体征作出鉴别诊断。

盆腔炎性疾病指上生殖道感染,一般由于下生殖道性传播感

from ascending sexually-acquired infection of the lower genital tract. Once pathogens gain access to the peritonitis may result. Common pathogens include chlamydia, *Neisseria gonorrhea* and anaerobic bacteria. Any sexually active woman is at risk of pelvic inflammatory disease, but precipitating factors include the intra-uterine contraceptive device, multiple sexual partners and instrumentation of the cervix in the presence of pathogenic organisms. The risk is reduced by the use of barrier methods of contraception and by limiting the number of sexual partners.

Early diagnosis and treatment is essential to prevent permanent damage to the fallopian tubes. This is sometimes difficult because infections can be asymptomatic and some women unfortunately become infertile. In severe cases the fimbrial ends of the tubes become occluded, allowing them to become distended with pus it is called a pyosolpinx. This indicates severe irreversible damage.

4.5.2　Clinical findings

Presentation is typically with bilateral lower abdominal pain and fever, accompanied by a vaginal discharge and deep dyspareunia. Examination reveals guarding and rebound tenderness over the lower abdomen and a tender uterus. Moving the cervix on vaginal examination causes severe pain called excitation. An adnexal mass with a high fever and leukocytosis suggests a pyosalpinx or tubo-ovarian abscess. Transperitoneal infection occasionally spreads to the upper abdomen, causing upper abdominal pain and perihepatic adhesions.

4.5.3　Symptoms and signs of acute pelvic inflammatory disease

1. Acute lower abdominal pain
2. Vaginal discharge
3. Fever

染上行引起,病原体导致腹膜炎即可形成。常见病原菌包括衣原体、奈瑟淋球菌和厌氧菌。任何性活跃女性都有患盆腔炎的风险,而易患因素包括宫内节育器,多性伴侣以及在致病菌环境下进行宫腔操作。但使用屏障避孕方法以及减少性伴侣能降低患病风险。

早期诊断和治疗盆腔炎对于防止输卵管永久性损伤非常必要。但有些情况下感染为无症状性,难以早期发现,从而这些女性不幸患上不孕症。严重时输卵管伞末端闭塞,输卵管扩张积脓,称为输卵管积脓,形成重度无法逆转的损伤。

4.5.2　临床表现

典型的症状为双侧下腹部疼痛,发热,阴道分泌物以及深部性交痛。查体发现下腹部肌紧张和反跳痛,子宫压痛。阴道检查时推动宫颈产生剧痛称为激惹。附件区包块伴有高热和白细胞增高提示输卵管积脓或输卵管-卵巢脓肿。经腹膜感染偶尔扩散到上腹部,可导致上腹部疼痛和肝周粘连。

4.5.3　急性盆腔炎的症状和体征

1. 急性下腹部疼痛
2. 阴道分泌物
3. 发热

4. Pelvic tenderness

5. Adnexal mass

4.5.4　Investigation of suspected acute pelvic inflammatory disease

A white cell count and erythrocyte sedimentation rate（ESR）should be taken together with swabs from the cervix, urethra, vagina and rectum. An important differential diagnosis here is ectopic pregnancy, so a pregnancy test should always be sent. If positive, ultrasound can help to distinguish between an ectopic and an intra-uterine gestation. Acute appendicitis, adnexal torsion and a bleeding corpus luteum cyst can all produce similar symptoms. Laparoscopy is therefore useful for diagnosis and is indicated in patients who do not respond to antibiotics. Laparoscopy allows assessment of tubal damage and culture of fluid from the fallopian tubes and pouch of Douglas. The typical findings in acute pelvic inflammatory disease are hyperemia of the fallopian tubes with edema and a sticky exudate on their peritoneal surface.

4.5.5　Treatment

Hospital admission is required for severe cases, for bed rest, intravenous antibiotics and analgesia. If an intra-uterine contraceptive device（IUCD）is present it should be removed. Combination antibiotic therapy is started immediately and is reviewed when bacteriological culture results are available. However, causative organisms are only isolated in about 30% of cases. Treatment is given for 10-14 days. A single intramuscular dose of 4.8 megaunits of procaine penicillin with 1 g oral probenecid will treat gonococcus.

4.5.6　Long-term morbidity from pelvic inflammatory disease

1. Recurrent attacks of infection

4. 盆腔触痛

5. 附件区包块

4.5.4　可疑急性盆腔炎的检查

应进行白细胞计数、红细胞沉降率以及宫颈、尿道、阴道和直肠拭子检查。一个重要的鉴别诊断是异位妊娠,因此通常应做妊娠试验,如阳性,超声可帮助区分宫内和宫外妊娠。急性阑尾炎、附件区扭转和黄体囊肿可有相似的症状。此时腹腔镜检查有助于诊断,且是抗生素治疗无效患者的适应证。腹腔镜检能评估输卵管损伤,并取出输卵管内液和子宫直肠陷凹积液行培养。腹腔镜下,急性盆腔炎的典型表现为输卵管充血水肿及其部位腹膜黏性渗出。

4.5.5　治疗

重症患者应住院治疗,卧床休息,静脉给予抗生素并镇痛。如有宫内节育器应取出。立即联合应用抗生素治疗,再根据细菌培养结果调整方案。然而,仅约30%的病例分离出致病菌。抗生素疗程为10～14天。单次肌内注射4.8兆单位普鲁卡因青霉素同时口服1 g丙磺舒可以治疗淋病。

4.5.6　盆腔炎性疾病的长期症状

1. 感染反复发作

2. Chronic pelvic pain

3. Dyspareunia

4. Ectopic pregnancy

5. Infertility

6. Menstrual disturbance

4.5.7 Chronic pelvic inflammatory disease

Recurrent attacks of pelvic inflammatory disease may result in chronic pelvic pain, menstrual disturbance, dyspareunia and infertility. The uterus and adnexa may become fixed due to tethering by adhesions. The best option for future fertility is by *in vitro* fertilization. Tubal reconstructive surgery is rarely of value. Relief from chronic pelvic pain and menstrual irregularity is often eventually sought by hysterectomy and bilateral salpingo-oophorectomy.

4.5.8 Pelvic abscess

4.5.8.1 Learning objectives

You should:

1. Understand the different pathophysiologies leading to a pelvic abscess.

2. Understand the principles of management of a pelvic abscess.

A collection of pus may accumulate in the pelvis to form an abscess. This is usually a tubo-ovarian abscess resulting from pelvic inflammatory disease. The features are a swinging fever, pelvic pain and a tender pelvic mass, with tenesmus if there is pressure on the rectum. Occasionally an abscess will spontaneously discharge into the posterior vaginal fornix or rectum, resulting in a prompt relief of pain. If there is no clinical improvement after 48 hours of intravenous antibiotics, drainage is required. This may be achieved by posterior colpotomy if the abscess is filling the pouch of Douglas. Otherwise, laparoscopic drainage and irrigation will be necessary. Major surgery to excise the pelvic organs

2. 慢性盆腔痛

3. 性交困难

4. 异位妊娠

5. 不孕症

6. 月经不调

4.5.7 慢性盆腔炎性疾病

盆腔炎性疾病反复发作可导致慢性盆腔痛,月经不调,性交困难和不孕症。子宫和附件可因粘附束带而位置固定。未来生育最好选择体外受精。输卵管重建手术很少有价值。慢性盆腔痛和月经不规则通常最终靠子宫切除术和双侧输卵管—卵巢切除术才能得到缓解。

4.5.8 盆腔脓肿

4.5.8.1 学习目标

你应该:

1. 理解盆腔脓肿的不同病理生理。

2. 理解盆腔脓肿处理原则。

盆腔脓液积聚可形成脓肿。通常为盆腔炎导致的输卵管-卵巢脓肿。特征包括高热,盆腔痛和触痛包块,如压迫直肠可伴里急后重。脓肿可偶然自发破溃入阴道后穹窿或直肠,从而导致疼痛很快缓解,如静脉用抗生素48 h后临床症状没有改善,需行引流。如脓肿位于子宫直肠陷凹,可行阴道后穹窿切开术引流。此外,有必要行腹腔镜手术引流和灌洗。不必要行大手术切除盆腔内器官,因为有肠管损伤和深部静脉血栓的风险。

is rarely necessary and carries a risk of bowel injury and deep vein thrombosis.

4.5.8.2　Causes of pelvic abscess

1. Pelvic inflammatory disease
2. Appendicitis
3. Postoperative
4. Induced abortion
5. Diverticulitis

4.5.9　HIV infection

You should：

1. Understand the implications of HIV infection.
2. Understand the principles of HIV prevention.
3. Be aware how disease presentation may vary.

The human immunodeficiency virus（HIV）is a retrovirus which causes acquired immune deficiency syndrome （ AIDS ）. It may be transmitted by unprotected penetrative sexual intercourse，infected blood，and from mother to baby during pregnancy，labor or by breast feeding. It selectively infects T lymphocytes with CD4 antigen，which decreases the host immune defences. Antibodies are produced 4-8 weeks after exposure，and are detectable in blood. Of those infected with HIV，50％ develop AIDS within 10 years. Many individuals will have acquired HIV infection unknowingly and can therefore be expected to develop AIDs in the future. Of the registered HIV-seropositive patients，11％ are female. As no cure or vaccine is currently available，disease prevention is the main method of controlling spread of HIV. Screening of blood，use of condoms and limiting the number of sexual partners all reduce the risk of infection.

Acute infection with HIV is usually subclinical，but there may be a transient non-specific illness. This is followed by a chronic infection，characterized in one third of patients by a persistent generalized

4.5.8.2　盆腔脓肿的原因

1. 盆腔炎性疾病
2. 阑尾炎
3. 手术后
4. 人工流产
5. 憩室炎症

4.5.9　人免疫缺陷病毒(HIV)感染

你应该：

1. 理解 HIV 感染的表现。
2. 理解预防 HIV 的原则。
3. 认识到疾病的临床表现不一。

人免疫缺陷病毒(HIV)是一种引起获得性免疫缺陷综合征(AIDS,艾滋病)的逆转录病毒,可通过未经保护的穿透性性交,感染的血液,妊娠分娩或哺乳期母婴之间传播。HIV 选择性感染 CD4 阳性 T 淋巴细胞,从而降低宿主的免疫防御。暴露 4～8 周后产生抗体,血液中可检测到。50％的 HIV 感染者在 10 年内发展为艾滋病。很多个体不知不觉获得 HIV 感染,因此可预期未来发展为艾滋病。在登记在案的 HIV 血清阳性患者中,11％为女性。因为目前艾滋病尚无治愈方法或疫苗,所以疾病预防是控制 HIV 传播的主要方法。血液筛查,使用避孕套和减少性伴侣都可以减少感染的风险。

急性 HIV 感染一般为亚临床型,但可能有一个短暂的非特异性病态,随后是一个慢性感染的过程,有三分之一的患者特征

lymphadenopathy. When this is accompanied by non-specific constitutional symptoms such as fever, weight loss and malaise, coupled with minor opportunistic infections such as oral candidiasis, it is called AIDS-related complex.

Full-blown AIDS develops after a median incubation period of 8-10 years. It is defined by the presence of certain reliably diagnosed diseases in the absence of any other cause of immune deficiency (Table 4-5-2). The patient will be seropositive. The clinical presentation varies according to the presenting disease. Symptoms include weight loss, dry cough, purple skin lesions of Kaposi's sarcoma, diarrhea, perianal ulceration, headache and dementia. Death occurs within 2 years of diagnosis. Treatment with zidovudine has been shown to improve survival and decrease the incidence of opportunistic infections.

Table 4-5-2　Disease indicative of cellular immune deficiency seen in AIDS

- Opportunistic infections
- Pneumocystic pneumonia
- Cryptococcosis
- Cytomegalovirus
- Herpes simplex virus
- Toxoplasmosis
- *Mycobacterium kansasii* or *avium*
- Candidiasis—esophageal or pulmonary
- Progressive multifocal leucoencephalopathy
- Malignancies
  — Kaposi's sarcoma
  — Primary cerebral lymphoma
  — Non-Hodgkin's lymphoma

4.5.10　Rare causes of pelvic sepsis

You should know:

1. That rare chronic granulomatous pelvic infections exist.

2. That TB and actinomycosis are rare causes of infertility.

性表现为持续性全身淋巴结病。当伴随非特异性全身症状如发热,体重减轻和全身乏力,加上机会性感染如口腔念珠病菌,总称为艾滋病相关综合征。

在一个 8～10 年的中位潜伏期后,就会发展为艾滋病发病。当出现一些确诊的疾病(如表 4-5-2 所示)而排除其他导致免疫缺陷的原因时,可定义为艾滋病发病。患者血清学检查阳性,根据存在的疾病不同,临床表现不一。症状包括体重减轻,干咳,卡波西氏肉瘤的紫色皮肤病变,腹泻,肛周溃疡,头痛和痴呆。确诊 2 年内死亡。用齐多夫定治疗可改善生存并降低机会性感染的机会。

表 4-5-2　提示 AIDS 中细胞免疫受损的疾病

- 机会性感染
- 肺囊虫性肺炎
- 隐球菌病
- 巨细胞病毒
- 单纯疱疹病毒
- 弓形虫病
- 堪萨斯分枝杆菌或鸟分枝杆菌
- 念珠菌病——食管或肺
- 进展性多病灶白质脑病
- 恶性肿瘤
  — 卡波西氏肉瘤
  — 原发性脑淋巴瘤
  — 非霍奇金淋巴瘤

4.5.10　盆腔败血症的罕见病因

你应该了解:

1.罕见慢性肉芽肿盆腔感染的存在。

2.结核病和放线菌病是不孕症的罕见病因。

Actinomycosis

Actinomycosis is caused by the anaerobic obligate fungal parasite *Actinomyces israeli*. It is a very uncommon cause of chronic pelvic infection, and thus rarely suspected on clinical grounds. It causes a characteristic granulomatous tissue reaction with the formation of hard masses and multiple discharging sinuses, which can result in bowel or ureteric obstruction. Extensive abdominal actinomycosis may occasionally be mistaken for malignancy, with the associated risk of inappropriate surgery. This emphasizes the fundamental importance of obtaining a tissue diagnosis prior to undertaking treatment. Diagnosis is made by anaerobic culture of pus, when typical yellowish "sulphur granule" colonies are seen. Treatment is with penicillin.

Actinomyces is sometimes reported in a cervical smear in a healthy woman in association with the IUCD. In such cases the coil can be changed and course of penicillin given.

Tuberculosis

Tuberculosis (TB) infects one third of the world's population. Pelvic tuberculosis is usually secondary to a primary lung infection, and it can be a cause of infertility. The fallopian tube is the most commonly affected site in the pelvis. It becomes thickened and filled with caseous material, with tubercles on the peritoneal surface. The diagnosis is rarely suspected on clinical grounds and is usually made on TB culture of uterine curettings. Treatment is with rifampicin, isoniazid and ethambutol.

Pyometra

Pyometra is a collection of pus in the uterus. It is usually secondary to a necrotic endometrial carcinoma or a cancer of the sigmoid colon which has eroded into the uterus.

Case report and analysis

✎A 38-year-old woman complains of an offensive

放线菌病

放线菌病是由专性厌氧的寄生真菌以色列放线菌引起的,是慢性盆腔感染非常罕见的病因,因此临床上很少考虑到。其特征为肉芽肿组织反应,硬块形成和许多排脓窦道,从而导致肠道或输尿管梗阻。广泛的腹部放线菌病偶尔可被误诊为恶性,有不当手术的相关风险。这样就强调了在采取治疗之前获取组织进行诊断的重要性。当看到典型淡黄色"硫黄颗粒"菌落时,进行脓液厌氧菌培养可做出诊断。治疗用青霉素。

有报道放线菌可在健康女性宫颈涂片中找到,与宫内节育器有关。对于这样的情况可更换线圈,并用青霉素治疗。

结核病

全世界有三分之一的人口感染结核。盆腔结核通常继发于肺部原发病灶,可成为不孕症的病因。盆腔结核通常继发于肺部原发病灶,可成为不孕症的病因。盆腔中最常受累的部位是输卵管,它变厚,充满干酪样物质,浆膜面出现结节。临床上较少怀疑该病,刮宫物行结核菌培养可诊断。治疗用利福平、异烟肼和乙胺丁醇。

宫腔积脓

宫腔积脓是宫腔内脓液积聚。通常继发于坏死的子宫内膜癌或侵蚀入子宫的异状结肠癌。

病例报道和分析

✎38 岁女性,主述性交后分泌物

odor after sexual intercourse. Examination reveals a greyish vaginal discharge. A sample of fluid is taken from the posterior fornix and mixed with 10% potassium hydroxide, which produces a fishy odor. On microscopy there are numerous squamous cells with stippled borders.

◇What are these cells called?

◇Name the diagnosis and the correct treatment.

☑ANSWERS

✓These are the so-called clue cells, which are epithelial cells with numerous bacteria adherent to them.

✓Together with the fishy odor on addition of potassium hydroxide, this is characteristic of *Gardnerella* infection. Treatment is with metronidazole.

✍A 18-year-old sexually active woman has a 10-day history of lower abdominal pain. Increased vaginal discharge and pain on micturition. On examination the cervix is hyperemic and there is tenderness on bimanual palpation. There is a low grade pyrexia.

◇ What is the differential diagnosis and what investigations are indicated?

☑ANSWERS

✓The symptoms and clinical findings are suggestive of infection with either chlamydia or gonorrhea. Endocervical and urethral swabs should be taken, and urine should be sent for culture to exclude a urinary tract infection. The patient should be immediately referred to a genito-urinary clinic for full STD screening and contact tracing.

Objective Structured Clinical Examniation（OSCE） questions

✍A 20-year-old woman has recently been treated in hospital for acute salpingitis. She now has a few questions for you:

(1)The hospital told her the swabs were all negative, so did she really have an infection?

(2)How could she have caught the infection?

异味。查体发现灰白色阴道分泌物。从阴道后穹窿取分泌物与10%氢氧化钾混合可产生腥臭味。显微镜下可见很多边界呈斑点状的鳞状细胞。

◇上述细胞叫做什么？

◇做出诊断和正确治疗。

☑答案

✓这些细胞被称为线索细胞，是很多细菌黏附于阴道上皮细胞形成的。

✓结合氢氧化钾试验有腥臭味，是加德那菌感染的特征。治疗用甲硝唑。

✍18岁性活跃女性，主述下腹痛10天，阴道分泌物增加且有尿痛。查体宫颈充血，双合诊触痛，有低热。

◇鉴别诊断是什么？应做哪些检查？

☑答案

✓症状和临床发现提示衣原体或淋球菌感染。应做宫颈内和尿道拭子，连同尿液一起做培养，以排除尿路感染。患者须立即到生殖泌尿专科做全套性传播疾病筛查和接触跟踪。

客观结构化临床考试(OSCE)问题

✍20岁女性有近期住院治疗急性输卵管炎的病史。她有一些问题想咨询：

(1)医院告诉她所有拭子都是阴性，她确实有感染吗？

(2)她是如何获得感染的？

（3）Why was she treated with three different antibiotics?

（4）Why was it necessary for the hospital to contact all her recent sexual partners?

（5）Is she likely to have difficulty getting pregnant in the future?

（6）Some of her friends want to know if there is any screening for chlamydia?

☑ANSWERS

（1）The sensitivity of currently available laboratory tests is such that a negative result does not exclude a diagnosis of acute salpingitis. Diagnosis and treatment is thus often based on clinical findings.

（2）The infection is usually sexually transmitted.

（3）A number of different organisms can cause acute salpingitis, such as *Chlamydia trachomatis*, *Neisseria gonorrhea* and anaerobes. A tetracycline such as doxycycline covers chalmydia, penicillin or a cephalosporin covers gonorrhea, and metronidazole covers the anaerobes, so three drugs are often given simultaneously.

（4）Contact tracing and treatment of sexual partners is vital to prevent reinfection and chronic salpingitis occurring.

（5）Although even one episode of acute salpingitis can result in tubal damage, with resultant infertility and increased risk of ectopic pregnancy, she should be reassured that prompt and appropriate antibiotic treatment reduces the risk.

（6）It is likely that screening and treating asymptomatic chlamydia infections in high risk groups, such as single women under the age of 35 years, would decrease the incidence of long-term complications such as infertility, ectopic pregnancy and pelvic pain. However, this is not possible currently, as there is a lack of a simple, cheap and rapid diagnostic test with sufficient sensitivity and specificity.

（3）为何用三种抗生素治疗？

（4）为什么有必要联系她近期的性伴侣？

（5）她未来受孕会有困难吗？

（6）她的一些朋友想知道有没有针对衣原体的筛查？

☑答案

（1）目前已有的实验室检测的敏感性决定了阴性的结果仍不能排除急性输卵管炎的诊断。因此，诊断和治疗常依据临床发现来进行。

（2）感染通常是性传播的。

（3）一些不同的病原微生物都可导致急性输卵管炎，如沙眼衣原体、奈瑟淋球菌和厌氧菌。四环素类如多西环素针对衣原体，青霉素或头孢菌素针对淋球菌，而甲硝唑针对厌氧菌，所以要同时使用三种药物。

（4）接触追踪和治疗性伴侣对预防复发和慢性输卵管炎非常重要。

（5）尽管一次急性输卵管炎发作就能引起输卵管损伤，结果导致不孕症和异位妊娠风险增高，但应告诉患者及时正确的抗生素治疗可以降低风险。

（6）对高危人群如 35 岁以下单身女性进行无症状衣原体感染的筛查和治疗，能降低长期并发症如不孕症、异位妊娠和盆腔痛的发生率。但是目前尚无一种简单、便宜和快速的检测方法可以兼具足够的敏感性和特异性。

A 21-year-old woman presents with genital warts. She wants to know：

(1) What treatments are available?

(2) Will treatment eradicate the virus from her?

(3) Will using condoms reduce her chances of further genital warts?

(4) Should her partners have any treatment?

☑ANSWERS

(1) Painting the warts with podophyllin solution or trichloracetic acid. · Cryotherapy using liquid nitrogen. Diathermy or surgical excision under anaesthetic for large warts, or those resistant to the other treatments.

(2) The virus is often found on histological examination of clinically normal tissue adjacent to the warts, and as such, it is unlikely that any physical treatment completely eradicates the virus.

(3) Although condoms do afford some protection from sexually transmitted diseases, they do not appear to reduce the risk of recurrence after treatment.

(4) Yes, her partner should be examined, and offered treatment if any warts are found.

4.6　Uterine Prolapse

Key words

1. uterine prolapse
2. vaginal pessary
3. Manchester operation
4. vaginal hysterectomy
5. pelvic floor reconstruction

4.6.1　Fast facts

1. Mostly in multiparous women.
2. Symptoms：sensation of vaginal fullness or

21 岁女性主述生殖器疣。她想了解：

(1) 有什么治疗方法?

(2) 治疗能够消除她携带的病毒吗?

(3) 使用避孕套能减少以后患生殖器疣的机会吗?

(4) 她的性伴侣需要治疗吗?

☑答案

(1) 将鬼臼树脂溶液或三氯乙酸涂抹患处。用液氮冷冻治疗。对于大范围或顽固性疣可用透热或手术切除。

(2) 对疣周围的临床上正常的组织进行组织学检查常可发现病毒。同样任何物理疗法都不可能完全清除病毒。

(3) 尽管避孕套对性传播疾病有一定预防作用,但不能减低治疗后复发的风险。

(4) 是的。她的性伴侣需要检查,如发现疣也需要治疗。

4.6　子宫脱垂

关键词

1. 子宫脱垂
2. 子宫托
3. 曼式手术
4. 阴式子宫切除术
5. 盆底重建

4.6.1　要点

1. 经产妇多见。
2. 症状:阴道充盈感或压力

pressure；lower abdominal pulling or aching；low backache.

3. Sometimes urinary tract infection，frequency and urgency，overflow voiding and incontinence.

4. Constipation and painful defecation in severe uterine prolapse.

5. Three degrees of uterine prolapse according to descending cervix.

First degree：Cervix palpable in lower third of vagin.

Second degree：Cervix projecting into or through the vaginal introitus.

Third degree： Cervix and entire uterus projecting through introitus. And large mass call be seen inthe perineum.

4.6.2　Etiology and pathgenesis

1. Multiparons.

2. Childbirth injury to endopelvic fascia.

3. Laceration of levator ani and perineal body muscles.

4. Congenital weakness in the pelvic fascia.

5. Systemic conditions： Obesity，asthma and COPD，etc，resulting in high abdominal pressure.

6. Local conditions：Ascites，pelvic tumor，sacral nerve disorders.

4.6.3　Treatment

1. Medical

（1）Vaginal pessary.

（2） Estrogen （systemically or vaginally） in postmenopansal patient.

（3）Treat systemic and local conditions：obesity，asthma，COPD，ascites，pelvic tumor，diabetes，*etc*.

（4）Prescribe laxatives or enemas for constipation.

2. Surgical

（1）Manchester operation for elongated cervix，

感；下腹牵拉感及疼痛；腰骶部疼痛。

3. 有时出现尿道感染，尿频、尿急，充盈性尿失禁。

4. 严重子宫脱垂时可出现便秘及排便疼痛。

5. 根据宫颈位置下降程度可分轻、中、重三度。

轻度：在阴道的下 1/3 可触及宫颈。

中度：宫颈脱出于阴道口。

重度：宫颈和宫体全部脱出，外阴可见包块。

4.6.2　病因及发病机制

1. 多产。

2. 分娩损伤盆底筋膜。

3. 提肛肌及会阴体的撕裂。

4. 盆底筋膜先天发育不良。

5. 肥胖、哮喘、慢性阻塞性肺病等造成腹内压增高的全身情况。

6. 局部疾病：腹水、盆腔肿瘤、骶神经病变。

4.6.3　治疗

1. 保守治疗

（1）子宫托。

（2）绝经后女性局部或全身使用雌激素。

（3）治疗全身及局部病变：肥胖、哮喘、慢性阻塞性肺病、腹水、盆腔肿瘤、糖尿病等。

（4）便秘者使用缓泻剂或灌肠剂。

2. 外科治疗

（1）曼式手术，适用于宫颈延

mild or moderale prolapse in young women.

(2) Vaginal hysterectomy.

(3) Pelvic floor reconstruction. including repairing actual or potential cystocele, rectocele, enterocele and repairing for relaxation of pelvic supports.

(4) Total abdominal hysterectomy and obliteration of any associated enterocele for contraindications to vaginal route.

(5) Le Fort operation (colpocleisis) for poor conditions or those having no sexual desire.

4.7　Cervical Cancer

Key words

1. postcoital spotting
2. malodorous
3. discharge
4. syphilis
5. costovertetral angle tenderness
6. genitalia
7. speculum
8. exophytic
9. Pap smear
10. presenting symptom
11. invasive cervical cancer
12. necrotic
13. flank tenderness
14. ureter
15. hydronephrosis
16. socioeconomic status
17. human papilloma virus, HPV
18. cervical intraepithelial neoplasia, CIN
19. atypia
20. incoporated
21. dysplasia
22. radical hysterectomy
23. radiation brachytherapy

长、轻、中度子宫脱垂的年轻女性。

(2) 阴式子宫切除术。

(3) 合并有盆底松弛患者,应行盆底重建术,包括修补已存在或潜在的膀胱、直肠、肠膨出和松弛的会阴等。

(4) 对于经阴道途径手术禁忌者,采用经腹途径全子宫切除术,同时修补存在的肠膨出。

(5) 阴道封闭术(适用于全身状况差及无性生活要求者)。

4.7　宫颈癌

关键词

1. 性交后点滴出血
2. 恶臭的
3. 分泌物、白带
4. 梅毒
5. 脊肋角压痛
6. 生殖器
7. 窥器
8. 外生的
9. 巴氏涂片
10. 主诉
11. 浸润性宫颈癌
12. 坏死的
13. 侧腹痛、肋胁痛
14. 输尿管
15. 肾积水
16. 社会经济状况
17. 人乳头瘤病毒
18. 宫颈上皮内瘤变
19. 不典型
20. 整合的
21. 发育异常
22. 根治性子宫切除术
23. 后装治疗的

24. radiation teletherapy		24. 远距离治疗的	
25. colposcopy		25. 阴道镜	
26. Soaked		26. 浸湿的	
27. acetic acid slotion		27. 醋酸溶液	
28. binocular		28. 双目镜的	
29. intraepithelial		29. 上皮内的	
30. acetowhite change		30. 醋白改变	
31. punctation		31. 镶嵌	
32. corkscew		32. 螺丝状	
33. hairpin		33. 发夹状	
34. papanicolaou test		34. 宫颈涂片检查(巴氏涂片)	
35. false-negative rate		35. 假阴性率	
36. carcinogenic subtype		36. 致癌亚型	
37. anesthesia		37. 麻醉	
38. intravenous pyelogram		38. 静脉肾盂造影	
39. proctoscopy		39. 直肠镜检查	
40. cystoscopy		40. 膀胱镜检查	
41. quadravalent vaccine		41. 四价疫苗	
42. adenomatous		42. 腺瘤的	
43. nulliparity		43. 未产妇	
44. conization of the cervix		44. 宫颈锥切	
45. condylomata acuminata		45. 尖锐湿疣	
46. agglutination		46. 凝集反应	
47. radiosenstiizer		47. 放疗增敏剂	

Case

A 50-year-old G_5P_5 woman complains of postcoital spotting over the past 6 months. Most recently, she complains of malodorous vaginal discharge. She states that she had syphilis in the past. Her deliveries were all vaginal and uncomplicated. She has smoked one pack of cigarettes per day for 20 years. On examination, her blood pressure is 100/80 mmHg, heart rate 80 bpm, and temperature 99 F. Heart and lung examinations are within normal limits. The abdomen reveals no masses, ascites, or tenderness. Back examination is unremarkable, and there is no costovertebral angle

病例

一 50 岁女性,G_5P_5,主诉性交后少量阴道出血 6 个月。近期阴道分泌物有异味。既往曾患梅毒。该妇全部为阴道分娩,顺产。有吸烟史 20 年,每天一包。查体:血压 100/80 mmHg,心率 80 次/分,体温正常,心肺检查未闻及异常,腹部检查无包块,腹水及压痛。盆腔检查:外生殖器无异常,阴道窥器检查发现宫颈前唇有 3 cm 外生型病变,双附件未扪及异常。

tenderness. Pelvic examination reveals normal external female genitalia. Speculum examination reveals a 3 cm exophytic lesion on the anterior lip of the cervix. No other masses are palpated.

1. What is your next step?

2. What is the most likely diagnosis?

ANSWERS TO CASE：Cervical cancer.

Summary：A 50-year-old $G_5 P_5$ women complains of 6 month history of postcoital spotting and malodorous vaginal discharge. She had a prior infection with syphilis, and she is a smoker. Speculum examination reveals a 3 cm exophytic lesion on the anterior lip of the cervix.

Next step：Biopsy of the cervical lesion.

Most likely diagnosis：Cervical cancer.

Analysis

Objectives

1. Understand that a cervical biopsy and not a Pap smear (which is actually a screening test) is the best diagnostic procedure when a cervical lesion is seen.

2. Know that postcoital spotting is a symptom of cervical cancer.

3. Know the risk factors for cervical cancer

Considerations

This 50-year-old $G_5 P_5$ woman with postcoital spotting. Abnormal vaginal bleeding is the most common presenting symtom of invasive cervical cancer，and in sexually active women, postcoital spotting is common. This patient's age is close to the mean age of presentation of cervical cancer, 51 years. She also complains of a malodorous vaginal discharge that is due to the large, necrotic tumor. Notably, the woman does not have flank tenderness. Which would be a result of metastatic obstruction of the ureter, leading to hydronephrosis. A cervical biopsy and not Pap smear is the best diagnosis test to evaluate a cervical mass. A Pap smear is a screening test and is

1. 下一步应该如何做？

2. 最有可能的诊断是什么？

答案：宫颈癌。

摘要：50 岁的女性，$G_5 P_5$，主诉性交后阴道少量出血伴异味阴道排液 6 个月，患者有梅毒病史，吸烟，阴道窥器检查发现宫颈前唇有 3 cm 外生型病变。

下一步处理：宫颈病变活检。

最有可能的诊断：宫颈癌。

分析

目的

1. 当宫颈有肉眼可见病灶时，应行宫颈活检而并非宫颈涂片（宫颈涂片实际上是筛查实验），宫颈活检是最好的诊断方法。

2. 了解性交后点滴出血为宫颈癌的症状之一。

3. 了解宫颈癌的发病高危因素。

考虑

患者，女性，50 岁，$G_5 P_5$，性交后出血。异常阴道出血为浸润性宫颈癌最常见的症状，在性活跃妇女，性交后阴道点滴出血很常见。该患者年龄接近于宫颈癌发病的平均年龄，51 岁。患者主诉阴道排液有恶臭，考虑因肿瘤大，组织坏死所致。显然，该患者没有明显疼痛，后者是，因肿瘤转移致输尿管梗阻，肾积水所致。宫颈活检而并非巴氏涂片是评估宫颈病变的最佳诊断方法。后者是筛查试验，适应于肉眼正

appropriate for a woman with a normal-appearing cervix.

Risk factors for cervical cancer in this woman include multiparity, cigarette smoking, and history of a STD(syphilis), and HIV infection (Table 4-7-1).

常宫颈的女性。

女性患宫颈癌的危险因素包括多产、吸烟、性传播疾病，如梅毒病史以及 HIV 感染史（见表 4-7-1）

Table 4-7-1　Risk factor for cervical
表 4-7-1　宫颈癌发病的危险因素

Early age of coitus 过早性生活	STD 性传播疾病
Early childbearing 早生育	Low socioeconomic status 较差社会经济状态
HPV 人乳头瘤病毒感染	HIV 艾滋病
Cigarette smoking 吸烟	Multiple sexual partners 多个性伴侣

4.7.2　Approach to cervical cancer

4.7.2.1　Definitions

CIN：Preinvasive lesions of the cervix with abnormal cellular maturation, nuclear enlargement, and atypia.

HPV：Circular, double-stranded DNA virus that can become incorporated into cervical squamous epithelium, predisposing the cells to dysplasia and/or cancer.

Radical hysterectomy：Removal of the uterus、supportive ligaments, such as the cardinal ligament, uterosacral ligament, and proximal vagina.

Radiation brachytherapy：Radioactive implants placed near the tumor bed.

Radiation teletherapy：External-beam radiation where the target is at some distance from the radiation source.

Clinical approach：When a woman presents with postcoital spotting or has an abnormal Pap smear, CIN or cancer should be suspected. An abnormal Pap

4.7.2　临床宫颈癌

4.7.2.1　定义

CIN：宫颈癌前病变,伴异常的细胞成熟,核增大及不典型性。

HPV：环状 双链 DNA 病毒能与宫颈上皮细胞 DNA 整合,致细胞癌变。

根治性子宫切除术：切除子宫、韧带,如主韧带、子宫骶骨韧带及近段阴道组织。

后装放射治疗：将放射源置于肿瘤病灶附近。

外照射放射治疗：外部电子束放射治疗,放射野与肿瘤病灶部位有一定距离。

临床路径：当妇女主诉性交后点滴阴道出血或巴氏图片有异常,应怀疑 CIN 或宫颈癌。细胞

smear usually is evaluated by colposcopy with biopsies, in which the cervix is soaked with 3% or 5% acetic acid solution. The colposcope is a binocular magnifying device that allows visual examination of the cervix. The majority of CIN and cancers arise near the SCJ of the cervix. Many times, CIN lesion turn white with the addition of acetic acid, the so-called "acetowhite change", along with the change in color, CIN lesions often have vascular changes, reflecting the more rapidly growing process. In fact, the vascular pattern usually characterizes the severity of the disease. An example of mild vascular pattern is punctations (vessels seen end-on) versus atypical vessels (e. g. corkscrew and hairpin vessels). A biopsy of the worst-appearing area should be taken during colposcopy for histologic diagnosis. Hence, the next step to evaluate an abnormal Pap smear is colposcpic examinations with directed biopsies.

When a woman presents with a cevical mass, biopsy of the mass, not a Pap smear, is appropriate. Because the Pap smear is a screening test used for asymptomatic women, it is not the best test when a mass is visible. The Pap test has a false-negative rate and may give false reassurance.

When cervical cancer is diagnosed, the next step is to stage the severity. Cervical cancer is staged clinically. Early cervical cancer (contained within the cervix) can be treated equally well with surgery (Piver Ⅲ, radical hysterectomy) or radiation therapy. However, advanced cervical cancer is best treated with radiotherapy, consisting of brachytherapy (implants) with teletherapy (whole-pelvis radiation radiation) along with chemotherapy, usually platinum based (cis-platinum), to sensitize the tissue to the radiotherapy. Because HPV is the etiologic agent in the vast majority of cervical cancer cases, research on vaccines against carcinogenic

学异常的患者,通常应用3%～5%的醋酸涂抹宫颈后进行阴道镜指导下活检。阴道镜为双目放大装置,可详细观察宫颈表面的病灶。大多数CIN及宫颈癌起源于宫颈鳞柱交界,通常CIN病变在应用醋酸后呈现白色改变,即所谓醋-白改变。CIN病灶有血管的异常,反映其快速的生长过程。事实上,宫颈表面血管的异常反映疾病的严重程度。如轻度的血管异常为镶嵌,不典型的血管如发夹状血管,活检在病灶最明显异常的区域进行,故进一步评估细胞学异常的步骤应是阴道镜下活检。

当女性诉宫颈肿块,应直接行活检,而不是行细胞学检查。因细胞学主要是针对无症状的女性所做的筛查。可肉眼可见明显病变,细胞学检查不是最佳的检查方法。细胞学检查有假阴性,从而遗漏患者的疾病。

当诊断宫颈癌后,接下来应对患者进行分期,以确定病变的严重程度。宫颈癌主要是临床分期,早期宫颈癌(病灶局限在宫颈)能很好地进行手术治疗(Piver Ⅲ,宫颈癌根治手术)或放射治疗。对晚期宫颈癌,主要是放疗,后装(局部植入放射源)及外照射(整个盆腔的放疗)同时行化疗,化疗方案主要是以顺铂为基础的联合化疗,可对放疗起增敏作用。因HPV与宫颈癌关系密切,研究高危型HPV疫苗给

subtypes of HPV holes promise.　　　　　　　　人们带来希望。

Table 4-7-2　Staging procedure for cervical cancer
表 4-7-2　宫颈癌的分期操作

Exmination under anesthesia	麻醉满意下检查
Intravenous pyelogram	静脉肾盂造影
Chest radiograph	胸片检查
Barium enema or proctoscopy	钡灌肠或乙状结肠镜检
Cystoscopy	膀胱镜检查

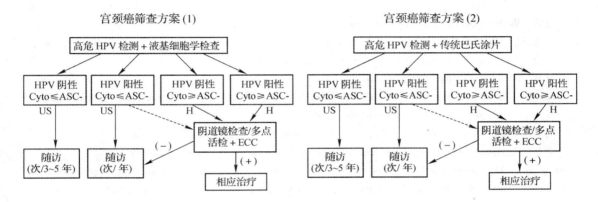

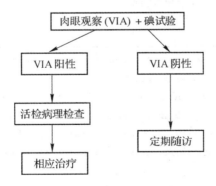

图 4-7-1　宫颈癌筛查方案

Table 4-7-3　Carcinoma of the cervix uteri

Stage Ⅰ　The carcinoma is strictly confined to the cervix (extension to the corpus would be disregarded)

  Ⅰ A　Invasive carcinoma which can be diagnosed only by microscopy, with deepest invasion ≤5 mm and largest extension ≥7 mm

    Ⅰ A1　Measured stromal invasion of ≤3.0 mm in depth and extension of ≤7.0 mm

    Ⅰ A2　Measured stromal invasion of >3.0 mm and not >5.0 mm with an extension of not >7.0 mm

  Ⅰ B　Clinically visible lesions limited to the cervix uteri or pre-clinical cancers greater than stage Ⅰ A

    Ⅰ B1　Clinically visible lesion ≤4.0 cm in greatest dimension

    Ⅰ B2　Clinically visible lesion >4.0 cm in greatest dimension

Stage Ⅱ　Cervical carcinoma invades beyond the uterus, but not to the pelvicwall or to the lower third of the vagina

  Ⅱ A　Without parametrial invasion

    Ⅱ A1　Clinically visible lesion ≤4.0 cm in greatest dimension

    Ⅱ A2　Clinically visible lesion >4 cm in greatest dimension

  Ⅱ B　With obvious parametrial invasion

Stage Ⅲ　The tumor extends to the pelvic wall and/or involves lower third of the vagina and/or causes hydronephrosis or non-functioning kidney

  Ⅲ A　Tumor involves lower third of the vagina, with no extension to the pelvicwall

  Ⅲ B　Extension to the pelvic wall and/or hydronephrosis or non-functioning kidney

Stage Ⅳ　The carcinoma has extended beyond the true pelvis or has involved (biopsy proven) the mucosa of the bladder or rectum. A bullous edema, as such, does not permit a case to be allotted to Stage Ⅳ

  Ⅳ A　Spread of the growth to adjacent organs

  Ⅳ B　Spread to distant organs

All macroscopically visible lesions, even with superficial invasion, are allotted to stage Ⅰ B carcinomas. Invasion is limited to a measured stromal invasion with a maximal depth of 5.00 mm and a horizontal extension of not >7.00 mm. Depth of invasion should not be N5.00 mm taken from the base of the epithelium of the original tissue, superficial or glandular. The depth of invasion should always be reported in mm, even in those cases with "early (minimal) stromal invasion" (∼1 mm). The involvement of vascular/lymphatic spaces should not change the stage allotment. On rectal examination, there is no cancer-free space between the tumor and the pelvic wall. All cases with hydronephrosis or non-functioning kidney are included, unless they are known to be due to another cause.

表 4-7-3　宫颈癌 2009 FIGO 分期

Ⅰ　肿瘤严格局限于宫颈(扩展至宫体将被忽略)

　　Ⅰ A　镜下浸润癌。间质浸润≤5 mm,水平扩散≤7 mm

　　　Ⅰ A₁　间质浸润≤3 mm,水平扩散＜7mm

　　　Ⅰ A₂　间质浸润＞3mm,且≤5 mm,水平扩散≤7mm

　　Ⅰ B　肉眼可见病灶局限于宫颈,或临床前病灶＞Ⅰ A 期*

　　　Ⅰ B₁　肉眼可见病灶最大径线≤4 cm

　　　Ⅰ B₂　肉眼可见病灶最大径线＞4 cm

Ⅱ　肿瘤超过子宫颈,但未达骨盆壁或未达阴道下 1/3

　　Ⅱ A　无宫旁浸润

　　Ⅱ B　有宫旁浸润

Ⅲ　肿瘤扩展到骨盆壁和(或)累及阴道下 1/3 和(或)引起肾盂积水或肾无功能者△

　　Ⅲ A　肿瘤累及阴道下 1/3,没有扩展到骨盆壁。

　　Ⅲ B　肿瘤扩展到骨盆壁和(或)引起肾盂积水或肾无功能

Ⅳ　肿瘤播散超出真骨盆或(活检证实)侵犯膀胱或直肠黏膜。泡状水肿不能分成Ⅳ期

　　Ⅳ A　肿瘤播散至邻近器官

　　Ⅳ B　肿瘤播散至远处器官

注:* 所有肉眼可见病灶甚至于仅仅是浅表浸润也都定为Ⅰ B 期。浸润癌局限于可测量的间质浸润,最大深度为 5 mm,水平扩散不超过 7 mm。无论从腺上皮或者表面上皮起源的病变,从上皮的基底膜量起浸润深度不超过 5 mm。浸润深度总是用毫米(mm)来报告,甚至在这些早期(微小)间质浸润(0～1 mm)。无论静脉或淋巴等脉管浸润均不改变分期。△直肠检查时肿瘤无盆腔间无肿瘤浸润间隙。任何不能找到其他原因的肾盂积水及肾无功能病倒都应包括在内。

Recently, the FDA is reviewing an application for a quadravalent vaccine for approval. Cervical cancer often spreads through the cardinal ligaments toward the pelvic side-walls. It can obstruct one or both ureters, leading to hydronephrosis. In fact, bilateral ureteral obstruction leading to uemia is the most common cause of death due to this disease.

最近,FDA 已批准四价疫苗应用于宫颈癌的预防,宫颈癌的播散通常是通过主韧带向盆壁浸润,可导致一侧或双侧输尿管阻塞,甚至肾盂积水。因此,双侧输尿管阻塞尿毒症是宫颈癌最常见的死因。

Comprehension Questions

1. Which of the following HPV subtypes most likely is associated with cervical cancer?　　（　）
   A. 6 and 11
   B. 16 and 18
   C. 55 and 57
   D. 89 and 92
2. Which of the following statements regarding

问题

1. 下列哪些 HPV 亚型最有可能与宫颈癌相关?　（　）
   A. 6 及 11
   B. 16 and 18
   C. 55 and 57
   D. 89 及 92
2. 关于宫颈癌,下列哪个陈述是

cervical cancer is true? 　　　　（　　）

A. The best therapy for advanced cervical cancer is surgical excision

B. Both brachytherapy and teletherapy are important in the treatment of cervical cancer

C. The main advantage of radiation therapy over radical hysterectomy in early stage cervical cancer is preservation of sexual function

D. The majority of cervical cancers are of adenomatous cell type

3. A 45-year-old woman is diagnosed with an early cervical cancer. Which of the following is a risk factor for cervical cancer? 　（　　）

A. Early age of coitus

B. Nulliparity

C. Obesity

D. Late menopause

4. A 33-year-old woman has a Pap smear showing moderately severe cervical intraepithelial neoplasia. Which of the following is the best next step? 　（　　）

A. Repeat Pap smear in 3 months

B. Conization of the cervix

C. Colposcopic-directed biopsies

D. Radical hysterectomy

5. A 40-year-old woman is referred for a Pap smear, which shows high-grade suamous intraepithelial lesions (HSIL). Which of the following statements is most accurate? 　（　　）

A. If HPV subtyping reveals no high-risk virus present, then routine cytology is recommended

B. If colposcopy demonstrates the entire transformation zone, then no further analysis is needed

C. If an endocervical curetting shows CIN, then an excisional procedure of the cervix is appropriate

D. Cervical cancer is highly unlikely because the Pap smear revealed only HSIL

对的? 　　　　（　　）

A. 晚期宫颈癌最佳治疗方法是手术切除

B. 后装及外照射是宫颈癌的重要治疗方法

C. 早期宫颈癌放射治疗及行宫颈癌根治术的优点可保留患者性功能

D. 宫颈癌病理类型大多为腺癌

3. 45岁女性,被诊断为早期宫颈癌,下列哪项是宫颈癌的危险因素? 　（　　）

A. 过早性生活

B. 未产

C. 肥胖

D. 晚绝经

4. 33岁女性,细胞学涂片显示CIN Ⅲ,最佳的处理方式是下列哪个?

A. 3个月后重复细胞学检查

B. 宫颈锥切术

C. 阴道镜指导下活检

D. 根治性全子宫切除术

5. 40岁女性行巴氏涂片,结果显示HSIL,下列陈述哪个是正确的? 　（　　）

A. 如果HPV分型未显示高危型病毒,可推荐行常规细胞学检查

B. 如阴道镜显示整个转化区,没有进一步检查的必要

C. 颈管搔刮显示CIN,宫颈锥切是适应证

D. 巴氏涂片仅显示HSIL,宫颈癌是最不可能出现的

Answers

1. B. HPV subtypes 6 and 11 are associated with condylomata acuminata，whereas subtype 16 and 18 are associated with CIN and cervical cancer.

2. B. Major advantages of radical hysterectomy over radiotherapy are preservation of sexual function （due to vaginal agglutination）and preservation of ovarian function. Radiotherapy can be performed on women who are poor operative candidates and is the best therapy for advanced disease，such as spread to the pelvic sidewalls or hydronephrosis.

3. A. Late menopause and obesity risk factors for endometrial cancer，not cervical cancer. HPV, usually from sexual exposure，is the main risk factor for cervical cancer.

4. C. Colposcopic examination with directed biopsies is the next step to evaluate abnormal cytology on Pap smear.

5. C. When HSIL is present，colposcopic examination is important. HPV typing has a role in triaging atypical cells of undetermined significance，but not HSIL. Demonstration of the entire transformation zone during colposcopy allows biopsy of the worse area. A cervical excisional procedure（LEEP）or CKC is indicated when there is the possibility of endocervical disease.

　　Further Reading：See chapter 4.7，American Cancer Society Guideline for the Early Detection of Cervical Neoplasia and Cancer.

4.8　Myoma

Key words

1. uterine myoma
2. intramural myoma
3. subserous myoma
4. submucous myoma

答案

1. B。HPV 6 及 11 型与宫颈湿疣有关,而 16 及 18 型与 CIN 及宫颈癌有关。

2. B。根治性子宫切除手术对放疗的主要优点是性功能的保留（因阴道的粘连融合）以及卵巢功能的保留,放射治疗主要针对那些不适合手术的晚期患者（如播散到盆壁或患者肾盂积水）,为最佳治疗方法之一。

3. A。晚绝经及肥胖为子宫内膜癌的危险因素,而不是宫颈癌的危险因素,HPV,通常性生活暴露,为宫颈癌的主要危险因素。

4. C。阴道镜指导下活检是进一步评估细胞学有异常的方法。

5. C。当细胞学显示 HSIL,阴道镜检查是重要的,HPV 分型应用于细胞学显示 ASCUS 的分型,而不应用于 HSIL,阴道镜下转化区的完全显示后行病灶活检。LEEP 及 CKC 为颈管有病变时的指征。

　　补充阅读:见 4.7 章节,美国癌症协会发布的早期发现宫颈肿瘤和宫颈癌的指南。

4.8　子宫肌瘤

关键词

1. 子宫肌瘤
2. 肌壁间肌瘤
3. 浆膜下肌瘤
4. 黏膜下肌瘤

5. hyaline degeneration

6. cystic degeneration

7. red degeneration

8. sarcomatous change

9. degeneration with calcification

10. myomectomy

4.8.1　Case

A 40-year-old P_5 woman complains of menorrhagia of 2-yr duration. She states that several years ago a doctor had told her that her uterus was enlarged. Her records indicate that 1 yr ago she underwent a uterine dilatation and curettage, with the tissue showing benign pathology. She takes ibuprofen but obtains no relief of her vaginal bleeding. On examination, her BP is 135/80 mmHg, P 80 bpm, and temperature 36.7 ℃. Heart and lung examinations are normal. Abdomen examination reveals a lower abdominal midline irregular mass. On pelvic examination, the cervix is anteriorly displaced. An irregular middle mass approximately 18 weeks' size seems to move in conjunction with the cervix. No adnexal masses are palpated. Her pregnancy test is negative. Her hemoglobin level is 90 g/L, leukocyte count $10 \times 10^9/L$, and platelet coun $160 \times 10^9/L$.

What is the most likely diagnosis?

What is your next step?

Answers to the case：Uterine leiomyomata.

Summary：A 40-year-old P_5 woman with a history of an enlarged uterus complains of menorrhagia and anemia despite ibuprofen therapy. A pior uterine dilatation and curettage showed benign patholoty. Examination revels an irregular midline mass approxamately 18 weeks' size that is seemingly contiuous with the cervix, and the cervix is anteriorly displaced.

Most likely diagnosis：Fibroid myoma of uterus.

4.8.1　病例

一位 40 岁生产过 5 胎的妇女,月经过多 2 年就诊,她说,几年前,医生曾告诉她,她的子宫增大。病历记录表明,1 年前,她接受了子宫刮宫,检查结果是良性组织改变。她服用了布洛芬,但阴道出血没有减少。查体:血压 135/80 mmHg,脉搏 80 bpm,体温 36.7℃,心肺检查正常。腹部检查示下腹中线不规则包块。盆腔检查:宫颈前倾位,盆腔中部触及一不规则包块,约 18 周妊娠大,似与子宫颈相连并移动,没有触及附件包块。妊娠试验阴性。血红蛋白 90 g/L,白细胞计数 $10 \times 10^9/L$,血小板计数 $160 \times 10^9/L$。

5. 玻璃样变

6. 囊性变

7. 红色样变

8. 肉瘤样变

9. 钙化

10. 肌瘤切除术

什么是最可能的诊断?

你的下一个步骤是什么?

案例的答案:子宫肌瘤。

摘要:子宫增大病史,40 岁的生产过 5 次的妇女,月经过多和贫血,应用布洛芬疗法无效。前次子宫刮宫表明良性组织表现。检查发现盆腔中部不规则包块,约 18 周大,似与宫颈相连,宫颈前倾位。

最可能的诊断:子宫肌瘤。

Next step：Hysterectomy.

4.8.2　Objectives

1. Understand that the most common reason for hysterectomy is symptomatic uterine fibroids.

2. Know that hysterectomy is reserved for syptomatic uterine fibroids that are refractory to an adequate trial of medical therapy.

3. Know that menorrhagia is the most common symptom of uterine leiomymata.

4.8.3　Considerations

This 40-year-old woman complains of menorrhagia. The physical examinaton is consistent with uterine fibroids because of the enlarged midline mass that is irregular and contiguous with the cervix. If the mass were lateral or moved apart form the cervix, another type of pelvic mass, such as ovarian, would be suspected. This patient complains of menorrhagia, which is the most common symptom of uterine fibroids. If she had inter menstrual bleeding, the clinician would have to consider other diseases, such as endometrial hyperplasia, endometrial polyp, or uterine cancer, in addition to the uterine leiomyomata. The patient has anemia despite medical therapy, which constitutes the indication for hysterectomy. If the uterus were smaller, consideration may be given toward another medical agent, such as medroxyprogesterone acetate (Provera). Also, a gonadotropin-releasing hormone (GnRH) agonist can be used to shrink the fibroids temporalily, correct the anemia, or facilitate surgery. The maximum shrinkage of fibroids usually is seen after 3 months of GnRH agonist therapy.

4.8.4　Approach to suspected uterine leiomyomata

4.8.4.1　Definitions

Leiomyomata：Smooth muscle, benign tumors,

下一步：子宫切除术。

4.8.2　学习目标

1. 了解子宫肌瘤是子宫切除术最常见的原因。

2. 明确子宫切除术是用于处理那些经过正规药物治疗无效并有明显临床症状的子宫肌瘤患者。

3. 了解月经过多是子宫肌瘤最常见的症状。

4.8.3　注意事项

这位 40 岁的妇女，主诉是月经过多。物理检查结果一致，支持子宫肌瘤诊断，因为有盆腔中部增大包块、不规则、与宫颈相连。如果包块是在侧方，或不与宫颈相连，要怀疑是其他部位的包块，如卵巢。患者主诉月经过多，是子宫肌瘤最常见的症状。如果她有月经间期出血，医生应当考虑其他疾病，如子宫内膜增生、子宫内膜息肉、子宫体癌或子宫肌腺病。该病人接受了药物治疗但仍然有贫血，这符合子宫切除术的适应证。如果患者的子宫较小（小于 18 周妊娠），可考虑应用其他药物疗法，如安宫黄体酮（孕酮）或促性腺激素释放激素（GnRH）激动剂，用于缩小肌瘤，纠正贫血，辅助手术（使手术更容易进行）。肌瘤的缩小通常是在应用 GnRH 激动剂治疗 3 个月后。

4.8.4　子宫肌瘤诊断方法

4.8.4.1　定义

肌瘤：发生于平滑肌，是子宫

usually of the uterus.

Leiomyosarcoma：Malignant, smooth muscle tumor, with numerous mitoses.

Submucous fibroid：Leiomyomata that are primarily on the endometrial side of the uterus and impinge on the uterine cavity.

Intramural fibroid：Leiomyomata that are primarily in the uterine muscle.

Subserosal fibroid：Leiomyomata that are primarily on the outside of the uterus, on the serosal surface. Physical examination may reveal a knobby sensation.

Pedunculated fibroid：Leiomyomata that is on the stalk.

Carneous degeneration：Change of the leiomyomata due to rapid growth; the center of the fibroid become red, causing pain.

4.8.4.2 Clinical approach

Uterine leiomyomata are the most common tumors of the pelvis and the leading indication for hysterectomy. They occur in up to 25% of women and have a variety of clinical presentations. The most common clinical manifestation is menorrhagia, or excessive bleeding during menses. The exact mechanism is unclear and may be due to an increased endometrial surface area or the disruption of hemostatic mechanisms during menses by the fibroids. Another speculated explanation is ulceration of the submucosal fibroid surfaces.

Many uterine fibroids are asymptomatatic and only require monitoring. Very rarely, uterine leiomyomata degenerate into leiomyosarcoma. Some signs of this process include rapid growth, such as an increase of more than 6 weeks' gestational size in 1 yr. A history of radiation to the pelvis is a risk factor.

If the uterine leiomyomata are sufficiently large, patients may also complain of pressure to the pelvis,

常见良性肿瘤。

平滑肌肉瘤：为平滑肌恶性肿瘤，有丝分裂活跃。

黏膜下肌瘤：发生在子宫内膜下的平滑肌瘤，向宫腔内突出。

子宫肌壁间肌瘤：主要位于子宫肌肉间的平滑肌瘤。

浆膜下肌瘤：向子宫浆膜层表面生长的子宫肌瘤。体检可能触及多个结节。

带蒂的肌瘤：有长柄的肌瘤。

红色样变：由于子宫肌瘤快速增长引起的组织改变，中心变成红色的，引起疼痛。

4.8.4.2 临床诊断

子宫肌瘤是最常见的肿瘤，是子宫切除术最多见的指征。高达25%的女性患有肌瘤，并有多种临床表现。最常见的临床表现为月经过多或月经期间失血过多。引发出血的确切的机制不明，可能是由于子宫内膜表面积增加或肌瘤的存在干扰了月经期间子宫的正常止血机制。另一种推测的解释是黏膜下子宫肌瘤表面溃疡。

许多子宫肌瘤是没有临床症状的，只需要监控观察。极少情况下，子宫肌瘤会恶变成平滑肌肉瘤。这个过程中的一些迹象，包括快速增长，如在1年增长超过6个孕周大小。盆腔内放射是恶变的一个危险因素。

如果子宫肌瘤足够大，患者可能会有骨盆、膀胱或直肠的压

bladder, or rectum. Rarely, the uterine fibroid on a pedicle may twist, leading to necrosis and pain. Also, a submucous leiomyomata can prolapse through the cervix, leading to labor-like uterine contraction pain.

The physical examination typical of uterine leiomyomata is an irregular, middline, firm, nontender mass that moves contiguously with the cervix. This initial treatment of uterine fibroids is medical, such as with nonsteroidal antiinflammatory drugs or progestin therapy. GnRH agonists lead to a decrease in uterine fibroid size, reaching maximal effect in 3 months. After discontinuation of this agent, the leiomyomata usually regrow to pretreatment size. Thus, GnRH agonist therapy is reserved for tumor shrinkage or correction of anemia prior to operative treatment.

Hysterectomy is considered the proven treatment for symptomatica uterine fibroids when pregnancy is undesired.

Uterine artery embolization is a technique performed by cannulizing the femoral artery, catheterizing both uterine arteries directly, and infusing embolization particles that preferentially float to the fibroid vessels. Fibroid infarction, subsequent hyalinization and fibrosis result. Although short-term results appear promising, long-term data are not yet available.

Myomectomy is still considered the procedure of choice for women with symptomatic uterine leiomyomata who desire pregnancy. The indication for surgery is persistent symptoms despite medical therapy. Significant menorrhagia often leads to anemia.

4.8.4.3　Comprehensive Questions

1. Which of the following types of uterine fibroids would most likely lead to recurrent abortion?　　　（　　）

    A. Submucosal　　　　　B. Intramural

迫症状。在极少数情况下，子宫肌瘤的蒂会扭转，导致坏死和疼痛。此外，黏膜下肌瘤可通过宫颈脱垂入阴道，导致像生产时一样的子宫收缩疼痛。

典型的子宫肌瘤体检表现，是不规则的、居骨盆中位、质硬、无压痛的包块，与宫颈相连并可移动。首选的治疗方法是非甾体类抗炎药物或孕激素治疗。GnRH 激动剂可导致子宫肌瘤体积缩小，在 3 个月内达到最大效应，但在停药后，肌瘤通常会恢复原来大小，因此，GnRH 激动剂只用于在手术前使肿瘤缩小或术前纠正贫血。

子宫切除术是治疗有临床症状且不再有生育要求的子宫肌瘤患者的有效方法。

子宫动脉栓塞术是经股动脉插管，直接置管于两侧的子宫动脉，注入血管栓塞颗粒，主要是堵塞子宫肌瘤血管，使子宫肌瘤梗死，随后发生玻璃样变和纤维化，从而达到治疗目的。虽然短期治疗效果较好，但远期的数据尚缺乏。

子宫肌瘤切除术是有临床症状并渴望怀孕的患者的选择。肌瘤切除术的指征是经药物治疗后临床症状持续，显著月经过多，或有贫血。

4.8.4.3　综合分析题

1. 以下哪种类型的子宫肌瘤最有可能导致习惯性流产？（　　）

    A. 黏膜下肌瘤　B. 肌壁间肌瘤

C. Subserous　　　　D. Parasitic

E. Pedunculated

2. Which of the following is the most common clinical presentation of uterine leiomyomata?　　（　　）

A. Infertility　　　　B. Menorrhagia

C. Ureteral obstruction　　D. Pelvic pain

E. Recurrent abortion

3. A 29-year-old G_2P_1 woman at 39 weeks' gestation previously had a myomectomy for inferlitility. While pushing during the second stage of labor, she is noted to have fetal tachycardia associated with some vaginal bleeding. The fetal head, which was previously at $+2$ station, is now toted to be -3 station. Which of the following is the most likely diagnosis?　　（　　）

A. Submucosal myomata

B. Umbilical cord prolapse

C. Uterine rupture

D. Placental abruption

E. Fetal congenital heart block

4. A 65-year-old woman is noted to have suspected uterine fibroids on physical examination. Over the course of 1 yr, she is noted to have enlargement of her uterus from approximately 12 weeks' size to 20 weeks' size. Which of the following is the best management?　　（　　）

A. Continued careful observation

B. Monitoring with ultrasound examinations

C. Exploratory laparotomy with hysterectomy

D. GnRH

E. Progestin therapy

Answers

1. A. Submucous fibroids are the fibroids most likely to be associated with recurrent abortion because of their effect on the uterine cavity.

2. B. Menorrhagia is the most common symptom of uterine fibroids.

C. 浆膜下肌瘤　D. 带蒂的肌瘤

E. 脱出的肌瘤

2. 下列哪项是最常见的子宫肌瘤的临床表现？　　（　　）

A. 不孕　　　　B. 月经过多

C. 输尿管梗阻　D. 盆腔疼痛

E. 复发性流产

3. 29 岁妇女，G_2P_1，孕 39 周，以前因不孕行子宫肌瘤剔除术。第二产程屏气用力时，发现胎心变慢并有少量的阴道流血。胎头位置由 $+2$ 上升到 -3。下列哪项是最可能的诊断？

（　　）

A. 黏膜下肌瘤

B. 脐带脱垂

C. 子宫破裂

D. 胎盘早剥

E. 胎儿先天性心脏传导阻滞

4. 一个 65 岁的妇女，体检怀疑有子宫肌瘤。在一年期间，发现肌瘤自 12 个孕周增大至 20 个孕周大小。下列哪项是最合适的治疗措施？　　（　　）

A. 继续严密观察

B. 应用 B 超进行监测

C. 腹腔镜探查行子宫切除术

D. 激素 GnRH 治疗

E. 孕激素治疗

答案

1. A. 黏膜下肌瘤. 黏膜下子宫肌瘤是与复发性流产密切相关联的，因为会对子宫腔内造成影响。

2. B. 月经过多是子宫肌瘤最常见的症状。

3. C. Extensive myomectomies sometimes necessitate cesarean delivery because of the risik of uterine rupture. Most practitioners use the rule of thumb that if the endometrial cavity is entered during myomectomy, a cesarean delivery should be performed with pregnancy.

4. C. The rapid growth suggests leiomyosarcoma; the diagnosis and treatment are surgical. Also, substantial growth of utertine fibroids in post-menopausal women is unusual.

4.8.4.4　Clinical pearls

The most common reason for hysterectomy is symptomatic uterine fibroids. The most common symptom of uterine fibroids is menorrhagia. The physical examination consistent with uterine leiomyomata is an irregular pelvic mass that is mobile, midline, and moves contiguously with the cervix.

Leiomyosarcoma rarely arises from leiomyoma; rapid growth or a history of prior pelvic irradiation should raise the index of suspicion. Significant growth in suspected uterine fibroids in postmenopausal women is unusual and generally requires surgical evaluation.

4.9　Endometrial Carcinoma

Key words

1. nulliparous
2. menopause
3. irregular menses
4. estrogen replacement therapy，ERT
5. diabetes mellitus
6. hypoglycemic agent
7. external genitalia
8. adnexal masses

3. C.巨大的子宫肌瘤剔除术史有时候需要剖宫产结束分娩，因为有子宫破裂的危险。大多数医生使用的经验法则是，如果在子宫肌瘤剔除术时进入到子宫腔,应行剖宫产。

4. C.肌瘤生长快速,提示可能为平滑肌肉瘤。诊断和治疗方案是手术。此外,在绝经后妇女肌瘤的快速增长是不正常的。

4.8.4.4　临床要点

子宫切除术的最常见原因是有临床症状的子宫肌瘤。子宫肌瘤最常见的症状是月经过多,子宫肌瘤体检典型发现,是不规则的盆腔包块,位置居中,移动,与宫颈相连且可移动。

极少数情况下,子宫肌瘤会恶变成平滑肌肉瘤。肌瘤快速增长或患者有盆腔照射史,应高度怀疑恶变可能。绝经后的妇女子宫肌瘤快速增长是不寻常的,一般需要手术治疗以明确诊断。

4.9　子宫内膜癌

关键词

1. 未产妇
2. 绝经
3. 月经不规律
4. 雌激素替代疗法
5. 糖尿病
6. 降糖药物
7. 外生殖器
8. 附件肿块

9.	postmenopausal vaginal bleeding	9.	绝经后阴道出血
10.	endometrial biopsy	10.	子宫内膜活检
11.	endometrial cancer	11.	子宫内膜癌
12.	risk factors	12.	高危因素
13.	malignant	13.	恶性的
14.	premalignant conditions	14.	癌前病变
15.	anovulation	15.	无排卵
16.	late menopause	16.	晚绝经
17.	aspiration	17.	抽吸
18.	flexible catheter	18.	可弯曲导管
19.	unopposed estrogen replacement therapy	19.	无拮抗的雌激素替代治疗
20.	surgical staging	20.	手术分期
21.	atrophic endometrium	21.	萎缩性子宫内膜
22.	blind sampling	22.	盲刮取样
23.	endometrial biopsy device	23.	子宫内膜活检器械
24.	hysteroscopy	24.	宫腔镜
25.	endometrial polyps	25.	子宫内膜息肉
26.	endometrial stripe	26.	子宫内膜线
27.	endometrial thickness	27.	子宫内膜增厚
28.	endometrial hyperplasia	28.	子宫内膜增生
29.	complex hyperplasia with atypia	29.	子宫内膜复杂增生伴不典型增生
30.	atrophic endometritis	30.	萎缩性子宫内膜炎
31.	vaginitis	31.	阴道炎
32.	hormone replacement therapy，HRT	32.	激素替代治疗
33.	vaginal sonography	33.	经阴道超声检查
34.	early menarche	34.	初潮过早
35.	obesity	35.	肥胖
36.	chronic anovulation	36.	慢性无排卵
37.	estrogen-secreting ovarian tumors	37.	分泌雌激素的卵巢肿瘤
38.	total abdominal hysterectomy	38.	经腹全子宫切除术
39.	bilateral salpingo-oophorectomy	39.	双侧卵巢输卵管切除术（双附件切除术）
40.	omentectomy	40.	大网膜切除术
41.	lymph node sampling	41.	淋巴结活检术
42.	peritoneal washings	42.	腹腔冲洗液
43.	polycystic ovarian syndrome	43.	多囊卵巢综合征

4.9.1　Case

A 66-year-old nulliparous woman who underwent menopause at age 55-years complain of a 2-week history of vaginal bleeding. Prior to menopause, she had irregular menses, She denies use of estrogen replacement therapy. Her medical history is significant for diabetes mellitus controlled with an oral hypoglycemic agent. On examination, she weighs 86 kg and 150 cm tall, Her blood pressure is 150/95 mmHg and temperature 37.2 ℃. Heart and lung examinations are normal. The abdomen is obese, and no masses are palpated. The external genitalia appear normal, and the uterus seems to be of normal size without adnexal masses.

What is the next step?

What is your conern?

ANSWERS TO QUESTION：Postmenopausal Bleeding.

Summary：A 66-year-old diabetic, nulliparous woman complains of postmenopausal vaginal bleeding. Prior to menopause, which occurred at age 55 years, she had irregular menses. She denies use of estrogen replacement therapy. Her examination is significant for obsesity and hypertension.

Next step：Perform an ednometrial biopsy.

Your concern：Endometrial cancer.

4.9.2　Objectives

1. Understand that postmenopausal bleeding requires endometrial sampling to assess for endometrial cancer.

2. Know the risk factors for endometrial cancer.

3. Know that endometrial cancer is staged surgically.

4.9.3　Considerations

This patient has postmenopausal vaginal bleeding, which always should be investigated,

4.9.1　病例

一位 66 岁的未产妇女，55 岁绝经，近两周出现阴道流血。绝经期之前，有月经不规则，否认使用雌激素替代疗法。既往有糖尿病史，口服降糖药控制血糖。查体：体重 86 kg，身高 150 cm，血压 150/95 mmHg，体温 37.2 ℃，心肺检查都正常，腹部脂肪肥厚，未触及包块。外生殖器检查正常，子宫正常大小，未发现附件包块。

下一步应当做什么？

你的意见是什么？

答案：绝经后出血。

摘要：一位 66 岁的糖尿病患者，未产妇女，出现绝经后阴道出血。55 岁绝经之前，有月经不规则史。未使用雌激素替代疗法。体检主要发现：肥胖和高血压。

下一步检查：子宫内膜活检。

你的意见：子宫内膜癌。

4.9.2　目标

1. 理解绝经后出血需要子宫内膜取样来评估是否患有子宫内膜癌。

2. 了解子宫内膜癌的危险因素。

3. 明确子宫内膜癌是根据手术来分期的。

4.9.3　注意事项

该患者有绝经后阴道出血，应当给予高度关注，因为这可能

because it can indicate malignant or premalignant conditons. The biggest concern should be endometrial cancer. She also has numerous risk factors for endometrial cancer, including obesity, diabetes, hypertension, prior anovulation (irregular menses), late menopause, and nulliparity. The endometrial sampling or aspiration can be performed in the office by placing a thin, flexible catheter through the cervix. It is the initial test of choice to assess for endometrial cancer. This patient is taking no unopposed estrogen replacement therapy, which should be another risk factor. If endometrial cancer were diagnosed, the patient would require surgical staging. If the endometrial sampling is negative for cancer, another care for postmenopausal bleeding, such as atrophic endometrium, is possible. A blind sampling of the endometrium, such as with the endometrial biopsy device, has 90% to 95% sensitivity for detecting cancer. If this patient, who has so many risk factors for endometrial cancer, were to have a negative endometrial sampling, many practitiioners would go to direct visualization of the endometrial cavity, such as hysteroscopy. If the clinician were to elect to observe this patient after the endometrial biopsy, any further bleeding episodes would necessitate further investigation.

4.9.4　Approach to postmenopausal bleeding

4.9.4.1　Definitons

Ednometrial smpling(biopsy)：Thin catheter is introduced through the cervix into the uterine cavity under some suction to aspirate endometrial cells.

Endometrial polyps：Growth of endometrial galnds and stroma, which projects into the uterine cavity, usually on a stalk; it can cause postmenopausal bleeding.

Atrophic endometrium：Most common cause of

是恶性肿瘤或癌前病变的表现。最先考虑的应该是子宫内膜癌。她有许多子宫内膜癌的高危因素,包括肥胖、糖尿病、高血压、排卵异常(月经不规则)、绝经延迟、未产。子宫内膜取样或吸宫可以通过宫颈插入细导管获取。这是评估子宫内膜癌的首选检查方法。该患者没有服用雌激素替代疗法,雌激素疗法是子宫内膜癌的另一个危险因素。如果子宫内膜癌的诊断确立,病人需要手术,然后根据手术结果进行分期;如果子宫内膜取样是阴性结果,那么,需考虑其他的病变,如子宫内膜萎缩。子宫内膜诊刮取样,有90%至95%的癌症检测的灵敏度。该病人有这么多的子宫内膜癌的危险因素,子宫内膜取样结果却是阴性,许多医生会直接进行宫腔镜下的直接可视化检查取样。如果医生选择对这个患者进行观察期待疗法,那么,任何再次出现的阴道流血情况,都要作进一步评估。

4.9.4　绝经后出血的诊断治疗

4.9.4.1　定义

子宫内膜活检(子宫内膜取样/活检)：细导管通过子宫颈到子宫腔,利用负压吸取子宫内膜细胞。

子宫内膜息肉：内膜腺体和基质增生,突向子宫腔,通常有蒂,可以引起绝经后出血。

萎缩性子宫内膜：绝经后出

postmenopausal bleeding is friable tissue of the endometrium or vagina because of low estrogen levels.

Endometrial stripe：Transvaginal sonographic assessment of the endometrial thickness；a thickness greater than 5 mm is abnormal in a postmenopausal woman.

4.9.4.2　Clinical approach

Postmenopausal bleeding always must be investigated because it can indicate malignant disorders and premalignant conditions. Such as endometrial hyperplasia. Notably, complex hyperplasia with atypia is associated with endometrial carcinoma in 30% to 50% of cases.

Approximately 20% of postmenopausal women not on hormonal therapy but complaining of vaginal bleeding will have an endometrial carcinoma. The most common etiology of postmenopausal bleeding is atrophic endometritis or vaginitis. In additoon, vaginal spotting can occur in a patient taking hormonal therapy. However, because endometrial malignancy can coexist with atrophic changes or in woment taking hormone replacement therapy, endometrial carcinoma must be ruled out in any patient with postmenopausal bleeding. Possible methods for assessment of the endometrium include endometrial sampling, hysteroscopy, and vaginal sonography.

Risk factors for endometrial cancer are listed in Table 4-9-1. They primarily include conditions of estrogen exposure without progesterone. Although endometrial cancer typically affects older women, a woman in her 30s with a history of chronic anovulation, such as polycystic ovarian syndrome, may be affected. When the endometrial sampling is unrevealing, the patient with persistent postmenopausal bleeding, or with numerous risk factors for endometrial cancer, should undergo

血的最常见的原因是由于雌激素水平低,子宫内膜或阴道组织脆弱易出血。

子宫内膜增厚：经阴道超声评估子宫内膜厚度。绝经后妇女内膜厚度超过 5 mm 为异常。

4.9.4.2　临床诊断

对绝经后出血必须高度重视,因为它可能是恶性疾病或/和癌前病变,如子宫内膜增生等的表现。值得注意的是,30% 至 50% 的子宫内膜癌病例中有复杂型增生与不典型增生同时存在。

大约 20% 的没有接受激素疗法的绝经后阴道出血妇女患子宫内膜癌。绝经后出血的最常见的病因是子宫内膜萎缩炎和阴道炎,另外,在服用激素治疗的病人可有阴道点滴出血。然而,因为子宫内膜癌可与子宫内膜萎缩性改变共存,也可发生在服用激素替代疗法的妇女,因此任何发生绝经后阴道流血的妇女都必须排除子宫内膜癌。子宫内膜的评估方法包括子宫内膜取样、宫腔镜下活检和经阴道超声检查。

子宫内膜癌的危险因素,见表 4-9-1。主要原因是无孕激素的雌激素暴露。虽然子宫内膜癌通常会出现在老年妇女,一个 30 岁有慢性无排卵史的年轻妇女,如患有多囊卵巢综合征,也有可能患子宫内膜癌。一个有多种子宫内膜癌危险因素的持续绝经后阴道出血的病人,如果子宫内膜取样结果是阴性的,应该接受进

further evaluation，such as hysteroscopy. Direct visualization of the intrauterine cavity can identify small lesions that may be missed by the office endometrial sampling device. Additionally, endometrial polyps can be identified by hysteroscopy.

一步的评估,如宫腔镜下直接可视化活检等。可以发现盲刮宫可能会错过的小病灶。此外,子宫内膜息肉也可以经过宫腔镜进行识别。

Table 4-9-1　Risk factors for endometrial cancer

表 4-9-1　子宫内膜癌的风险因素

Early menarche 初潮早	Late menopause 晚绝经
Obesity 肥胖	Chronic anovulation 慢性无排卵
Estrogen-secreting ovarian tumors 分泌雌激素的卵巢肿瘤	Ingestion of unopposed estrogen 不反对雌激素的摄入
Hpyertension 高血压	Diabetes mellitus 糖尿病
Personal or family history of breast or ovarian cancer 乳腺癌或卵巢癌的个人或家族史	

Endometrial carcinoma is the most common female genital tract malignancy. Although endometrial cancer is not the most common cause of postmenopausal bleeding, it usually is the one of most concern. Fortunately, endometrial cancer usually is detected at an early stage because it is associated with an early symptom, postmenopausal bleeding. Once diagnosed, endometrial cancer is staged surgically.

子宫内膜癌是最常见的女性生殖道恶性肿瘤。虽然子宫内膜癌不是绝经后出血的最常见的原因,它通常是最受关注之一。幸运的是,子宫内膜癌通常在早发现阶段发现,因为绝经后出血是其早期症状,一旦确诊,就需行手术治疗。子宫内膜癌的分期程序如表 4-9-2 所示。

Table 4-9-2　Staging procedure for endometrial cancer

表 4-9-2　子宫内膜癌的分期程序

Total abdominal hysterectomy, bilateral salpingo-oophorectomy 经腹全子宫切除术,双侧输卵管卵巢切除术	Omentectomy 大网膜切除术
Lymph node sampling 淋巴结取样	Peritoneal washings 腹腔冲洗

Carcinoma of the endometrium(FIGO,2009)：

Stage Ⅰ Tumor confined to the corpus uteri

　　Ⅰ A No or less than half myometrial invasion

　　Ⅰ B Invasion equal to or more than half of the myometrium

子宫内膜癌的分期(FIGO,2009)：

Ⅰ 肿瘤局限于子宫体

　　Ⅰ A 肿瘤浸润深度<1/2 肌层

　　Ⅰ A 肿瘤浸润深度≥1/2 肌层

Stage Ⅱ Tumor invades cervical stroma, but does not extend beyond the uterus

Stage Ⅲ Local and/or regional spread of the tumor

　　Ⅲ A Tumor invades the serosa of the corpus uteri and/or adnexae

　　Ⅲ B Vaginal and/or parametrial involvement

　　Ⅲ C Metastases to pelvic and/or para-aortic lymph nodes

　　　　Ⅲ C1 Metastases to pelvic lymphnodes

　　　　Ⅲ C2 Metastases to para-aortic lymphnodes

Stage Ⅳ Tumor invades the mucosa of bladder or rectal and/or distant organ.

　　Ⅳ A Tumor invades the bladder mucosa and rectal mucosa.

　　Ⅳ B Metastases to distant organ including inguinal lymph nodes, *etc.*

4.9.5　Comprehension questions

1. A 60-year-old woman is diagnosed with endometrial cancer. Which of the following is a risk factor for endometrial cancer?　　（　　）

　　A. Mulitiparity

　　B. Herpes simplex infection

　　C. Diabetes mellitus

　　D. Oral contraceptive use

　　E. Smoking

2. A 48-year-old postmenopausal woman undergoes Pap smear examination, which reveals atypical glandular cells. Which of the following is the best next step?

　　A. Repeat Pap smear in 3 months　　（　　）

　　B. Colposcopy, endocervical curettage, endometrial sampling

　　C. Hormone replacement therapy

　　D. Vaginal sampling

3. A 57-year-old postmenopausal woman with hypertension, diabetes, and a history of polycystic ovaian syndrome complains of vaginal

Ⅱ 肿瘤侵犯宫颈间质,但无宫体外蔓延

Ⅲ 肿瘤局部和(或)区域扩散

　　Ⅲ A 肿瘤累及浆膜层和(或)附件

　　Ⅲ B 阴道和(或)宫旁受累

　　Ⅲ C 盆腔淋巴结和(或)腹主动脉旁淋巴结转移

　　　　Ⅲ C1 盆腔淋巴结阳性

　　　　Ⅲ C2 腹主动脉旁淋巴结阳性和(或)盆腔淋巴结阳性

Ⅳ 肿瘤侵及膀胱和(或)直肠黏膜,和(或)远处转移

　　Ⅳ A 肿瘤侵及膀胱或直肠黏膜

　　Ⅳ B 远处转移,包括腹腔内和(或)腹股沟淋巴结转移

4.9.5　理解问题

1. 一个 60 岁的妇女被诊断出患有子宫内膜癌。下列哪一个是子宫内膜癌的危险因素?　（　　）

　　A. 多次生产

　　B. 单纯疱疹病毒感染

　　C. 糖尿病

　　D. 使用口服避孕药

　　E. 吸烟

2. 一位 48 岁的绝经后妇女进行子宫颈抹片检查,发现非典型腺细胞。下列哪项是最好的下一步检查项目?　（　　）

　　A. 在 3 个月重复抹片

　　B. 阴道镜检查,宫颈管搔刮宫,子宫内膜取样

　　C. 激素替代疗法

　　D. 阴道活检

3. 一个 57 岁的绝经后妇女患有高血压、糖尿病和多囊卵巢综合征,阴道出血 2 周。子宫内

bleeding for 2 weeks. The endometrial sampling shows a few fragments of atrophic endometrium. Estrogen replacement therapy is begun. The patient continues to have several episodes of vaginal bleeding 3 months later. Which of the following is the best next step? (　　)

A. Continued observaton and reassurance

B. Unopposed estrogen replacement therapy

C. Hysteroscopic examination

D. Endometrial ablation

E. Serum cancer antigen 125(CA-125) testing

4. Which of the following is the most important therapeutic measure in the treatment of stagel (confined to the uterus) endometrial cancer? (　　)

A. Radiation therapy

B. Chemotherapy

C. Immunostimulation therapy

D. Progestin therapy

E. Surgical therapy

Answers

1. C. Diabetes mellitus is associated with endometrial cancer. Progestin use will decrease the risk of endometrial cancer.

2. B. A typical galandular cells on the Pap smear may indicate endocervical or endometrial cancer. Therefore, an colaposcopic examination of the cervix, curetage of the endocervix and endometrial sampling are indicated.

3. C. Persistent postmenopausal bleeding, especially in a woman with risk factors for endometrial cancer, must be pursued. Hysteroscopy is one of the best methods for assessing the uterine cavity.

4. E. Surgical treatment is a fundamental aspect of the treatment. Radiotherapy is used as an adjunctive treatment for possible spread.

膜取样显示子宫内膜萎缩,开始雌激素替代疗法。3个月后病人持续有阴道出血。下列哪项是最好的下一步检查项目? (　　)

A. 继续观察

B. 单一雌激素替代疗法(无孕激素抵抗)

C. 宫腔镜检查

D. 子宫内膜消融术

E. 血清癌胚抗原-125(CA-125)检测

4. 下列哪项是1期子宫内膜癌(局限在子宫内)最重要的治疗措施? (　　)

A. 放射治疗

B. 药物化疗

C. 免疫刺激疗法

D. 孕激素治疗

E. 手术治疗

答案

1. C. 糖尿病与子宫内膜癌发病有关。孕激素的使用会减少子宫内膜癌的风险。

2. B. 子宫颈抹片发现腺样细胞可能表明宫颈或子宫内膜癌。因此,要进一步行阴道镜检查、宫颈刮片和子宫内膜活检检查。

3. C. 持续性绝经后出血,特别是在有子宫内膜癌的危险因素的妇女,必须引起关注。宫腔镜下活检是评估子宫腔的最好方法之一。

4. E. 手术治疗是子宫内膜癌的基本治疗方法。放疗作为辅助治疗,用于可能有扩散的病人。

4.9.6　Clinical pearls

- An endometrial sampling should be performed in a woman with postmenopausal bleeding to assess for endometrial carcinoma.
- Unopposed estrogen is generally the biggest risk tactor for development of endometrial cancer.

- Endometrial cancer is staged surgically, and surgery is a fundamental part of its treatment.

- Persistent postmenopausal bleeding warrants further investigation(e. g hysteroscopy)even after a normal endometrial sampling.

    Note 1　Menopausal vaginal bleeding (postmenopausal vaginal bleeding)：Vaginal bleeding after menopause refers to menopause a year, and abnormal reproductive tract bleeding. According to the clinical manifestations and causes of postmenopausal bleeding by the following factors have led to：genital tract inflammation, endocrine disease, benign and malignant tumors. Genital tract inflammation, most (including atrophic vaginitis, cervicitis, atrophic endometritis, the IUD caused by foreign body inflammation, etc.), followed by the female reproductive tract (including cervical cancer, endometrial cancer, ovarian cancer, breast cancer after tamoxifen treatment, etc.).

    Note 2　Endometrial cancer risk factors (risk factors for endometrial cancer)：According to the causes of endometrial cancer and the pathological type can be divided into two types：a class of hormone-dependent tumors (type Ⅰ) occurred in the circuit postmenopausal women, the general endometrial adenocarcinoma; prognosis is good; other special type of endometrial cancer (type Ⅱ), occurs in older women endometrial atrophy in postmenopausal pathology mostly clear cell carcinoma、serous adenocarcinoma for the gene

4.9.6　临床要点

- 绝经后出血的妇女应当进行子宫内膜取样以排除子宫内膜癌。
- 无孕激素对抗的单一雌激素替代疗法,是子宫内膜癌发生的最大的危险因素。
- 子宫内膜癌是根据手术结果进行分期的,手术治疗是其治疗的基本方法。
- 持续性绝经后出血的病人要进一步检查,即使在子宫内膜取样(如宫腔镜)结果正常后。

    注 1　绝经后阴道流血 (postmenopausal vaginal bleeding)：绝经后阴道流血指绝经 1 年后出现的异常生殖道出血。根据临床表现和病因,绝经后阴道流血可由以下因素导致:生殖道炎症、内分泌疾病、良性肿瘤和恶性肿瘤。其中生殖道炎症最多(包括萎缩性阴道炎、宫颈炎、萎缩性子宫内膜炎、宫内节育器造成的异物性炎症等),其次是女性生殖道恶性肿瘤(包括子宫颈癌、子宫内膜癌、卵巢癌、乳腺癌术后的三苯氧胺治疗等)。

    注 2　子宫内膜癌高危因素 (risk factors for endometrial cancer)：根据子宫内膜癌的发生原因和组织病理类型可分为两种类型:一类为激素依赖性肿瘤(Ⅰ型),多发生于围绝经女性,一般为子宫内膜样腺癌,预后好;另一类为特殊类型的子宫内膜癌(Ⅱ型),多发生于绝经后老年女性萎缩的子宫内膜,病理多为透明细胞癌、浆液性腺癌,其发生为基因

mutation due to poor prognosis.

Papillary serous adenocarcinoma (papillary serous adencarcinoma) the high degree of malignancy can easily invade the myometrium, vascular and peritoneal dissemination.

Note 3　Staging surgery (surgical staging) of endometrial cancer. Surgical staging of endometrial cancer clinical staging (FIGO, 1971) and surgical stage (FIGO, 2009) standards, according to the size of the uterus, myometrium and infiltration of the neck, cell differentiation, select different type and scope of surgery and postoperative adjuvant therapy.

4.9.7　Clinical stage (FIGO, 1971)

0　Complex hyperplasia or carcinoma in situ

Stage Ⅰ　Limited to the body of uterus

Ⅰa　Uterine length ≤ 8 cm

Ⅰb　Uterine length > 8 cm

Stage Ⅱ　Of violations of the cervical

Stage Ⅲ　Of pelvic or less

The pelvic outside of stage Ⅳ

Ⅳa　Nearby organs, rectum, bladder

Ⅳb　Of distant metastasis

Note 4　Endometrial complex atypical hyperplasia (complex hyperplasia with atypia): Of endometrial cancer occurrence and development of a long-term progressive pathological process of development, endometrial hyperplasia (simple hyperplasia, SH), complex hyperplasia (complex hyperplasia, CH), dysplasia (atypical hyperplasia, AH, precancerous lesions) to the development of endometrial cancer.

1987 International Association of gynecologic pathology (International Society of Gynecological Pathologist, ISGP) atypical endometrial hyperplasia is divided into the simple type of atypical hyperplasia (simple atypical hyperplasia, SAH) and the

突变所致,预后差。浆液性乳头状腺癌为高度恶性肿瘤,易浸润给肌层血管,并发生腹腔播散。

注 3　手术病理分期(surgical staging):子宫内膜癌的分期是根据子宫内膜癌临床分期(FIGO,1971)和手术病理分期(FIGO,2009)标准,按照子宫大小、肌层和颈管浸润程度、细胞分化程度,选择不同类型和范围的手术及术后辅助治疗。

4.9.7　临床分期(FIGO,1971)

0 期　复杂性增生或原位癌

Ⅰ期　限于宫体

Ⅰa 期　宫腔长度≤8 cm

Ⅰb 期　宫腔长度>8 cm

Ⅱ期　侵犯宫颈

Ⅲ期　盆腔以内

Ⅳ期　盆腔以外

Ⅳa 期　附近器官、直肠、膀胱

Ⅳb 期　远处转移

注 4　子宫内膜复杂性不典型增生(complex hyperplasia with atypia):子宫内膜癌的发生和发展是一个长期渐进性病理发展过程,即由子宫内膜单纯性增生(simple hyperplasia, SH)、复杂增生、(complex hyperplasia, CH)、不典型增生(atypical hyperplasia, AH,癌前病变)发展为子宫内膜癌。

1987 年国际妇科病理协会(International Society of Gynecological Pathologist, ISGP)将子宫内膜不典型增生分为单纯性不典型增生(simple atypical hyperplasia,

complexity of atypical hyperplasia （complex, hyperplasia with atypia, CAH）, based on the degree of dysplasia is divided into mild, moderate, and severe. The complexity of endometrial atypical hyperplasia （complex hyperplasia with atypia） are precancerous lesions of the endometrium, its chance to co-exist or develop endometrial cancer is as high as 17%-43%, it should cause doctors attached great importance to timely diagnosis and treatment.

Note 5　Hormone replacement therapy （Hormone Replacement Therapy, HRT）: Hormone replacement therapy aims to maximize the physical fitness of perimenopausal women, to improve the mental state of mind, to improve the quality of life and social activity, prevention and treatment of perimenopausal symptoms and diseases of aging to make them healthy, safe and smooth through the golden dusk of life. Hormone replacement therapy is a medical interventions, there are strict indications, relative contraindications and contraindications, should follow the principle of "people-oriented and evidence-based medicine", follow the principle of individualized, individualized risk/benefit than the assessment, patients with informed consent. It must be pointed out that, for primary and secondary prevention of women's cardiovascular disease, postmenopausal hormone replacement therapy can not be used.

Note 6　Polycystic ovary syndrome （polycystic ovarian syndrome, PCOS; Stein-leventhal syndrome. Sclerocystic ovary disease）: Polycystic ovary syndrome is characterized by HPO axis endocrine dysfunction, insulin resistance, hyperinsulinemia, hyperandrogenism, aovulation, amenorrhea, or menstrual thin hair, infertility and ovarian polycystic change. PCOS has recently aroused anovulation, amenorrhea, hirsutism, obesity and infertility, long-term PCOS may cause endometrial cancer, breast

SAH）和复杂性不典型增生（complex hyperplasia with atypia, CAH），根据不典型增生程度又分为轻度、中度、重度。子宫内膜复杂性不典型增生（complex hyperplasia with atypia）属于子宫内膜癌前病变，其并存或发展为子宫内膜癌的概率高达 17%～43%，故应引起医生高度重视并及时诊治。

注 5　激素替代治疗（Hormone Replacement Therapy, HRT）: 激素替代治疗的目的是最大限度地延长围绝经期妇女的体能，改善精神心理状态，提高生活质量和社会适应能力，防治围绝经相关症状和衰老性疾病，使她们健康、安全顺利度过人生的金色黄昏。激素替代治疗是一种医学干预措施，有严格的适应证、相对禁忌证和禁忌证，应遵照"以人为本"和循证医学原则，遵循个体化原则，以个体化风险/受益比评估为依据，在患者知情同意的情况下进行。必须指出，激素替代治疗不能用于绝经后妇女心血管疾病的一级和二级预防。

注 6　多囊卵巢综合征（polycystic ovarian syndrome, PCOS; Stein-leventhal syndrome, sclerocystic ovary disease）: 多囊卵巢综合征是以 H-P-O 轴内分泌功能失调、胰岛素抵抗、高胰岛素血症、高雄激素血症、无排卵、闭经或月经稀发、不孕和卵巢多囊改变为特征的综合征。PCOS 近期引起无排卵、闭经、多毛、肥胖

cancer, diabetes and cardiovascular disease. Incidence of PCOS in women of childbearing age is 4%, accounting for 8% of the gynecological endocrine diseases, 0.6%-4.3% of the total number of infertility, anovulatory infertility, 30%-40%.

Note 7　cancer antigen 125：CA-125 is an ovarian cancer cell surface glycoprotein secreted protein, an important indicator of epithelial ovarian cancer diagnosis, treatment, follow-up and evaluation of prognosis. Normal < 35 mIU/ml, clinical observations, about 90% of ovarian cancer and tumors contain epithelial components CA-125 expression, the majority of serous carcinoma, endometrial adenocarcinoma and clear cell carcinoma, elevated CA-125, but mucinous carcinoma of the lower. CA-125 is not ovarian cancer specific tumor markers. Non-neoplastic varian diseases, including endometriosis, adenomyosis, menstrual phase, proliferative phase endometrium, pelvic inflammatory disease sequelae; neoplastic diseases, including endometrial cancer, colon cancer, stomach cancer, breast cancer, liver cancer, kidney cancer, lung cancer can also be elevated.

4.9.8　Case

Patients 66 years old, older women, aged 55, menopause, nearly two weeks of bleeding vaginal bleeding. Patients with nulliparous premenopausal menstrual irregularities, deny the application of estrogen replacement therapy. And suffering from severe diabetes, are oral antidiabetic drug therapy. Examination：the patient was obese body weight 86 kg, height 150 cm, BP 150/95 mmHg, T 37.2 ℃, heart and lung check without exception. Abdominal obesity, no palpable mass. Gynecological examination：normal external genitalia, uterus like a normal size, the attachments were not palpable mass.

和不孕,远期则引起子宫内膜癌、乳腺癌、糖尿病和心血管疾病。育龄妇女 PCOS 的发生率为4%,占妇科内分泌疾病的8%,占不孕症总数的0.6%～4.3%,占无排卵不孕的30%～40%。

注7　癌抗原-125（cancer antigen CA-125）：CA-125 是一种卵巢癌细胞分泌的表面糖蛋白,是上皮性卵巢癌诊断、治疗、随访和评价预后的重要指标。正常值<35 mIU/ml,临床观察发现,约90%卵巢癌和含有上皮成分的肿瘤均存在 CA-125 表达,多数为浆液性癌、子宫内膜样腺癌和透明细胞癌 CA-125 升高,但黏液性癌 CA-125 表达较低。CA-125 并非为卵巢癌特异性肿瘤标志物。非卵巢肿瘤性疾病,包括子宫内膜异位症、子宫腺肌病、月经期、增生期子宫内膜、盆腔炎性疾病后遗症等;肿瘤性疾病,包括子宫内膜癌、结肠癌、胃癌、乳腺癌、肝癌、肾癌、肺癌等也可升高。

4.9.8　点评

患者66岁,老年女性,55岁绝经,近2周出现阴道出血。患者从未生育,绝经前月经不规则,否认应用过雌激素替代治疗。并患有严重糖尿病,现口服降糖药物治疗。查体:患者呈肥胖体态,体重 86 kg,身高 150 cm,BP 150/95 mmHg,T 37.2 ℃,心肺检查无异常。腹部肥胖,未触及肿块。妇科检查:外生殖器正常,子宫似正常大小,附件未触及肿块。

Abnormal vaginal bleeding, postmenopausal patients 11 years with endometrial cancer risk factors, including premenopausal menstrual disorders, late menopause, never childbirth, obesity, diabetes and hypertension, should be highly alert to the reproductive tract, especially the uterus endometrial cancer, this should be the diagnostic curettage, and take the endometrium for histopathological examination.

The diagnosis of endometrial cancer in addition to relying on history, symptoms, signs and gynecological examination, it is important that diagnostic curettage for endometrial pathological diagnosis. Curettage before passing through the vaginal ultrasound Doppler detection of endometrial thickness and myometrial changes are necessary, the study suggests that postmenopausal endometrial thickness <4 mm, no need to line the endometrial biopsy, endometrial thickness >4 mm, endometrial check. Such as blind scraping can not obtain endometrial specimens, should be selected in open hysteroscopic biopsy. Can not obtain endometrial samples such as blind scraping, and the choice of observation, during any vaginal bleeding again, have to be further examination. Application of a single long-term estrogen (without progesterone resistance) treatment, including long term use of tamoxifen in the treatment of women with breast cancer, endometrial thickness endometrial biopsy in the normal range (5-12 mm). B-Tip endometrial thickness $\geq$ 12 mm, exclude pregnancy-related curettage to rule out the potential of endometrial lesions.

In addition, pelvic CT and MRI in the diagnosis of pelvic tumors and endometrial cancer also has an important role in endometrial cancer should be identified with the following diseases, including atypical endometrial hyperplasia, endometrial hyperplasia and polyps, uterine mucosa, muscle

根据患者绝经 11 年出现异常阴道出血,同时具有子宫内膜癌的高危因素,包括绝经前月经失调、晚绝经、未曾生育、肥胖、糖尿病和高血压,应高度警惕生殖道恶性肿瘤,特别是子宫内膜癌,为此应进行诊断性刮宫,取子宫内膜进行组织病理学检查。

子宫内膜癌的诊断除依靠病史、症状、体征和妇科检查外,重要的是通过诊断性刮宫,获取子宫内膜进行病理诊断。诊刮前行经阴道超声多普勒检测子宫内膜厚度和肌层变化是必要的,研究认为,绝经后子宫内膜厚度<4 mm,无必要行子宫内膜活检,子宫内膜厚度>4 mm,应进行子宫内膜检查。如盲刮不能获取子宫内膜标本,则应选择宫腔镜下直视活检。如盲刮不能获取子宫内膜标本而选择观察,期间的任何再次阴道出血,都必须进一步检查。长期应用单一雌激素(无孕激素抵抗)治疗,包括长期应用三苯氧胺治疗的乳腺癌妇女,即使子宫内膜厚度在正常范围(5-12 mm)也应该进行子宫内膜活检。B 超提示子宫内膜厚度≥12 mm,排除与妊娠相关后,应进行诊刮,以排除潜在的内膜病变。

此外,盆腔 CT 和 MRI 在诊断盆腔肿瘤和子宫内膜癌中也具有重要作用,子宫内膜癌应与下列疾病鉴别,包括子宫内膜不典型增生、子宫内膜增生和息肉、子宫黏膜下肌瘤、子宫肉瘤和子宫

tumor, uterine sarcoma and uterine adenomyosis, rely on pathological examination.

　　Comprehensive treatment of endometrial cancer surgery, according to the clinical (FIGO, 1970) and surgical pathologic staging (FIGO, 2009) administration of different types and extent of surgery, advanced endometrial cancer (Ⅲ, Ⅳ period) confirmed pelvic lymph node metastases should be given chemotherapy and radiation therapy after surgery. Synthetic progestin, MPA, megestrol acetate, 17-hydroxyl caproic acid progesterone and 18-norgestrel, antiprogestins (RU486) can be used as an adjuvant treatment of endometrial cancer.

腺肌病,均依靠组织病理检查。

　　子宫内膜癌主要采用以手术为主的综合治疗,即根据临床(FIGO,1970)和手术病理分期(FIGO 2009)施行不同类型和范围的手术,晚期子宫内膜癌(Ⅲ、Ⅳ期),手术后证实盆腔淋巴结转移者应给予化疗和放射治疗。合成孕激素、MPA、醋酸甲地孕酮、17-羟己酸孕酮和18-甲基炔诺酮、抗孕激素(RU486)可作为子宫内膜癌的辅助性治疗。

4.10　Ovaian Tumor

4.10　卵巢肿瘤

Key words

关键词

1. parous
2. palpitations
3. weight loss medications
4. immature teratomas
5. afebrile
6. malignant teratomas
7. proptosis
8. unilateral salpingo-oophorectomy
9. lid lag
10. peritoneal implant
11. bowel sounds
12. grade
13. sonography
14. combination chemotherapy
15. adnexal mass
16. magnetic resonance imaging, MRI
17. tachycardia
18. mucinous tumors
19. hyperthyroidism
20. pseudomyxoma peritonei
21. exploratory laparotomy

1. 经产妇
2. 心悸
3. 减肥药
4. 未成熟畸胎瘤
5. 无发热的
6. 恶性畸胎瘤
7. 眼球突出
8. 单侧输卵管卵巢切除术
9. 眼睑下垂
10. 腹膜种植
11. 肠鸣音
12. 级别/分化程度
13. 超声
14. 联合化疗
15. 附件肿块
16. 磁共振成像
17. 心动过速
18. 黏液瘤
19. 甲状腺功能亢进症
20. 腹膜假黏液瘤
21. 剖腹探查

22. ovarian cystectomy
23. intra-abdominal cavity
24. goiter
25. endometrial carcinoma
26. dermoid cyst
27. serous
28. extensive surgery
29. endometroid
30. frozen section
31. Brenner tumor
32. cystic teratoma
33. celar cell
34. corpus luteal

22. 卵巢囊肿切除术
23. 腹腔内
24. 甲状腺肿
25. 子宫内膜癌
26. 皮样囊肿
27. 浆液性
28. 广泛性手术
29. 内膜样的
30. 冰冻切片
31. 纤维上皮瘤
32. 囊性畸胎瘤
33. 透明细胞
34. 黄体

4.10.1 Case

A 22-year-old parous woman complained of a 3-month history of weight loss, nervousness, palpitations, and sweating. She denied a history of thyroid disease and was not taking any weight loss medications. She denied abdominal pain, nausea vomiting, and fever. On examination, she had BP 110/60 mmHg and heart rate 110 bpm, and she was afebrile. Her thyroid gland is normal to palpation. She did not have proptosis or lid lag. Her abdomen was nontender and had normal bowel sounds. She was noted to have a fine tremor. Her uterus was normal in size. A mobile nontender with 9-cm mass was plapated on the right side of the pelvis, which on sonography had the appearance of an adnexal mass with solid and cystic components.

What is the most likely diagnosis?

What is your management of this patient?

Answers to the case：Ovarian Tumor（Struma Ovarti）.

Summary：A 22-year-old parous woman without a history of thyroid disease cmplains of a 3-month history of weight loss, nervousness, palpitations, and sweating. She has tachycardia, but her thyroid gland is normal to plapation. She does not have

4.10.1 病例

一位 22 岁的经产妇女,主诉近 3 月体重下降,紧张,心悸和出汗。无甲状腺疾病史,未服用任何减肥药物。无腹痛、恶心呕吐、发烧或眼前发花等症状。查体:血压 110/60 mmHg,心率 110 bpm,无发烧,甲状腺触诊正常。无突眼或眼睑下垂症状。腹部无压痛,肠鸣音正常。手指有细震颤。子宫大小正常。盆腔扣诊触及一 9 cm 大小包块,无压痛,可移动,居盆腔右侧,超音波检查显示为附件包块,质地囊实性。

最可能的诊断是什么?

如何处理该病人?

此案的解答:卵巢肿瘤(卵巢甲状腺肿)。

摘要:一位 22 岁的经产妇女,无甲状腺病史,近 3 月出现体重减轻,紧张,心悸和出汗。心动过速,但甲状腺触诊正常。无突眼或眼睑下垂。发现有一移动、

proptosis or lid lag. She is noted to have a mobile nontender with 9-cm mass, which on sonography has solid and cystic components.

　　Most likely diagnosis：Hyperthyroidism caused by a benign cystic teratoma containing thyroid tissue (struma ovarti).

　　Management of this patient：Exploratory laparotomy with ovarian cystectomy.

4.10.2　Objectives

　　1. Know that benign cystic teratomas (dermoid cysts) are the most common ovarian tumor in women younger than 30 years.

　　2. Understand that dermoid cysts sometimes contain thyroid tissue and cause hyperthyrodism.

　　3. Know that surgical therapy is the treatment of choice for ovarian tumors.

　　4. Understand how to evaluate and manage adnexal masses in the various age groups.

4.10.3　Considerations

　　This 22-year-old woman has symptoms of hyperthyroidism with weight loss, palpitations, and nervousness. The most common cause of hyperthyroidism is Graves' disease, but the paitent has no history of thyroid disease, and her thyroid is normal to palpation, A patient with Graves' disease usually has a nontender goiter and many times eye-related symptoms (proptosis or lid lag). She has an ovarian mass, which on sonography is noted to be comple, that is, it has both solid and cystic components. There is no mention of ascites in the abdomen; the presence of ascites would be consistent with ovarian cancer. In a young woman (<30 years old) with a unilateral comple ovarian mass, the most likely diagnosis is a cystic teratoma or dermoid cyst. These tumors sometimes contain thyroid tissue and may cause hyperthyroidism. The treatment of choice

无压痛、9 cm 的盆腔肿块，超音波检查为囊实性成分。

　　最可能的诊断：由卵巢良性囊性含甲状腺组织畸胎瘤（卵巢甲状腺肿）引起的甲状腺功能亢进症。

　　病人管理：剖腹探查、卵巢囊肿切除术。

4.10.2　学习目标

　　1. 明确良性囊性畸胎瘤（皮样囊肿）是年龄小于 30 岁妇女中最常见的卵巢肿瘤。

　　2. 了解皮样囊肿有时会含有甲状腺组织并导致出现甲状腺机能亢进症状。

　　3. 明确手术治疗是卵巢肿瘤的首选方法。

　　4. 理解如何评估和处理在各年龄组的附件包块。

4.10.3　注意事项

　　该 22 岁的妇女，有甲亢症状，消瘦，心悸和不安。最常见的甲状腺功能亢进症的原因是 Graves 病，但病人无甲状腺病史，甲状腺触诊正常，患 Graves 病的病人通常有甲状腺无压痛性包块和眼相关症状，常见的是眼球突出或眼睑下垂。该病人有卵巢肿块，超声检查显示为复合性，也就是说，兼有囊实性成分。腹腔无腹水，如果有腹水存在，提示为卵巢癌。在一个年轻的妇女（小于 30 岁）有复合性单侧卵巢肿块，最可能的诊断是囊性畸胎瘤或皮样囊肿。这些肿瘤有时含有甲状腺组织，并可能导致甲状腺功能亢进症。如果肿瘤是良性

for ovarian nioplasm is exploratory laparotomy with ovarian cystectomy, if benign, or more extensive surgery, if malignant. At the time of surgery, the excised cyst is sent for frozen section to determine if it is benign (no further surgery needed) or malignant (surgical staging needed).

4.10.4　Approach to adnexal masses

Germ cell tumors represent approximately one fourth of all ovarian tumors and are the second most frequent type of ovarian neoplasms. They are found mainly in young women, usually in the second and third decades of life. The most common tumor is the benign cystic teratoma (dermoid). A germ cell tumor usually presents as a pelvic mass and causes pain dure to its rapidly enlarging size. Because of these symptoms, 60%-70% of patients present at stage Ⅰ, with tumor limited to one or both ovaries.

Definitions

Cystic teratoma：Benign germ cell tumor that may contain all three germ cell layers.

Struma ovarii：Benign cystic teratoma containing thyroid tissue, which can cause symptoms of hyperthyroidism.

Ovarian neoplasm：Abnormal growth (either benign or malignant) of the ovary; most will not regress.

Epithelial ovarian tumor：Neoplasm arising from the outer layer of the ovary, which can imitate the other epithelium of the gynecologic or urologic system. This is the most common type of ovarian malignancy, ususlly occurring in older women.

Functional ovarian cyst：Physiologic cysts of the ovary, which occur in reproductive-aged women of follicular, corpus lutea or the corpus lutein in origin.

4.10.4.1　Dermoid cysts

Teratomas

Mature benign cystic teratomas (dermoid cysts)

4.10.4　卵巢囊肿诊断治疗

生殖细胞瘤约占所有卵巢肿瘤的 1/4,是第二个最常见的卵巢肿瘤的类型。主要发生于年轻妇女,通常在 20～30 岁之间发现。最常见的肿瘤是良性囊性畸胎瘤(皮样囊肿)。生殖细胞肿瘤通常表现为盆腔肿块,因迅速增大引起疼痛。由于有这些症状,60%～70%的患者会在 1 期就诊被发现,肿瘤局限于一侧或双侧卵巢。

定义

囊性畸胎瘤:良性生殖细胞肿瘤可能包含所有三个胚层的细胞。

卵巢甲状腺肿:良性囊性畸胎瘤含有甲状腺组织,可能会导致甲状腺功能亢进症的症状。

卵巢肿瘤:卵巢异常赘生物(可能为良性或恶性性);多数不会自行消失。

卵巢上皮性肿瘤:源于卵巢外层发生的新生物,组织来源与生殖或泌尿系统上皮相接近。这是最常见的卵巢恶性肿瘤,通常发生在老年妇女。

功能性卵巢囊肿:卵巢生理性囊肿,发生在育龄妇女,可为卵泡或黄体囊肿或黄素囊肿。

4.10.4.1　皮样囊肿

畸胎瘤

成熟的良性囊性畸胎瘤(皮

constitute more than 95% of all ovarian teratomas. They make up 15% to 25% of all ovarian tumors, especially in the second and third decades of life. The most common elements are ectodermal derivatives, such as skin, hair follicles, and sebaceous or sweat glands. However, they can also contain tissues of the three embryonic layers, including mesoderm and endoderm. Ultrasound features of dermoid cysts include a hypoechoic area or echoic bandlike strand.

Torsion is the most frequent complication, with severe acute abdominal pain as the typical initial symptom. This is more commonly seen during pregnancy and puerperium. Torsion is also more common in children and younger patients. Rupture is an uncommon compliction and presents as shock or hemorrhage. A chemical peritonitis can be caused by spill of the contents of the tumor into the peritoneal cavity. The treatment is usually a cystectomy or unilateral oophorectomy with inspection of the contralateral ovary.

Immature teratomas contain all three germ layers, as well as immature or embryonal structures. They are uncommon and comprise less than 1% of ovarian cancers. They occur primarily in the first and second decades of life and are basically unknown after menopause. Malignant teratomas contain immature neural elements, and that quantity alone determines the grade. They are almost always unilateral. The prognosis is direcly related to the stage and the celluar immaturity. The treatment is a unilateral salpingo-oophorectomy with wide sampling of peritoneal implants.

Struma Ovarii

Struma ovarii is a teratoma in which thyroid tissue has overgrown the other elements. They are usually unilateral, occurring more frequently in the right adnexa, generally with a diameter of less than 10 cm. Preoperative clinical or radiologic diagnosis is very difficult. Patients only rarely develop thyrotoxicosis. On magnetic resonance imaging,

样囊肿）占卵巢畸胎瘤的 95%。占全部卵巢肿瘤的 25%，尤多见于 20～30 岁年龄组。最常见是外胚层衍生物，如皮肤、毛囊、皮脂腺或汗腺。也可以包含三胚层组织，包括中胚层和内胚层组织。皮样囊肿的超声特点包括囊状低回声区或带状回声区。

囊肿蒂扭转是最常见的并发症，以严重急性腹痛为典型的首发症状。孕期和产褥期较常见，也常发生于儿童和年轻患者。破裂是少见的并发症，可导致休克或出血。破裂使肿瘤的内容溢出进入腹腔，可引起化学性腹膜炎。治疗方法是卵巢囊肿切除术或单侧卵巢切除术，并行对侧卵巢活检。

未成熟的畸胎瘤包含所有三个胚层的组织，包括不成熟或胚胎结构，是罕见的肿瘤，只占卵巢癌的 1%。主要发生在 10～20 岁年龄组，绝经后少见。恶性畸胎瘤含有未成熟的神经元，单纯从神经元数目上可以决定肿瘤的分级，肿瘤几乎全部是单侧的。预后与分级和神经元的成熟程度直接相关。治疗方法是单侧输卵管卵巢切除术，并对腹腔内种植物进行广泛取样检查。

卵巢甲状腺肿

卵巢甲状腺肿是一种含甲状腺组织为主的畸胎瘤。通常是单侧的，右侧多见，一般直径小于 10 cm。术前临床或放射学诊断是非常困难的。只有少数患者会出现甲状腺中毒症状。磁共振成像显示为复杂性的较厚的隔断的

these tumors appear as complex multilobulated masses with thick septa, thought to represent multiple large thyroid follicles. Most of these tumors are benign, but approxiamtely 10% can have malignant changes. They rarely produce sufficient thyroid hormone to induce hyperthyroidism. The treatment is usually cystectomy or salpingo-oophorectomy.

Epithelial Tumors

The most common ovarian tumors in women older than 30 years are of epithelial origin (Table 4-10-2), The serous subtype is the most common and more often bilateral. Mucinous tumors are characterized by their large size and, if ruptured, may lead to pseudomyxoma peritonei, in which the mucinous material spills out into the intraabdominal cavity. Endometrioid tumors of the ovary may coexist with a primary enndometrial carcinoma of the uterus.

Treatment of epithelial tumors is surgical, and, if malignancy is confirmed, cancer staging is indicated. Treatment of epithelial ovarian cancer involves surgical staging, optimal debulking, followed by combination chemotherapy. Malignant ascites is common in cancer cases. When the ascites is spread to the small bowel and omentum, lymphatic extension may be seen. The tumor marker cancer antigen-125(CA-125) is elevated in most epithelial ovarian tumors and is more specific in post-menopausal women, because a variety of diseases can elevate the CA-125 level during the reproductive years.

多房肿块,类似甲状腺泡。大部分肿瘤是良性的,但大约 10% 会恶性变。它们很少产生足够的甲状腺激素诱发甲亢。通常的治疗是囊肿切除术或输卵管卵巢切除术。

上皮性肿瘤

上皮来源的卵巢肿瘤在大于 30 岁女性中常见(见表 4-10-2),浆液性最常见,常为双侧性。黏液性肿瘤的特点是体积较大,如果破裂,黏液物质泄漏进入腹腔可形成腹膜假性黏液瘤。卵巢子宫内膜样肿瘤也可能与子宫内膜癌并存。

治疗方法是手术,术中确诊为恶性时,进行手术病理分期。上皮性卵巢癌的治疗方法包括手术、优化肿瘤减灭术和随后的联合化疗。恶性腹水在癌症中多见,如果已经蔓延到小肠及大网膜,要进行扩大的淋巴清扫。大多数上皮性肿瘤中可出现肿瘤标志物癌抗原-125(CA-125)升高,在绝经后妇女中敏感性更强,因为在生育年龄,有多种疾病可导致 CA-125 水平升高。

Table 4-10-2 Epithelial ovarian tumors

表 4-10-2 卵巢上皮性肿瘤

Serous 浆液性	Mucinous 黏液性
Endometrioid 子宫内膜样	Brenner 移行细胞
Clear cell 透明细胞	

Adnexal Massses

Evaluation of adnexal masses is guided by the suspicion of neoplasm (benign or malignant). At the extremes of ages, there are few functional ovarian cysts, and the management is straightforward (Table 4-10-3). During the reproductive years, functional ovarian cysts, such as follicular and corpus luteal cysts, sometimes make the evaluation difficult.

In general, any adnexal mass larger than 8 cm is likely a tumor and should be explored. Any adnexal mass smaller than 5 cm suggests a functional cyst. Between 5 and 8 cm, the sonographic features may help to distinguish functional ovarian cyst from neoplasm. Septations, solid components, or excrescences (growth on surface or inner lining) are consistent with a neoplastic process, whereas a simple cyst is more suggestive of a functional cyst. Sometimes a practitioner chooses to observe an adnexal mass that is between 5 and 8 cm in size for 1 month and operate if the mass is persistent.

附件肿块

在发现附件包块后要对其评估以确定良恶性。在极小的年龄段，很少会有功能性卵巢囊肿，处理方法是直接手术（见表 4-10-3）。在生殖年龄段，会有一些功能性的包块，如卵泡或卵巢囊泡或黄素瘤等，造成诊断困难。

一般情况下，任何超过 8 cm 的附件包块很可能是一个肿瘤，应当剖腹检查。任何小于 5 cm 的附件包块有可能是功能性囊肿。在 5 和 8 cm 之间的包块，声像图特征可能有助于区分肿瘤的性质。多房的、实质性内容物或有赘生物（向表面或内层生长）常提示为肿瘤新生物，而一个简单的囊肿常常是功能性囊肿。有时，医生会对 5～8 cm 之间的附件包块观察 1 个月，如果肿块持续存在，进行手术。

Table 4-10-3　Evaluttion of adnexal masses tased on age

表 4-10-3　手术方法

Ace group 年龄组	Ovarian size(cm) 卵巢大小（厘米）	Plan 计划
Prepubertal 青春期	>2	Operate 手术
Reproductive age 育龄期	<5	Observe 观察
	5～8	Sonogram: if septations, solid compoments or excrescences, then operate, observe for 1 month B 超检查，若有分隔、实性成分或赘生物，则观察 1 个月后手术
	>8	Operate 手术
Menopausal 更年期	>4～5	Operate 手术

Comprehension Question

1. Which of the followings is an epithelial cell tumor

理解性问题

1. 下列哪项是卵巢上皮细胞肿

of the ovary? 　　　　　　　　　（　　）

    A. Benign cystic teratoma (dermoid)

    B. Endodermal sinus tumor

    C. Brenner bumor

    D. Choriocarcinoma

2. A 66-year-old woman undergoes ovarian cancer surgical staging, Both ovaries have enlargement, papillary cecrescences, and nodular metastasis on the peritoneum. Which of the followings is the most likely associated? 　　　（　　）

    A. Ascites

    B. Metastasis to the stomach

    C. Pulmonary metastasis

    D. Ureteral obstruction

3. Which of the followings is the best treatment of a suspected dermoid cyst found in an 18-year-old mulliparous woman? 　　　　（　　）

    A. Total abdominal hysterectomy

    B. Unilateral salpingo-oophorectomy

    C. Ovarian cystectomy

    D. Observation

Match the following sonographic findings (A-D) to the ovarian tumor type (4-6) 　（　　）

    A. Completely solid

    B. Simple cyst

    C. Complex

    D. Ascites is commonly seen

4. Granulosa cell tumor 　　　　　　（　　）

5. Benign cystic teratoma (dermoid cyst) 　（　　）

6. Follicular cyst 　　　　　　　　　（　　）

7. A 44-year-old woman is noted to have a 30-cm tumor of the ovary. Which of the following is the most likely cell type? 　　　　（　　）

    A. Dermoid cyst

    B. Granulosa cell tumor

    C. Serous tumor

    D. Mucinous tumor

瘤? 　　　　　　　　　　（　　）

    A. 良性囊性畸胎瘤（皮样）

    B. 内胚窦瘤

    C. 布伦纳（Brenner）瘤

    D. 绒癌

2. 一位 66 岁的女人进行了卵巢癌的手术,双侧卵巢肿大,乳头状增生,腹膜结节性转移灶。下列哪项是最可能的诊断? 　　　　　　　　　（　　）

    A. 腹水

    B. 转移至胃

    C. 肺转移

    D. 输尿管梗阻

3. 一位 18 岁未生育女性,发现疑似皮样囊肿的最佳治疗方法是 　　　　　　　　　（　　）

    A. 经腹全子宫切除术

    B. 单侧输卵管卵巢切除术

    C. 卵巢囊肿切除术

    D. 期待观察

找出下列超声表现（A～D）与卵巢肿瘤类型(4～6)的相互关联性: 　　　　　　　（　　）

    A. 完全实质性

    B. 单纯囊肿

    C. 复合性

    D. 腹水常见

4. 颗粒细胞瘤 　　　　　　　（　　）

5. 良性囊性畸胎瘤(皮样囊肿)（　　）

6. 卵泡囊肿 　　　　　　　　（　　）

7. 一位 44 岁的妇女,发现有一个 30 cm 大的卵巢肿瘤。下列哪项是最有可能的细胞类型? 　（　　）

    A. 皮样囊肿

    B. 颗粒细胞瘤

    C. 浆液性肿瘤

    D. 黏液性肿瘤

Answers

1. C. A Brener is tumor an epithelial type of ovarian neoplasm.
2. A. Ascites commonly is associated with malignant ovarian tumor, particularly of the epithelial variety. Ureteral obstruction is more likely in cervical cancer.
3. C. Ovarian cystectomy is the best treatment of benign cystic teratomas.
4. A. Granulosa cell tumors and Sertoli-Leydig cell tumors are usually solid on ultrasound and may secrete sex hormones. Typically, granulosa theca cell tumors produce estrogen, whereas Sertoli-Leydig cell tumors make androgens.
5. C. Dermoids usually have both solid cystic components.
6. B. Follicular cysts are generally simple cysts without septations or solid parts.
7. D. Mucinous tumors are characterized by their large size.

4.10.5　Clinical pearls

◆ The most common ovarian tumor in a woman younger than 30 years is a benign cystic teratoma (dermoid cyst). The best treatment of a dermoid in a young woman is ovarian cystectomy.

- The most common ovarian tumor in a woman older than 30 years is epithelial in origin, most commonly serous cystadenoma.

- An ovarian mass larger than 5 cm in a postmenopausal woman most likely represents an ovarian tumor and generally should be removed. An ovarian mass larger than 2 to 3 cm in a prepubertal girl likewise should be investigated and many times require removal.
- During the reproductive years, functional ovarian

答案

1. C. 布伦纳（Brener）瘤是上皮发生的卵巢肿瘤。
2. A. 腹水通常与恶性卵巢肿瘤有关,特别是上皮来源的肿瘤。输尿管梗阻常发生在宫颈癌病人。
3. C. 卵巢囊肿切除术是良性囊性畸胎瘤最好的治疗方法。
4. A. 颗粒细胞瘤和睾丸间质细胞瘤通常在超声波中显示为实质性,可分泌性激素。如颗粒细胞瘤产生雌激素,而睾丸间质细胞瘤产生雄激素。
5. C. 皮样囊肿通常有实质性和囊性两种组织成分。
6. B. 卵泡囊肿是一种单纯的囊肿,没有间隔,没有实质部分。
7. D. 黏液性肿瘤的特点是体积较大。

4.10.5　临床要点

- 年龄超过 30 岁的女人最常见的卵巢肿瘤是良性囊性畸胎瘤（皮样囊肿）。年轻妇女患皮样囊肿的最好的治疗方法是卵巢囊肿切除术。

- 在 30 岁以上的妇女最常见的卵巢肿瘤是起源于上皮细胞的肿瘤,最常见的是浆液性囊腺瘤。

- 绝经后妇女大于 5 cm 的卵巢肿块,大部分是卵巢肿瘤,一般应手术切除。在青春期女孩大于 2～3 cm 的卵巢肿块要高度关注,通常需要手术切除。

- 在生育年龄,功能性卵巢囊肿

cysts are common and are usually smaller than 5 cm in diameter. Any ovarian cyst larger than 8 cm in a reproductive-aged woman is probably a neoplasm and should be excised.

- The tumor marker cancer antigen-125 and HE4 is most specific for ovarian cancer in postmenopausal women.

- Mucinous tumors of the ovary can grow to be very large. If they rupture intraabdominally, they may cause pseudomyxoma peritonei, which leads to repeated bouts of bowel obstruction.

◆ Ascites is a common sign of ovarian malignancy.

Ovarian cancer surgery consists of total abdominal hysterectomy, bilateral salmping-oophorectomy, omentectomy, peritoneal biopsies, peritoneal washings or sampling of ascitic fluid, and lymphadenectomy.

Note 1　Graves' disease: the most common hyperthyroidism (hyperthyroidism referred to as hyperthyroidism) also known as diffuse toxic goiter, Graves' disease or Base Du disease (Basedow disease). Graves' disease has a familial tendency, women with a high incidence, and more on the basis of genetic factors, trauma infection, drugs (amiodarone), environment, pregnancy and stress factors induced belong to the suppression of T lymphocyte functional defects, organ-specific systemic autoimmune diseases.

Note 2　germ cell tumors: accounted for 20%-40% of the primary ovarian tumor derived from primordial germ cells of the embryonic gonad, it had a hand into the potential of a variety of organizations, including: ① simple reproductive cell tumors teratoma, dysgerminoma, embryonal carcinoma, endodermal sinus tumor, choriocarcinoma, and multi-blastoma and so on. Which teratoma including mature and immature categories, cystic, solid, or

是常见的,通常是小于直径 5 cm。在育龄妇女任何超过 8 cm 大的卵巢囊肿可能是一个肿瘤,必须切除。

- 肿瘤标志物癌抗原 125 和 HE4 在绝经后妇女对于诊断卵巢癌具有较高的特异性。

- 黏液性肿瘤卵巢能够生长到非常大。如果它们在腹腔内破裂,可能会导致腹膜假性黏液瘤,从而导致肠梗阻反复发作。

- 腹水是卵巢恶性肿瘤的常见表现。

卵巢癌的手术类型包括经腹全子宫切除术、双侧输卵管卵巢切除术、大网膜切除、腹膜活检、腹水的腹腔冲洗或取样、淋巴结清扫等。

注 1　格拉夫斯病(Graves病)是最常见的甲状腺功能亢进(hyperthyroidism,甲亢),也称为毒性弥漫性甲状腺肿、突眼性甲状腺肿或巴塞杜病(Basedow disease)。Graves 病具有家族遗传倾向,女性发病率高于男性,多在遗传因素基础上,由感染、精神创伤、药物(乙胺碘呋酮)、环境、妊娠和应激因素所诱发,属于抑制性 T 淋巴细胞功能缺陷性、器官特异性全身免疫性疾病。

注 2　生殖细胞肿瘤(germ cell tumor)占卵巢原发性肿瘤的20%～40%,来源于胚胎性腺的原始生殖细胞,它有分化为多种组织的潜能,包括:①单纯性生殖细胞肿瘤,如畸胎瘤、无性细胞瘤、胚胎癌、内胚窦瘤、绒毛膜癌和多胚瘤等。其中畸胎瘤包括成熟型和未成熟型两类,可为囊性、

solid and cystic tumor. Teratoma single mesoderm highly specific differentiation of tumors, including ovarian goiter (tumor), carcinoid tumors, goiter-like carcinoid tumor. ② mixed germ cell tumors, gonadal cell tumors and mixed germ cell-sex cord Leydig cell tumor.

Note 3 ovarian thyroid tumor (Struma ovarii): mesoderm rare ovarian single, highly-specific differentiation of the teratoma. The tumor was composed of all or substantially all thyroid substantive organization, it is also known as ovarian goiter. For unilateral growth, diameter < 10 cm, pathological examination of tumor tissue and normal thyroid tissue, nodular goiter or thyroid tumors similar, and the secretion of thyroid hormone function, showing about 25%-35% of patients with hyperthyroidism the clinical manifestations. The majority of struma ovarii are benign, a handful of malignant goiter, including follicular thyroid carcinoma and papillary carcinoma.

Note 4 ovarian tumors (ovarian neoplasm): ovarian tumors of female genital common tumors, including ovarian benign, borderline and malignant tumors. Accordance with the WHO, 1999 to develop ovarian tumor histopathology classification, primary ovarian tumors are divided into four categories: ① epithelial tumors (benign, borderline and malignant), accounting for 50%-70%; ② The sex cord stromal tumors, accounting for 5%-10%; ③germ cell tumor, accounting for 20%-40%; ④non-specific interstitial tumor; ⑤ metastatic ovarian tumors.

Note 5 of the functional ovarian cysts (functional ovarian cyst): women of childbearing age, physiologic ovarian cysts include follicular cysts luteum cyst, luteinized cyst and unruptured luteinized follicle. The formation of functional ovarian cysts and ovarian endocrine dysfunction

实性或囊实性肿瘤。畸胎瘤中单胚层高度特异性分化的肿瘤,包括卵巢甲状腺肿(瘤)、类癌、甲状腺肿样类癌;②混合性生殖细胞肿瘤,包括性腺细胞瘤和混合性生殖细胞-性索间质细胞瘤。

注 3 卵巢甲状腺肿 (Struma ovarii)为较少见的卵巢单胚层、高度特异性分化的畸胎瘤。肿瘤全部或绝大部分由甲状腺实质性组织组成,故也称为卵巢甲状腺肿。多为单侧生长,直径<10 cm,组织病理检查示,肿瘤组织与正常甲状腺组织、结节性甲状腺肿或甲状腺瘤相似,并具有分泌甲状腺激素功能,约25%~35%病人呈现甲状腺功能亢进的临床表现。卵巢甲状腺肿多数为良性,极少数为恶性甲状腺肿,包括甲状腺滤泡状癌和乳头状癌。

注 4 卵巢肿瘤(ovarian neoplasm):卵巢肿瘤为女性生殖器官常见肿瘤,包括卵巢良性、交界性和恶性肿瘤。按照 WHO 1999 年制定的卵巢肿瘤组织病理分类法,原发性卵巢肿瘤分为四类:①上皮性肿瘤(良性、交界性和恶性),约占 50%~70%;②性索间质肿瘤,约占 5%~10%;③生殖细胞瘤,约占 20%~40%;④非特异性间质肿瘤,约占1%~5%;⑤卵巢转移性肿瘤。

注 5 功能性卵巢囊肿 (functional ovarian cyst)即育龄妇女卵巢生理性囊肿,包括卵泡囊肿、黄体囊肿、黄素化囊肿和未破裂黄素化卵泡等。功能性囊肿的形成与卵巢内分泌功能失调相

associated with the menstrual cycle hormone fluctuations，and more natural healing and rarely malignant transformation. Smaller functional cysts can be followed up，the larger and complications (infection，reverse the malignant transformation) who should be treated surgically and sent to histopathological examination.

Note 6　Brenner tumors (Brenner tumors)：sources of rare ovarian cells (the body cavity epithelial ovarian network and ovarian stromal) tumors，accounting for 2% of ovarian tumors，mostly (99%) were benign，very few borderline or malignant tumors. The conventional wisdom is not that the Brenner tumor of endocrine function，recently observed，Brenner tumor may also cause post-menopausal women with endometrial hyperplasia and bleeding，caused by the reports of female masculine.

Note 7　HE4：HE4 is a new tumor marker found in the human epididymis in 1991. It was initially thought to be a mature sperm protease inhibitors，4-disulfide (WFDC) protein belongs to the whey acidic family，with the characteristics of the suspected trypsin inhibitor. Other proteins in this family also include the SLPI，Elafin and PS20 (WFDC1). HE4 gene encodes a 13 kD protein, and its mature glycosylated form is 20-25 kD and includes a single-chain of two WFDC domains. It has been reported that HE4 expression both in the number of normal tissues (including respiratory and reproductive tissues，and ovarian carcinoma)，intraepithelial Is expressed not only at the cellular level，HE4 was confirmed as a ovarian cancer serum marker in 2002. HE4 for ovarian cancer early detection to the U. S. Food and Drug Administration and the European Union approved in 2008，and began in the United States and the European Union The state put into clinical application.

关，与月经周期性激素波动相关，多可自然消退而很少发生恶变。体积较小的功能性囊肿可随访观察，体积较大和出现并发症（感染、扭转、恶性变）者则应行手术治疗并送病理组织学检查。

注 6　勃伦纳瘤（Brenner瘤）为卵巢罕见的多细胞（体腔上皮、卵巢网和卵巢间质）来源的肿瘤，约占卵巢肿瘤的 2%，99%为良性，极少数为交界性或恶性肿瘤。传统观念认为，勃伦纳瘤无内分泌功能，而近来观察发现，勃伦纳瘤也可引起绝经后妇女子宫内膜增生和出血，也有引起女性男性化的报道。

注 7　HE4：HE4 是一种新的肿瘤标志物，1991 年在人附睾中发现，并且最初认为与精子成熟相关的蛋白酶抑制剂，属于乳清酸性 4-二硫化中心（WFDC）蛋白家族，具有疑似胰蛋白酶抑制剂的特性。此家族中的其他蛋白还包括 SLPI、Elafin 和 PS20（WFDC1）。HE4 基因编码一段长度为 13 kD 的蛋白，尽管在其成熟的糖基化形式时，此蛋白大概为 20～25 kD，并且包括含有两个 WFDC 结构域的一条单链。一直以来有报道认为，HE4 在多个正常组织（包括呼吸道和生殖道组织，以及卵巢癌组织）的上皮内均有所表达。不仅在细胞水平上有所表达，2002 年 HE4 被证实为卵巢癌的血清标志物，2008年 HE4 用于卵巢癌早期检测获得美国食品药品管理局和欧盟的批准，并开始在美国和欧盟多个国家投入临床应用。

4.10.6　Review

The patient was a 22-year-old young women, who complained of weight loss, nervousness, heart palpitations and sweating for three months. She denied that she had the history of thyroid disease, nor has the weight-loss drugs, denied there had been abdominal pain, malignant and vomiting, fever, exposed to radiation.

Physical examination：BP 110/60 mmHg, HR 110 bpm, the temperature is normal, normal thyroid palpation, no exophthalmos and lagophthalmos. . Abdominal xamination is soft, no tendernessnd normal bowel. Patients (finger) is a slight tremor phenomenon. The gynecological examination: normal size uterus, the right accessories can reach a diameter of about 9 cm, activities, painless mass. Ultrasound examinations showed right attachment area mass was solid and cystic.

According to the signs and symptoms of patients with progressive emergence of the recent March of hyperthyroidism, the thyroid examination is normal, gynecological examination and ultrasound examination revealed the ovarian tumors, patients with symptoms of hyperthyroidism should be linked to ovarian cancer, further checks whether the ovarian thyroid tumors(or ovarian goiter).

For ovarian thyroid tumor, surgical resection (laparoscopic or open surgery) should be performed, and intraoperative rapid pathological examination should be done to determine the nature of the tumor. In case of benign tumor, simple cystectomy or oophorectomy can be performed. In case of malignant tumor, cytoreductive surgery and postoperative chemotherapy should be used. Given endocrine changes and clinical symptoms of serum thyroxine therapy after surgery.

4.10.6　点评

患者为 22 岁年轻经产妇女，主诉体重减轻、神经过敏、心悸和多汗 3 个月，否认曾患甲状腺疾病史，也未曾服用减肥药，否认曾出现过腹痛、恶性和呕吐、发热、接触放射线等。

体格检查：BP 110/60 mmHg，HR 110 bpm，体温正常，甲状腺触诊检查正常，无突眼和眼睑闭合不全。腹部检查柔软、无压痛、肠鸣正常。患者（手指）轻微震颤现象。妇科检查：子宫正常大小，右附件可触及直径约 9 cm、活动、无痛性肿块。超声检查提示右附件区肿块为囊实性。

根据患者近 3 月来渐进出现的甲状腺功能亢进症状和体征，甲状腺检查正常，但妇科检查和超声检查发现卵巢肿瘤，因此应将患者甲亢症状与卵巢肿瘤联系起来，进一步检查是否为卵巢甲状腺瘤（或卵巢甲状腺肿）。

卵巢甲状腺瘤应手术切除（腹腔镜或开腹手术），术中快速病理检查确定肿瘤性质。如肿瘤为良性，可行单纯肿瘤剥除术或附件切除术。如为恶性，应行肿瘤细胞减灭术和术后化疗。手术后根据血清甲状腺素的变化和临床症状给予相应的内分泌治疗。

4.11 Polycystic Ovary Syndrome

Key words

1. polycystic ovarian syndrome，PCOS
2. insulin resistance and insulin recptor
3. sex hormone-binding globulin，SHBG

4.11.1 Learning objectives

1. Understand the hormone changes in polycystic ovarian syndrome.

2. Be able to recognize the biochemical features.

3. Understand the principles of diagnosis and treatment.

POCS is a syndrome with disfunction of preproductive function and glycometablism. It's main charactors are overproduction of androgen and increased LH pulse frequency. The main clinical symptoms are menstrual irregularity，hirsutism，and infertility，25% of patients are of obsity. A theca cell hyperplasia. The ovaries then become typically enlarged. The characteristic appearance on ultrasound examination is multiple small peripherally placed follicles. Androgen hypersecretion increases the sensitivity of the pituitary to GnRH. This results in increased pulsatile LH secretion and elevated serum LH levels. LH causes further androgen secretion from ovarian theca cells. A vicious circle is thus established. Hypersecretion of LH is associated with both anovulation and an increased risk of miscarriage. A raised fasting insulin and increased insulin responses to oral glucose are seen in many individuals with polycystic ovarian syndrome. Hyperinsulinaemia is the key to the pathogenesis of PCOS，as insulin stimulates androgen secretion by the ovarian stroma and appears to affect the normal development of ovarian follicles.

4.11 多囊卵巢综合征

关键词

1. 多囊卵巢综合征，PCOS
2. 胰岛素抵抗和胰岛素受体
3. 性激素结合球蛋白

4.11.1 学习目标

1. 掌握多囊卵巢综合征的激素变化。

2. 熟悉多囊卵巢综合征的生化表现。

3. 掌握多囊卵巢综合征的诊断与治疗。

多囊卵巢综合征是一种生殖功能障碍与糖代谢异常并存的内分泌紊乱综合征,主要特征是卵巢过度分泌雄激素以及黄体生成素(LH)的脉冲式分泌增加。常见临床表现包括月经失调,多毛症和不孕。25%的患者有肥胖。持续增高的 LH 分泌导致卵巢膜细胞的增生,进而导致卵巢增大。B 超下的典型表现为卵巢边缘有多个小的卵泡。雄激素过度分泌导致垂体对 GnRH 的敏感性增高,这会导致 LH 脉冲式分泌增多,血清 LH 水平增高。LH 会使卵巢膜细胞分泌雄激素进一步增多,从而导致恶性循环。LH 的过度分泌导致不排卵和流产的风险增高。许多 PCOS 患者空腹胰岛素水平增高,且口服葡萄糖后反应性胰岛素水平也增高。高胰岛素血症是 PCOS 致病的关键因素,因为胰岛素通过刺激卵巢基质使雄激素分泌增多,并且影响正常的卵泡发育。

4.11.2 Clinical features of polycystic ovarian syndrome

1. oligomenorrhoea
2. hirsutism
3. acne
4. amenorrhea
5. infertility
6. obesity

4.11.3 Biochemical features

1. Increased LH/FSH ratio.
2. Raised serum androgen index.
3. Decreased sex hormone binding globulin (SHBG).
4. Increased prolactin.
5. Increased serum insulin.

4.11.4 Treatment

Weight loss is the cornerstone of management in obese women. This is usually associated with improvement in both menstrual irregularity and acne, together with a normalisation of the hormone profile. In women of normal weight, the low dose oral contraceptive pill is useful for cycle control. If infertility is the presenting feature, ovulation can be induced with clomiphene. About 20% of such women will not ovulate in response to clomiphene alone and will require more potent ovarian stimulation using gonadotrophins. For clomiphene resistant cases, laparoscopic ovarian surgery is a useful measure which can bring about a reduction in serum LH concentrations and thereby restore regular ovulation. The surgery consists of partial ovarian destruction, using laser or diathermy.

4.11.5 Clinical case

Female, 28 years old. Married for 5 years and no pregnant post abortion due to arrested embryo

4.11.2 多囊卵巢综合征的临床表现

1. 月经稀发
2. 多毛症
3. 痤疮
4. 闭经
5. 不育
6. 肥胖

4.11.3 生化特征

1. LH/FSH 比值增高。
2. 血清雄激素指数增高。
3. 性激素结合蛋白(SHBG)降低。
4. 催乳素增高。
5. 血清胰岛素增高。

4.11.4 治疗

对于肥胖的患者,减轻体重是治疗的关键。这会改善月经不调和痤疮的症状,且使激素水平趋于正常。对于体重正常的患者,可以口服小剂量的避孕药,对于控制月经周期有效。如果不孕症是主要表现,则可给予克罗米芬促排卵。约有 20% 的患者单独使用克罗米芬不能排卵,此时需要联合使用更强有力的促排卵药物,即促性腺激素。对于克罗米芬抵抗的病例,腹腔镜下卵巢手术将是一个有效的办法,能够降低血清 LH 的水平,从而恢复有规律的排卵。术式包括用激光或电热使部分卵巢破坏。

4.11.5 临床病例

女,28 岁。因"结婚 5 年流产后不孕 1 年多"于 2006 年 1 月

development with a previous pregnancy by ovulation induction. Visited in January 2006. Usually has irregular menstruation cycles from 36 to 40 days with the longest one up to 2 months. Menstrual periods are 4 to 6 days, without dysmenorrhea. Often acanthosis nigricans. PE: Height 158 cm, WT 70 kg. No lactating and gynecological examination was normal. Auxiliary examination. Basal body temperature showed single-phase curve. Ultrasound showed that there were more than 12 follicles with diameter less than 8 mm in both ovaries. Tubal patent test showed patency. Hormone tests at day 30 of menstruation cycle with single-phased basal body temperature, estradiol 620 pmol/L, progesterone 2.67 nmol/L, luteinizing hormone 23 U/L, follicle stimulating hormone 8.45 U/L, prolactin 0.91 nmol/L, testosterone 1.7 nmol/L and thyroid stimulating hormone 1.94 mU/L. Blood lipids and transaminases were normal. Anticardiolipin antibodies IgG, IgM and antinuclear antibodies were negative. Fasting glucose was 5.81 mmol/L and fasting insulin was 17.84 mU/L. Both male and female partner's karyotype were normal.

Quastion

1. What is the diagnosis?
2. How to treat the patient?

Answer

1. Diagnosis:
(1) PCOS;
(2) Infertility.
2. Treatment:
(1) Weight loss;
(2) Treat hyperinsulinemia;
(3) Cycle control;
(4) Ovulation.

4.11.6　Test

1. Regarding the polycystic ovarian syndrome:

来我院妇科门诊就诊。患者平时月经不规律，周期 36～40 日，最长达 2 个月，经期 4～6 日，无痛经。常需口服甲羟孕酮月经才来潮。体格检查：身高 158 cm，体重 70 kg（体重指数 28），呈腹部肥胖型（腰围/臀围＞0.85）。毛发分布正常，无黑棘皮征，乳腺无泌乳，妇科检查无异常。辅助检查：基础体温单相曲线；B 型超声检查：双卵巢内均有 12 个以上直径＜8 mm 的卵泡；输卵管通液术通畅；激素检查：基础体温单相的月经第 30 日：雌二醇 620 pmol/L、孕酮 2.67 nmol/L、黄体生成激素 23 U/L、卵泡刺激素 8.45 U/L、催乳激素 0.91 nmol/L、睾酮 1.7 nmol/L、促甲状腺激素 1.94 mU/L；血脂及转氨酶正常、抗心磷脂抗体 IgG、IgM 及抗核抗体均阴性；空腹血糖 5.81 mmol/L，空腹胰岛素 17.84 mU/L；男女染色体核型均正常。

问题

1. 该病例的诊断是什么？
2. 该病例的治疗原则是什么？

答案

1.诊断：
(1)PCOS；
(2)不孕症。
2.治疗原则：
(1)减轻体重；
(2)治疗高胰岛素血症；
(3)调控月经周期；
(4)诱发排卵。

4.11.6　测验

1. 关于多囊卵巢综合征

a. SHBG levels are increased

b. Androgens are increased

c. LH secretion is decreased

d. Galactorrhoea is a feature

e. Menstrual irregularity is a common feature

Answer

a. False. SHBG levels are suppressed by the excess testosterone.

b. True. There is excess androgen secretion which causes hirsutism and acne.

c. False. LH secretion is increased.

d. False.

e. True. Menstrual irregularity reflects disordered ovarian function.

4.12 Menopause

Key words

1. menopause

2. hot flushes

3. perspiration

4. atrophic vaginitis

5. incontinence

6. hormone replacement therapy，HRT

4.12.1 Fast facts

1. Average age at menopause in Chinese women is 49.5 yr.

2. Ovarian failure.

3. Spontaneous cessation of menses.

4. Mark the transition from reproductive to nonreproductive phase of Life.

5. Estrogen deficiency.

4.12.2 Symptoms and signs of estrogen deficiency

1. Hot flushes and perspiration.

2. Atrophic vaginitis，lack of vaginal secretions

a. SHBG 水平增高

b. 雄激素水平增高

c. LH 降低

d. 溢乳是一个特征

e. 月经紊乱是共同特征

答案

a. 错。过高的睾酮抑制了 SHBG 水平。

b. 正确。雄激素增高引起多毛和痤疮。

c. 错。LH 分泌增高。

d. 错。

e. 正确。月经紊乱是排卵障碍的表现。

4.12 绝经

关键词

1. 绝经

2. 潮热

3. 出汗

4. 萎缩性阴道炎

5. 尿失禁

6. 激素替代治疗（HRT）

4.12.1 要点

1. 我国妇女绝经平均年龄为 49.5 岁。

2. 卵巢功能衰退。

3. 自发性月经终止。

4. 标志由生育期过渡到无生育能力的阶段。

5. 雌激素缺乏。

4.12.2 雌激素缺乏的症状和体征

1. 潮热、出汗。

2. 萎缩性阴道炎、阴道分泌

and dyspareunia.

3. Stress incontinence，urethral caruncles and bladder stimulation symptoms.

4. Regression of mammary glands and atrophy of breast tissue.

5. Skin changes，such as loss of tension，elasticity and thickness.

6. Psychologic changes，depression，anxiety，sleep disturbance，loss of memory，fatigue，*etc*.

7. Loss of libido.

8. Osteoporesis and increased fractures.

9. Increased risk of cardiovasclar disease.

4.12.3　Hormone replacement therapy(HRT)

1. Low-dose estrogen treatment，if no contraind-icatious exist，will relieve menopausal symptoms.

2. Discuss the complications and contraindicatious of HRT with patients before therapy and obtain informed consent.

3. HRT complications：

①Endometrial cancer.

②Breast cancer.

③Hypertension.

④Thromboembolic disease.

⑤Lipid metabolism disturbance.

4. HRT contraindications：

①Undiagnosed vaginal bleeding.

②Cancer of endometrium or breast.

③History of thromboembolic disease.

④Acute liver disease.

⑤Chronic impaired liver function.

5. Adverse effects of HRT：

①Uterine bleeding.

②Generalized edema.

③Mustodynia and breast swelling.

④Abdominal distension.

⑤Headaches.

⑥Excessive cervical mucus.

物缺乏和性交痛。

3.压力性尿失禁、尿道肉阜和膀胱刺激症状。

4.乳腺退化、乳房组织萎缩。

5.皮肤改变,如失去弹性和变薄。

6.心理学变化:精神抑郁、焦虑、睡眠障碍、记忆力减退、疲劳等。

7.性欲减退。

8.骨质疏松和骨折增加。

9.心血管疾病的风险增加。

4.12.3　激素替代治疗(HRT)

1.如果无禁忌证,低剂量雌激素治疗能减轻绝经期症状。

2.治疗前必须和患者讨论HRT 的并发症和禁忌证,并取得知情同意。

3.HRT 的并发症:

①子宫内膜癌。

②乳腺癌。

③高血压。

④血管栓塞性疾病。

⑤脂代谢紊乱。

4.HRT 的禁忌证:

①诊断不明的子宫出血。

②子宫内膜癌、乳腺癌。

③血管栓塞性疾病史。

④急性肝病。

⑤慢性肝功能损害。

5.HRT 的副作用:

①子宫出血。

②全身性水肿。

③乳房疼痛和肿胀。

④腹胀。

⑤头痛。

⑥宫颈黏液过多。

6. HRT indications：

Risks and benefits must be evaluated for each patient. Individual designed.

7. Methods of HRT：

Estrogen and progesterone therapy. Oral，skin or vaginal administration are available. Either periodically or continuously sequential or combined therapy are used.

Test：The contraindications of HRT?

Answer：

1. Undiagnosed vaginal bleeding.
2. Cancer of endometrium or breast.
3. History of thromboembolic disease.
4. Acute liver disease.
5. Chronic impaired liver function.

4.13　Amenorrhea

Key words

1. primary amenorrhea
2. secondary amenorrhea
3. imperforate hymen
4. vaginal atresia
5. pituitary tumor
6. Asherman syndrome

4.13.1　Definition

4.13.1.1　Primary amenorrhea

1. No menses by age 16 but with normal second sexual characteristics.

2. No menses by age 14 with absence of secondary sexual characteristics.

4.13.1.2　Secondary amenorrhea

No menses for 6 months or longer after previous regular menses.

---

6. HRT 的适应证：

评估 HRT 对每一位病人的危险性和益处。个体化选择。

7. HRT 的治疗方法：

雌、孕激素治疗。口服、贴皮或阴道用药。可以周期性序贯或联合治疗；或连续性联合或序贯治疗。

测试题：HRT 有哪些禁忌证?

答案：

1. 诊断不明的子宫出血。
2. 子宫内膜癌、乳腺癌。
3. 血管栓塞性疾病史。
4. 急性肝病。
5. 慢性肝功能损害。

4.13　闭经

关键词

1. 原发性闭经
2. 继发性闭经
3. 无孔处女膜
4. 阴道闭锁
5. 垂体肿瘤
6. Asherman 综合征

4.13.1　定义

4.13.1.1　原发性闭经

1. 年龄超过 16 岁，第二性征已发育，无月经来潮者。

2. 年龄超过 14 岁，第二性征尚未发育，无月经来潮者。

4.13.1.2　继发性闭经

正常月经建立后月经停止 6 个月以上者。

4.13.1.3　Physiological amenorrhea

(1) Before menarche.

(2) Pregnancy.

(3) Lactation (breast feeding).

(4) Post-menopause.

This is a normal physiologic status.

4.13.2　Etiology

4.13.2.1　Primary amenorrhea (rare disease)

1. Mullerian agenesis syndrome：

(1) Congenital absence of the uterus.

(2) Imperforate hymen.

(3) Vaginal atresia.

(4) Cervical stenosis.

2. Gonadal dysgenesis：

(1) Turner's syndrome. XO genotype，with dwarfism and webbing of neck.

(2) Hermaphroditism.

(3) Male pseudo-hermaphroditism.

Also named：Androgen insensitivity syndrome. Phenotype is female genitalia with male gonads (46, XY).

4.13.2.2　Secondary amenorrhea (common)

1. Surgical intervention：

Oophorectomy

Hysterectomy

Over-irradiation

2. Pelvic disease：

e. g. Endometrial tuberculosis.

3. Endocrine causes：

55% hypothalamus

20% pituitary

20% ovary

5% uterus

4.13.1.3　生理性闭经

(1)月经初潮前。

(2)妊娠期。

(3)哺乳期。

(4)绝经期后。

生理性闭经属于正常生理状态。

4.13.2　病因

4.13.2.1　原发性闭经(少见)

1.米勒管发育不全综合征：

(1)先天性子宫缺如。

(2)无孔处女膜。

(3)阴道闭锁。

(4)宫颈狭窄。

2.性腺发育不全：

(1)特纳综合征，XO 基因型,伴身材矮小和颈蹼。

(2)两性畸形。

(3)男性假两性畸形。

临床称为雄激素不敏感综合征。表型为女性外生殖器,性腺为睾丸(46,XY)。

4.13.2.2　继发性闭经(常见)

1.手术干预：

卵巢切除

子宫切除

过量照射

2.盆腔疾病：

如子宫内膜结核。

3.内分泌原因：

下丘脑、垂体、卵巢、子宫原因导致的闭经分别占 55%、20%、20%及 5%。

4.13.2.3　Hypothalamic amenorrhea

Most common.

Common causes：

（1）Emotional stress and psychologic disorder.

（2）Weight loss and lack of nutrition.

（3）Drug history：perphenazine, reserpine, OCp, *etc*.

4.13.2.4　Pituitary amenorrhea

（1）Pituitary tumor：Hyperprolactinemia accompanied with amenorrhea and galactorrhea.

（2）Pituitary necrosis：Sheehan's syndrome, following postpartum massive hemorrhage, shock and infection and causing ischemic necrosis of the pituitary.

4.13.2.5　Ovarian amenorrhea

（1）Premature ovarian failure.

（2）Oophorectomy or over-irradiation.

（3）Ovarian functional tumours.

Arrhenoblastoma of ovary, androgen producing tumour.

（4）Polycystic ovarian syndrome（PCOS）：Elevated LH/FSH ratio（＞2）, increased androgens, amenorrhea, infertility, hirsutism and obesity.

4.13.2.6　Uterine amenorrhea

（1）Asherman's syndrome：Over-curettage, endometritis, and intrauterine synechiae.

（2）Hysterectomy.

（3）Radiation of uterus.

4.13.2.3　下丘脑性闭经

最常见的一类闭经。

常见原因：

（1）精神紧张或心理障碍。

（2）体重下降和营养缺乏。

（3）长期服用某些药物,例如奋乃静、利血平及避孕药等。

4.13.2.4　垂体性闭经

（1）垂体肿瘤:高泌乳素血症伴有闭经、泌乳。

（2）垂体坏死:希恩综合征。继发于分娩时大出血、休克、感染,导致产后垂体的局部缺血坏死。

4.13.2.5　卵巢性闭经

（1）卵巢早衰。

（2）卵巢切除或放疗破坏卵巢组织。

（3）卵巢功能性肿瘤。

卵巢睾丸母细胞瘤、雄性激素分泌性肿瘤。

（4）多囊卵巢综合征:LH/FSH 比率高于正常（＞2）。雄性激素产生过多。闭经、不孕、多毛和肥胖。

4.13.2.6　子宫性闭经

（1）Asherman 综合征:刮宫过度、子宫内膜炎、宫腔粘连。

（2）子宫切除。

（3）子宫放疗后。

4.13.3　Diagnosis procedure

4.13.3　诊断步骤

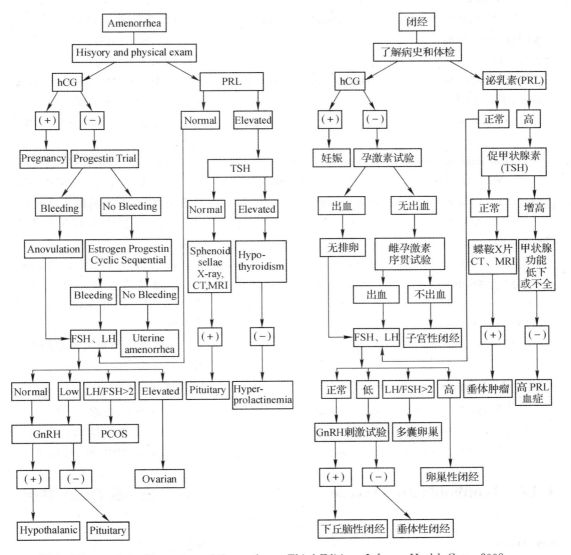

Clinical Protocols in Obstetrics and Gynecology. Third Edition. Informa Health Care，2008

4.13.4　Treatment

The prognosis of most amenorrhea is good.

4.13.4.1　General physical therapy

（1）Resolve anxiety and nervousness.

（2）Supply with full nutrition and keep standard weight.

4.13.4　治疗

多数闭经治疗的预后是良好的。

4.13.4.1　全身治疗

（1）消除精神焦虑和紧张情绪。

（2）供给足够营养、保持标准体重。

4.13.4.2　Medical therapy

According to hormone profile.

(1) Management of patients desiring pregnancy—Ovulation induction.

Including：

1）Patients with amenorrhea-galactorrhea and with/without adenomas.

2）Patients with hypothyroidism.

3）Patients with premature ovarian failure.

4）Patients with hypoestrogenic，hypothalamic amenorrhea（progestin challenge negative）.

5）Patients who bleed in response to progestin challenge.

(2) Patients not desiring pregnancy.

Hypoestrogenic patient should be treated to maintain bone density and prevent genital atrophy.

Oral contraceptives are good replacement therapy for most women.

4.13.4.3　Surgical treatment

(1) Removal of the pituitary adenoma.

(2) Hymenectomy.

(3) Incision of congenital atresia of vagina.

4.14　Trophoblastic Disease

Key words

1. clinical diagnosis
2. nonmetastatic
3. metastatic
4. local(pelvic)
5. extra-pelvic
6. morphologic diagnosis
7. hydatidiform mole
8. noninvasive mole
9. invasive mole

4.13.4.2　药物治疗

药物治疗依据体内激素状况。

（1）希望获得妊娠者的治疗目的——诱发排卵：

包括下列情况：

1）患者闭经伴有泌乳，同时伴有/不伴有垂体腺瘤。

2）患者闭经伴有甲状腺功能低下。

3）患者闭经伴有卵巢早衰。

4）患者伴有低雌激素性下丘脑性闭经（孕激素刺激无反应）。

5）患者孕激素刺激有撤退出血。

（2）无妊娠要求患者的治疗：

低雌激素患者给予激素治疗，以保持骨密度和预防生殖器官萎缩。

口服避孕药对大多数妇女是很好的替代治疗。

4.13.4.3　手术治疗

（1）垂体瘤切除。

（2）处女膜切开。

（3）先天性阴道闭锁切开。

4.14　妊娠滋养细胞肿瘤

关键词

1. 临床诊断
2. 无转移
3. 转移性
4. 局部（盆腔）
5. 盆腔外
6. 形态学诊断
7. 葡萄胎
8. 非侵蚀性葡萄胎
9. 侵蚀性葡萄胎

10. choriocarcinoma

11. uncertain

Gestational trophoblastic neoplasia（GTN）represents a unique spectrum of diseases that includes benign gydatidiform mole；invasive mole which can metastasize；and choriocarcinoma. The majority （80％ to 90％）of GTN have a benign course，with their disease remitting spontaneously. Most patients with metastatic disease can be effectively cured with chemotherapy. This diverse group of diseases has a sensitive tumor marker，hCG，which is secreted by all of these tumors and allows accurate follow-up and assessment of the disease.

4.14.1　Classification

The benign form of GTN is called hydatidiform mole. Although this entity is usually confined to the uterine cavity，trophoblastic tissue can occasionally embolize to the lungs.

The malignant forms of GTN are invasive mole and choriocarcinoma. Invasive mole is usually a locally invasive lesion，but it can be associated with metastases. This lesion accounts for the majority of patients who have persistently decreasing hCG titers following molar evacuation.

Choriocarcinoma is the frankly malignant form of GTN.

10. 绒癌

11. 不确定

GTN 代表一类独特的疾病，包括葡萄胎、侵蚀性葡萄胎和绒癌。大多数（80％～90％）GTN 为疾病能自然缓解的良性过程。大多数发生转移的患者通过化疗能有效治愈。这类不同的疾病都能分泌一种敏感的肿瘤标志物：hCG，因而能准确随访和评估病情。

4.14.1　分类

良性的 GTN 称为葡萄胎。虽然，病变通常局限于宫腔内，滋养细胞组织偶可发生肺栓塞。

恶性类型为侵蚀性葡萄胎和绒癌，侵蚀性葡萄胎可伴有转移，但病变一般为局部侵润，大部分侵蚀性葡萄胎患者发生于葡萄胎清宫后，hCG 滴度持续不降。

绒癌为高度恶性。

Table 4-14-1　Clinical features of metastatic GTN with prognosis

Modified WHO Prognostic Scoring System	0	1	2	4
Age	<40	≥40	—	—
Antecedent pregnancy	mole	abortion	term	—
Interval months from index pregnancy	<4	4-6	7-12	>12
Pretreatment serum hCG （IU/L）	$<10^3$	$10^3\text{-}10^4$	$10^4\text{-}10^5$	$>10^5$
Largest tumor size （including uterus）	<3	3-4 cm	≥5 cm	—
Site of metastases	lung	spleen，kidney	gastrointestinal	liver，brain
Number of metastases	—	1-4	5-8	>8
Previous failed chemotherapy	—	—	single drug	≥2 drugs

In this scoring system，women with a score of 7 or greater are considered at high risk.

表 4-14-1　转移性 GTN 临床特征

评分	0	1	2	3
年龄（岁）	＜40	≥40	—	—
前次妊娠	葡萄胎	流产	足月产	—
距前次妊娠时间（月）	＜4	4～6	7～12	＞12
治疗前血 hCG（mIU/ml）	＜10^3	10^3～10^4	10^4～10^5	＞10^5
最大肿瘤大小（包括子宫）	＜3	3～4 cm	≥5 cm	—
转移部位	肺	脾、肾	胃肠道	肝、脑
转移病灶数目	—	1～4	5～8	＞8
先前失败化疗	—	—	单药	两种或两种以上联合化疗

预后评分总分≤6 分为低危，＞7 分为高危。

表 4-14-2　妊娠滋养细胞肿瘤解剖学分期（FIGO，2000 年）

Ⅰ期	病变局限于子宫
Ⅱ期	病变扩散，但仍局限于生殖器官（附件、阴道、阔韧带）
Ⅲ期	病变转移至肺，有或无生殖系统病变
Ⅳ期	所有其他转移

表 4-14-3　完全性和部分性葡萄胎核型和病理特征比较

特征	完全性葡萄胎	部分性葡萄胎
核型	46,XX（90%）和 46,XY	三倍体
胎儿组织	缺乏	存在
胎膜、胎儿红细胞	缺乏	存在
绒毛水肿	弥漫	局限
扇贝样轮廓绒毛	缺乏	存在
滋养细胞增生	弥漫	局限
滋养细胞异型性	弥漫	局限

4.14.2　Hydatidiform mole

4.14.2.1　Histologic features of complete molar pregnancy

1）Trophoblast proliferation.

2）Villi interstitial edema.

3）Disappearance of fetal origin capillary.

A partial mole has some hydropic villi, whereas

4.14.2　葡萄胎

4.14.2.1　完全性葡萄胎的组织病理学特征

1）滋养细胞增生；

2）绒毛水肿；

3）缺乏胎儿血管

部分性葡萄胎含有一些水肿

other villi are essentially normal. Fetal vessels are seen in a partial mole, and the trophoblastic tissue exhibits less striking hyperplasia.

Histologically, choriocarcinoma consists of sheets of malignant cytortophoblasts and syncytiotrophoblasts with no identifiable villi.

4.14.2.2　Clinical presentations of hydatidiform mole

1) Bleeding postamenorrhea (most common): Most patients with hydatidiform mole present with irregular or heavy vaginal bleeding during the 1st or early 2nd trimester of pregnancy.

2) Uterus usually large than expected uterine date/size discrepancy in two thirds of patients.

3) Luteinizing cyst.

4) Severe nausea and vomiting.

5) Pregnancy induced hypertension.

6) Clinical hyperthyroidism.

The standard therapy for hydatidiform mole is suction evacuation followed by sharp curettage of the uterine cavity, regardless of the duration of pregnancy. This should be performed in the operating room with general or regional anesthesia.

Intravenous oxytocin is given simultaneously to help stimulate uterine contractions and reduce blood loss.

4.14.2.3　Preventive chemotherapy

1) Age more than 40;

2) Level of serum hCG increased significantaly (more than 100 kIU/L);

3) Titer of hCG has not returned to normal after 12 weeks postevacuation;

4) Re-elevated hCG level;

5) Uterus larger than expected;

6) Diameter of luteinizing cyst more than 6 cm;

7) Trophoblast hyperproliferation after second curettage;

Has no condition to follow-up.

绒毛,但其他绒毛基本正常。部分性葡萄胎可见胎儿血管,滋养细胞增生不显著。

组织学上,绒癌由片状恶性滋养细胞和合体滋养细胞组成,无可辨认的绒毛。

4.14.2.2　葡萄胎的临床表现

1) 闭经后阴道出血(最常见)。多数葡萄胎患者表现为妊娠早期或中期妊娠不规则或大量阴道出血。

2) 子宫增大大于孕周,2/3患者子宫增大不明显。

3) 黄素囊肿。

4) 严重的恶性及呕吐。

5) 妊娠期高血压。

6) 甲状腺功能亢进的临床表现。

葡萄胎的标准治疗为:无论妊娠时间长短,一旦确诊,行吸引清宫、后刮宫腔。手术应在手术室内全身或区域麻醉下进行。

同时,静脉给予缩宫素,刺激子宫收缩、减少出血。

4.14.2.3　葡萄胎的预防性化疗

1) 年龄＞40 岁;

2) hCG 明显增高(100 kIU/L);

3) 葡萄胎排出后 12 周 hCG未恢复正常;

4) hCG 再次升高;

5) 子宫增大超过孕周;

6) 黄素囊肿直径＞6 cm;

7) 第二次清宫后病理显示:滋养细胞过度增生;

无随访条件。

Follow-up：

Pelvic examination，ultrasound examination.

Assessment of hCG：

Serum quantitative hCG level every 1 week until three normal results.

Every 1 week(three months).

Every 2 weeks(three months).

Every 1 month(half year).

Every half year(one year).

Contraception for 1 year.

葡萄胎患者的随访：

随访内容：盆腔检查，阴道超声。

hCG 的测定：

每周测一次，直至连续 3 次正常；

每周 1 次，连续 3 个月；

每 2 周测一次，连续 3 个月；

每月测 1 次直至半年；

每半年测 1 次直至 1 年；

避孕 1 年。

4.14.3　Choriocarcinoma

About one half of patients with gestational choriocarcinoma have had a preceding molar pregnancy. In the remaining patients，the disease is preceded by a spontaneous or induced abortion， ectopic pregnancy, or normal pregnancy. The tumor has a tendency to disseminate hematogenously, particularly to the lungs, vagina, brain, liver, kidneys, and gastrointestinal tract.

4.14.3　绒癌

约半数绒癌患者有前次葡萄胎病史，其他患者可继发于自然或人工流产、异位妊娠或正常妊娠。肿瘤倾向于血行转移，特别是肺、阴道、脑、肝、肾和胃肠道。

4.14.3.1　Symptoms

Most patients with choriocarcinoma present with symptoms of metastatic disease，

1. Vaginal bleeding.

2. Hemoptysis, cough, or dyspnea may occur as a result of lung metastasis.

3. Headaches, dizzy spells and blacking out.

4. Rectal bleeding or dark stool.

4.14.3.1　症状

大多数绒癌患者具有转移灶症状、阴道出血；如肺转移患者可出现咯血、咳嗽或呼吸困难。头痛、头晕小发作、一时性晕厥；直肠出血或黑大便。

4.14.3.2　Signs

Acute abdomen because of rupture of the enlarged uterus. Neurologic signs, such as partial weakness or paralysis, dysphasia, aphasia, or unreactive pupils, indicate probable central nervous system involvement.

4.14.3.2　体征

子宫增大，因破裂出现急腹症。神经体征，如局部虚弱或麻痹、言语困难、失语或瞳孔无反应，提示肿瘤累及中枢神经系统。

4.14.3.3　Diagnosis

Choriocarcinoma is a great imitator of other diseases. In females of reproductive age, a hCG measurement to screen for choriocarcinoma should be

4.14.3.3　诊断

绒癌与其他疾病非常相似，生育年龄女性如果出现任何罕见症状和体征，应检测 hCG，筛查

performed when any unusual symptoms or signs develop.

Investigations hCG，because simultaneous evaluation of the β-hCG level in the cerebrospinal fluid and serum may allow detection of early cerebral metastases. The β-subunit does not readily cross the blood-brain barrier. A ratio of serum to cerebrospinal fluid β-hCG levels of less than 40∶1 suggests central nervous system involvement. CT and MRI scan.

4.14.3.4　Treatment of gestational trophoblastic neoplasia

The chemotherapy most often employed is either MTX or actinomycin D. MTX is usually given as a daily dose for 5 consecutive days or every other day for 8 days，alternating with folinic acid.

Actinomycin D is given for 5 consecutive days intravenously or every other week as a single dose.

In appropriately selected patients，hysterectomy may be the primary therapy for invasive hydatidiform mole and choriocarcinoma.

4.14.3.5　Treatment

For patients with disease having a poor prognosis combination chemotherapy is always used. MAC/EMA-CO.

In patients with disease metastatic to the brain or liver，radiation is often employed to these areas in conjunction with chemotherapy. If necessary，operation or intervene therapy may be needed.

4.14.3.6　Case∶trophoblstic disease

History∶A 25-year-old gravida 1, para o of Hispanic background presented at the prenatal clinic for obstetrical care fourteen weeks after her last menstrual period. The presenting complaints were irregular dark brown vaginal spotting, nausea and vomiting, edema of the lower extremities, fatigue and lethargy.

Examination∶The patient was a poorly nourished woman with a blood pressure of 150/100 and

绒癌。

hCG，因同时检测脑脊液和血清 β-hCG 水平能发现早期脑转移。因 β-hCG 水平不易通过血脑屏障,如血清/脑脊液水平比值＜40∶1,则提示中枢神经系统转移。CT,MRI 扫描。

4.14.3.4　滋养细胞疾病的治疗

最常用的化疗方案为 MTX,每日 1 次连用 5 天,或隔日 1 次共 8 日,与叶酸交替使用。

放线菌素 D 连用 5 日,或单剂量隔周使用。

选择合适的病例行子宫全切术作为侵蚀性葡萄胎及绒癌的治疗方式之一。

4.14.3.5　治疗

预后差的患者常使用联合化疗。用 MAC 或 EMA-CO 方案。

脑肝转移患者一般采用放疗联合化疗,必要时手术治疗或介入栓塞治疗。

4.14.3.6　病例:滋养细胞疾病

病史:患者,25 岁,孕 1 产 0,西班牙人,因停经 14 周,在产前门诊作产科检查。主诉为阴道不规则暗红色点滴出血、恶性呕吐、下肢水肿、疲劳及嗜睡。

检查:患者营养不良,血压150/100 mmHg,脉率 100/min。

pulse rate of 100/min. Abdominal examination revealed the fundus to be about two fingers below the umbilicus. No fetal heart tones were heard by ultrasonic doppler instrument. On pelvic examination, the cervix was soft and closed. There was noticeable brownish vaginal discharge; the uterus was soft and boggy. The ovaries were palpable and cystic bilaterally. Extremities: 1+ edema of both legs.

Laboratory data:

A routine prenatal work-up revealed the followings:

Urinalysis: +2 albumin

Hb: 85 g/L

Hct: 26%

WBC: 10×10^9/L

Hemagglutination inhibition pregnancy test: positive.

Questions:

1. What is the probable diagnosis?

2. Which investigations could confirm the diagnosis? What is the biologic basis of their use in this pathologic entity?

3. What is the pathophysiology of gestational trophoblastic disease?

4. What is the current classification of GTD?

5. What is the etiology of GTD?

6. What is the prognosis of hydatidiform mole?

7. What are the basic invasive mole and choriocarcinoma?

Answers:

1. Amenorrhea followed by irregular vaginal spotting or bleeding, emesis, and the findings of toxemia of pregnancy early in gestation, anemia, and a uterus larger than expected, from the menstrual history, with absence of fetal heart tones suggest the diagnosis of molar pregnancy. However, threatening abortion, multiple gestation, mistaken dates and hydramnios all have some similar features and should be considered in the differential diagnoses.

2. Clinical diagnosis of hydatiform molar can be

腹部检查子宫底约在脐下两指，超声多普勒仪未闻及胎心。盆腔检查宫颈软，宫口闭，可见带棕色阴道分泌物；子宫柔软有泥沼感。可触及双侧卵巢，双下肢浮肿+。

实验室资料：

产前常规检查结果如下：

尿液分析：白蛋白++

血红蛋白：85 g/L

红细胞压积：26%

白细胞：10×10^9/L

血液凝集抑制妊娠试验：阳性。

问题：

1. 可能的诊断是什么？

2. 哪些检查能证实此诊断？在此病理过程中，这些检查的生物学基础是什么？

3. GTD 的病理生理学如何？

4. GTD 如何分类？

5. GTD 病因学是什么？

6. 葡萄胎的预后如何？

7. 侵蚀性葡萄胎和绒癌基本组织学和病理学区别是什么？

答案：

1. 闭经后出现不规则阴道出血、呕吐；孕早期妊娠期高血压疾病的表现、贫血、子宫较孕周大以及无胎心，均提示葡萄胎。然而先兆流产、多胎妊娠、孕期计算错误及羊水过多均有某些相似，鉴别诊断应加以考虑。

2. 葡萄胎的临床诊断可由下

confirmed by the following investigations：

(1) Hormone assays：Trophoblastic tumor cells retain the ability of synthesizing the steroidal and polypeptide hormones normally produced by the placenta. The frequent appearance of galactorrhea, hyperthyroidism, theca lutein cysts, and amenorrhea reflects the fact that trophoblastic tumors are active endocrinologically. The polypeptide hormones include hCG, placental lactogen and TSH. The steroid hormones are estrogen and progesterone.

(2) Radiographic and sonographic methods：Definitive diagnosis of molar pregnancy prior to evacuation can be usually obtained by B-ultrasound.

3. Hydatidiform mole has been shown to be associated with pathologic conceptus in which the embryo is absent or dead prior to the time of establishment of fetal circulation. In the absence of vascular channels, the villous connective tissue stroma becomes hydropic and swollen.

The main pathologic changes that characterize mole are described above.

The criteria for diagnosis of invasive mole are：① An inordinate degree of trophoblastic overgrowth. ② Undue penetration of the trophoblastic villi into the uterine wall.

In choriocarcinoma, villi are replaced by proliferating trophoblastic cells consisting of varying proportions of syncytial and Langhans elements. There is no recognizable villous pattern.

4. International Classification has the advantage of a dual system of clinical and morphologic diagnosis.

5. The cause of hydatidiform mole and choriocarcinoma is unknown. It is far more common in the Far east than in the Western countries. The ratio of benign mole to pregnancy varies from 1：82 to 1：700 in Asia compared to about 1：2000 in the United States. The cause of this difference is not known.

There is no significant relationship between the

列检查证实：

(1) 激素测定：滋养细胞肿瘤细胞保持着正常时由胎盘产生的甾体及多肽激素的合成能力。患者出现溢乳、甲状腺功能亢进、卵泡膜黄素囊肿及闭经，这些均反映滋养细胞肿瘤在内分泌学上是活跃的。多肽激素包括 hCG、PRL 及 TSH。甾体激素为雌激素及孕酮。

(2) 影像学及超声检查方法：通过 B 超等影像学检查可诊断。

3. 已表明葡萄胎与病理性妊娠有关，该妊娠物胚胎存活或在胎儿循环建立前已经死亡。当缺乏血管通道时，绒毛结缔组织水肿。

葡萄胎的主要病理变化如前所述。

侵蚀性葡萄胎的诊断标准为：① 滋养细胞不同程度的过度增生；② 滋养层绒毛过度穿入子宫肌层。

在绒癌，绒毛被增生的滋养层细胞所代替，由不同比例的合体细胞及朗罕氏细胞构成，无可识别的绒毛结构。

4. 国际分类法的优点在于具有临床和形态学诊断的双重系统。

5. 葡萄胎及绒癌病因不明，在远东比西方国家常见。葡萄胎和妊娠的比例在亚洲由 1：82 至 1：700 不等，而在美国大约为 1：2000，这种差别的原因不明。

葡萄胎发病率与患者经产次

incidence of hydatidiform mole and the parity of the patient, but the entity is more prevalent in the higher reproductive age groups. Etiologic similarities among a group of reproductive abnormalities which included early spontaneous abortion, ectopic pregnancy, placenta previa and accreta, fetal developmental defects and chromosome anomalies as well as hydatidiform mole have been described. In an analysis of 400 consecutively treated cases of hydatidiform mole, the malignancy rate at and above 40 years of age was 36.6 percent in contrast to 15-20 percent in the general population. In the same study, the malignancy rate was 14.3 percent for women with three or more children in contrast to 3.8 percent for women of lower parity.

Choriocarcinoma is preceded by hydatidiform mole in about 50%, by abortion in 25%, by normal pregnancy in 22.5% and by ectopic pregnancy in 2.5% of the cases.

6. About 80% of the cases of hydatidiform mole have a benign course. One-half of the patients become pregnant subsequently. About 16% of hydatidiform moles become invasive moles and some 2.5% progress into choriocarcinoma.

7. In invasive hydatidiform mole, molar villi invade the myometrium, the blood vessels or both. Choriocarcinoma is an an tumor of the embryonic chorion. Within the uterus, it shows a red granular hemorrhagic surface which may be discrete or diffuse throughout the cavity. Metastases occur early and are widespread. Chorionic villi are not seen. Microscopically, there is a typical plexiform pattern of pure trophoblast, blood clot, and fragments of necrotic decidua or myometrium. The most common sites for metastasis are the lungs, vagina, brain, liver, and kidney. Choriocarcinoma should be suspected in patients with persistent bleeding after termination of a normal pregnancy, hydatidiform mole, abortion, or if evidence of metastasis such as

数间无显著关系，但高龄产妇更容易发生葡萄胎，在一组生殖异常中包括早期自然流产、异位妊娠、前置胎盘及胎盘植入，胎儿发育缺陷和染色体异常以及葡萄胎的病因学相似点已有描述，在400例连续性葡萄胎病例分析中，40岁及40以上患者的恶变率为36.6%，而总恶变率为15%～20%。在同一研究中，生育3胎或3胎以上者恶性率为14.3%，相反，经产次数较少的妇女恶变率为3.8%。

绒癌病例发生于葡萄胎后约占50%，流产约占25%，正常妊娠约占22.5%，而异位妊娠约占2.5%。

6. 大约80%的葡萄胎病例为良性病程，其中半数患者以后妊娠，大约16%的葡萄胎为侵蚀性葡萄胎，约2.5%发展为绒癌。

7. 在侵蚀性葡萄胎，绒毛侵入子宫肌层或血管或两者皆有。绒癌为胚胎绒毛恶性肿瘤，在子宫内表现为红色颗粒状出血面，可稀疏或弥漫至整个宫腔。转移发生早而广泛，见不到滋养层绒毛。镜下可见典型的丛状纯滋养细胞、血凝块及坏死的蜕膜碎片或子宫肌层。最常见的转移部位为肺、阴道、脑、肝及肾。正常妊娠终止后，葡萄胎或流产后患者持续出血，或在hCG滴度高时出现咯血、偏瘫等转移征象应高度怀疑绒癌。诊断性刮宫有助于诊断。

hemoptysis, hemiplegia, etc. Is seen in the presence of high hCG titers. A diagnostic curettage may be helpful in making the diagnosis.

Outcome: The suspected diagnosis of GTD was confirmed by sonographic demonstration of characteristic patterns of molar tissue. The same investigation failed to demonstrate the presence of a fetal head. Quantitative tests for urinary hCG levels revealed an hCG concentration of 500 000 IU/24 hrs of collected urine. The patient was prepared for surgery. The night before the operation she received 2 units of whole blood following which the hemoglobin was 103 g/L and the hematocrit 33%. An additional 4 units of blood was X-matched. Under general anesthesia the cervix was dilated to 12 mm and the uterus was evacuated by suction curettage, while syntocinon was infused in IV drip at a rate of 40 drops/min. A substantial amount of molar tissue was removed. Blood loss during the procedure was moderate. The uterus was gently curetted at the end of the procedure. The patient made a good postoperative recovery and she was ready to leave the hospital on the 3rd postoperative day. Pathological report received the same morning confirmed the diagnosis of hydatidiform mole. Appropriate measures were taken for further follow-up in the outpatient clinic.

4.15　Endometriosis and Adenomyosis

Key words

1. endometriosis
2. adenomyosis
3. chronic pelvic pain
4. hysterectomy
5. salpingoooophorectomy
6. pseudopregnancy therapy

结局：妊娠滋养细胞疾病的可疑诊断通过超声检查显示葡萄胎的特征性征象而证实。同样的检查未能证实胎头的存在。尿 hCG 定量测定显示浓度为 500 000 IU/24 h。患者准备手术，术前该患者输了 2 单位红细胞悬液，此后，血红蛋白为 103 g/L，红细胞压积为 33%，另 4 单位交叉配血。在全麻下将宫口扩张至 12 mm，以吸刮术排空子宫。其间以 40 滴/min 的速度静点缩宫素，清除了多量葡萄胎组织，术中失血量中等，手术结束时轻轻搔刮子宫。患者术后恢复好，术后第 3 天准备出院。病理回报提示：葡萄胎。在门诊进一步随访。

4.15　子宫内膜异位症和子宫腺肌病

关键词

1. 子宫内膜异位症
2. 子宫腺肌症
3. 慢性盆腔痛
4. 全子宫切除术
5. 输卵管卵巢切除术
6. 假孕疗法

7. pseudomenopause therapy

8. danazol

9. GnRH-α

10. mirene (levonorgestrel releasing IUD)

11. dMPA (medroxyprogesterone acetate)

4.15.1 Endometriosis

Endometriosis is a benign condition in which endometrial glands and stroma are present outside the uterine cavity and walls. It has benign condition with malignant behavior. It is locally infiltrative, invasive, and widely disseminated.

4.15.1.1 Incidence

It is estimated that 5%-15% of women have some degree of the disease. The typical patient with endometriosis in her 30s, nulliparous, and infertile. Occasionally, endometriosis may occur in infancy, childhood, or adolescence, but it is usually associated with obstructive genital anomalies at these early ages.

4.15.1.2 Pathogenesis

The pathogenesis of endometriosis is not understood.

1. The retrograde menstruation theory of Sampson.

2. The mullerian metaplasia theory of Meyer.

3. The lymphatic spread theory of Halban.

Most authorities today believe that several factors are involved in the initiation and spread of endometriosis, including retrograde menstruation, coelomic metaplasia, immunologic changes and genetic predisposition.

4.15.1.3 Sites of occurrence

Endometriosis occurs most commonly in the dependent portions of the pelvis. Specifically, implants can be found on the ovaries, the broad ligament, bhe peritoneal surfaces of the cul-de-sac and the rectovaginal septum.

7. 假绝经疗法

8. 丹那唑

9. 促性腺激素释放激素-激动剂

10. 曼月乐(左炔诺孕酮释放宫内节育装置)

11. 醋酸甲地孕酮

4.15.1 子宫内膜异位症

子宫内膜异位症是子宫内膜腺体和间质出现在子宫腔和肌层以外的位置的良性疾病。良性疾病,恶性行为。该疾病在局部浸润、侵袭,广泛播散。

4.15.1.1 发病率

据估计有 5%～15% 的妇女不同程度患病。典型的子宫内膜异位症患者年龄为 30 多岁,未产、不孕。子宫内膜异位症偶见于婴儿、儿童或青少年。多与阻塞性生殖道畸形相关。

4.15.1.2 机制

其发病机制不清。

1. 经血逆流理论。

2. 苗勒氏管化生学说。

3. 淋巴转移理论。

现在大多数专家认为,多个因素参与子宫内膜异位症的发生和播散,包括经血逆流、体腔上皮化生、免疫改变和遗传倾向。

4.15.1.3 发生部位

子宫内膜异位症多发生于盆腔支撑组织。具体而言,子宫内膜异位症病灶可见于卵巢、阔韧带、直肠子宫凹陷腹膜和直肠阴道隔。

Endometriosis is occasionally seen in laparotomy scars, especially after a cesarean section or myomectomy. Two third of women with endometriosis have ovarian involvement.

4.15.1.4　Pathology

Islands of endometriosis respond cyclicly to ovarian steroidal hormone production. It induces a profound inflammatory response resulting appearance of endometriosis depends on the site of the implant, activity of the lesion, day of the menstrual cycle, and the time since implantation.

Lesion may be raised and flat with red, black, or brown coloration; fibrotic scarred areas are yellow or white in hue; or vesicles are pink, clear, or red. Newer implants tend to be red, blood-filled active lesions, while older lesions tend to be scarred with a puckered appearance.

Endometriomas of the ovary are cysts filled with thick, chocolate-colored fluid that some times has the black color and tarry consistency of crankcase oil.

Histologically, two of four characteristics must be found in the specimen to confirm the diagnosis-endometrial epithelium, endometrial glands, endometrial stroma, and hemosiderin-laden macrophages.

4.15.1.5　Symptoms

The characteristic triad of symptoms associated with endometriosis is dysmenorrhea, dyspareunia, and dyschezia. There is no clear relationship between the stage of endometriosis and the frequency and severity of pain symptoms.

Dyspareunia is generally associated with deep thrust penetration during intercourse and occurs mainly when the CUL-DE-SAC, uterosacral ligaments, and portions of the posterior vaginal fornix are involved.

Dyschezia is experienced with uterosacral, cul-

子宫内膜异位症偶见于剖腹疤痕,尤其是剖宫产术后或子宫肌瘤剔除术后。2/3 患者的病变累及卵巢。

4.15.1.4　病理

子宫内膜异位症对周期性的卵巢分泌的甾体类激素起反应。它导致继发的疼痛和长期的纤维化,病灶的大体外观取决于种植的部位、病灶的活动程度、月经周期的天数以及种植时间的长短。

病灶可突起或平坦,外呈红色、黑色或棕色;纤维疤痕区域呈黄色或白色;或粉红色、透明或红色小泡。新鲜种植灶多为红色、充血性活动病灶,陈旧病灶多为外表皱褶的疤痕。

卵巢内膜样囊肿为稠厚巧克力样液体,有时会有类似黑色焦油样物质。

组织学诊断时标本必须具备以下 4 个特征中的 2 个:子宫内膜上皮、子宫内膜腺体、子宫内膜间质和富含铁血黄素的巨噬细胞。

4.15.1.5　症状

子宫内膜异位症的三联症:包括痛经、性交痛和大便困难。

子宫内膜异位症分期和疼痛的严重程度、频率没有明显的相关性。

性交痛常与性交时插入较深有关,病变累及子宫直肠陷窝、宫骶韧带和阴道后穹窿。

大便困难发生在病变累及宫骶韧带、直肠子宫凹陷和直肠乙状结肠者。粪便通过宫骶韧带之间时,可引起典型的大便困难。

de-sac, and rectosigmoid colon in involvement. As the stool passes between the uterosacral ligaments, the character dyschezia is experienced.

Premenstrual and postmenstrual spotting is a characteristic symptom of endometriosis.

4.15.1.6　Signs

Characteristically, a tender, fixed adnexal mass is appreciated on bimanual examination. The uterus is fixed and retroverted in a substantial number of women with endometriosis. Occasionally, no signs at all are appreciated on physical examination.

4.15.1.7　Diagnosis

The diagnosis of endometriosis should be suspected in an afebrile patient with the characteristic triad of pelvic pain, a firm, fixed, tender adnexal mass, and tender nodularity in the cul-de-sac and uterosacral ligaments. The characteristic sharp, firm, exquisitely tender barb felt in the uterosacral ligament is the diagnostic sinequanon of endometriosis.

An ultrasonic evaluation may indicate an adnexal mass of complex echogenicity, with internal echoes consistent with old blood. CA-125 are frequently elevated in women with endometriosis.

The definitive diagnosis is generally made by the characteristic gross and histologic findings obtained at laparoscopy or laparotomy.

4.15.1.8　Treatment

The management of endometriosis depends on certain key considerations:

1) the certainty of the diagnosis.
2) The severity of the symptoms.
3) The extent of the disease.
4) The desire for future fertility.
5) The age of the patient.
6) The threat to the gastrointestinal or urinary tract.

Treatment is indicated for endometriosis

经前或经后点滴出血是子宫内膜异位症的典型症状。

4.15.1.6　体征

典型的体征是双合诊时触及附件区固定、压痛包块。子宫后位,固定、后屈。偶尔患者体检时没有任何体征。

4.15.1.7　诊断

没有发热,有典型的盆腔疼痛三联症,坚硬、固定、压痛的附件包块,直肠子宫凹陷和宫骶韧带触痛结节的患者,应怀疑子宫内膜异位症。在宫骶韧带触及典型尖锐、质硬,触痛结节是诊断子宫内膜异位症的必要条件,超声检查可发现附件区混合性回声包块,内部回声与陈旧性血液一致,CA-125 水平常升高。

一般子宫内膜异位症的确诊依赖于腹腔镜或剖腹探查时典型的大体和组织学检查。

4.15.1.8　治疗

子宫内膜异位症的治疗需考虑以下几点:

1) 诊断的准确性。
2) 症状的严重程度。
3) 病变范围。
4) 对生育的渴望程度。
5) 患者年龄。
6) 对胃肠道或泌尿道的影响。

对有盆腔疼痛、痛经、性交

associated pelvic pain, dysmenorrhea, dyspareunia, abnormal bleeding, ovarian cysts, and infertility due to gross distortion of tubal and ovarian anatomy.

Surgical intervention is required for an endometrioma larger than 3 cm gross distortion of pelvic anatomy, involvement of bowel or bladder, and adhesive pathological changes.

1. Surgical treatments

The most comprehensive surgery includes total abdominal hysterectomy, bilateral salpingoooophorectomy with destruction of all peritoneal implants, and dissection of all adhesions.

The desire for future fertility often precludes this surgical option. In this situation, laparoscopic or open surgery is designed to destroy all endometriotic implants and remove all adhesive lesions. This usually involves excision of all adhesions and laser ablation or electrocautery of suspected implants.

Preoperative treatment with medical agents, e. g. GnRH agonists for 3 to 6 months, can improve surgical success.

There is a risk of recurrence of endometriosis throughout a woman's life. DMPA and mirene are all attractive long-term options.

2. Medical treatments

For relief of pelvic pain, short-term treatment may be used, and either a GnRH-α or danazol appears to be equally effective.

Danzol is an androgenic derivative that may be used in a pseudomenopause regimen to suppress symptoms of endometriosis if fertility is not a present concern. It is given over a period of 6 to 9 months and daily doses of 600 to 800 mg are generally necessary to suppress menstruation.

GnRH-α causes a temporary medical castration, thereby bringing about a marked, albeit temporary, regression of endometriosis. The disadvantages of these agonists are high price, hot flashes calcium loss

痛、异常阴道出血、卵巢囊肿、输卵管和卵巢解剖结构破坏较大所致不孕的子宫内膜异位症患者需要治疗。

手术指征：内膜样囊肿大于 3 cm，盆腔解剖结构异常，累及膀胱或肠道，粘连性病变。

1. 手术治疗

最全面的手术包括经腹全子宫切除术＋双附件切除术，破坏所有腹膜病灶，分解所有粘连。

对希望生育的患者，多不考虑行根治术。腹腔镜或开腹手术的目的在于破坏所有异位症病灶，去除所有粘连病灶。通常包括去除所有粘连病灶和激光或电凝可疑病灶。

术前给予药物如 GnRH-α 3～6 个月，可提高手术成功率。

在妇女一生中都有子宫内膜异位症复发的风险。DMPA、曼月乐成为有效的长期措施。

2. 药物治疗

采用短期治疗缓解盆腔疼痛，GnRH-α 或丹那唑效果似乎相近。

丹那唑是雄激素的衍生物，如患者无生育要求，可采用假绝经疗法控制子宫内膜异位症的症状。给药 6～9 个月，通常需要每天 600～800 mg 的剂量来抑制月经。

GnRH-α 引起暂时的药物去势，因此会导致显著地，虽然是短暂的，子宫内膜异位症消退。它的缺点是价格昂贵，潮热、骨钙丢

from bone and an unfavorable lipid profile.

If treatment with a GnRH-α is effective in relieving chronic pelvic pain and surgery is not indicated, low-dose estrogen progestin add-back therapy can permit longer-term use of GnRH-α by eliminating the estrogen deficiency impacts without reducing the efficacy of GnRH-α.

Oral contraceptives and oral medroxyprogesterone acetate are more effective in treating endometriosis associated pelvic pain than placebos. The levonorgestrel releasing IUD reduces dysmenorrhea.

4.15.2　Adenomyosis

Adenomyosis is defined as the extension of endometrial glands and stroma into the uterine musculature more than 2.5 mm beneath the basalis layer. About 15% of patients with adenomyosis have associated endometriosis.

4.15.2.1　Pathology

Generally, the gross appearance of the uterus consists of diffuse enlargement with a thickened myometrium containing characteristic glandular irregularities, with implants containing both glandular tissue and stroma.

4.15.2.2　Symptoms

Although many women are asymptomatic, those who suffer from this condition typically complain of severe secondary dysmenorrhea and menorrhagia.

4.15.2.3　Signs

On pelvic examination, the uterus is generally symmetrically enlarged and somewhat boggy and tender if the examination is conducted premenstrually.

4.15.2.4　Treatment

Conservative management with NSAIDS and hormonal control of the endometrium are mainstays of therapy. Combination oral contraceptives or hormone containing patches and vaginal rings may be

失和血脂改变。

如果 GnRH-α 缓解慢性盆腔疼有效、又无手术指征,加用雌-孕激素反加疗法可消除雌激素缺乏的影响,同时不降低 GnRH-α 的疗效。

口服避孕药和口服醋酸甲羟孕酮治疗子宫内膜异位症相关的盆腔疼痛比安慰剂有效。曼月乐可减少痛经。

4.15.2　子宫腺肌病

子宫腺肌病定义为:子宫内膜腺体和间质蔓延至内膜基底下大于 2.5 mm 的子宫肌层。约15%子宫腺肌病患者合并子宫内膜异位症。

4.15.2.1　病理

通常,子宫外观呈弥慢性增大,肌层增厚、内含不规则腺体,种植灶含有腺体和间质两种成分。

4.15.2.2　症状

很多妇女没有症状,但有症状患者的典型主诉是严重的继发性痛经和月经过多。

4.15.2.3　体征

盆腔检查可见子宫通常呈对称性增大,如在经前检查感觉质软而有弹性,伴压痛。

4.15.2.4　治疗

采用非类固醇抗炎药和激素控制子宫内膜的保守治疗是其主要的治疗方法。复合口服避孕药或含有激素的贴片和阴道环可用

used to reduce cyclic blood loss and menstrual pain，DMPA，Levonorgestrel IUD，and continuous oral contraceptive pills can be used to try to achieve amnorrhea. If the woman is not a candidate for any of these medical interventions or if medical treatments do not sufficiently control her symptoms，hysterectomy may be indicated. Endometrial ablation to control the bleeding is another option.

Case 1

History：A 33-year-old nulliparous woman complains of pelvic pain during menstruation for four years but has become progressively worse over the years，with pre and postmenstrual spotting. The dyspareunia and pain during defecation began six months ago，but has gotten worse. There was no change in the color or caliber of her stool. The woman is sexually active only with her husband. They do not use birth control，as they have been trying to get pregnant for the last 3.5 years. The patient takes no medications and has no other health problems. She had a normal pap smear 6 months ago.

Pelvic examination：Fixed, retroverted uterus. There is tender nodularity of the uterosacral ligaments bilaterally. Both ovaries are somewhat tender and mildly enlarged.

1. What is the diagnosis of the patient?
2. Which steps do you take?
3. How to treat it?

Case 2

History：A 41-year-old woman complains of increasing colicky pain during menstruation that has become almost intolerable，and she needs ibuprofen during menstruation. The patient states that over the last several months，her volume of menstrual flow has increased steadily，though her cycles continue to be regular. The patient denies vaginal discharge or fever. The patient had a Pap smear and dilation and

于减少经量和缓解经期疼痛。DMPA、曼月乐和连续口服避孕药可致停经。如果患者不适合这些药物治疗或药物治疗无法控制症状，可行全子宫切除术。也可采用子宫内膜消融术控制出血。

病例 1

病史：33 岁未产妇，主诉经期盆腔痛 4 年，逐渐加重。伴经前或经后点滴出血，6 月前出现排便疼痛及性交痛，逐渐加重，大便的颜色正常，该患者性生活活跃，未避孕，过去 3.5 年一直希望妊娠，该患者未用药，平素体健，6 个月前行宫颈刮片正常。

盆腔检查：子宫后屈、固定，双侧宫骶韧带有痛性结节，双侧卵巢似乎有压痛轻度增大。

1. 该患者的诊断是什么？
2. 进一步需做何检查？
3. 如何治疗？

病例 2

病史：41 岁女性，主诉经期逐渐加重的下腹痛不能忍受，需服用止痛药，该患者诉近几个月月经延迟，经量增多，周期基本正常，患者无阴道排液或发热。2 个月前行宫颈刮片及诊断性刮宫无异常。

curettage performed 2 months ago, which were both negative.

　　Pelvic examination: Reveals a symmetrically enlarged, smooth uterus with a boggy consistency that is somewhat tender during palpation. No adnexal masses are appreciated.

　　Laboratory findings: Hemoglobin 110 g/L.

1. What is the diagnosis of the patient?
2. Which steps do you take?
3. How to treat it?

4.16　Infertility

Key words

1. infertility
2. hypothalamic-pituitary-ovarian axis
3. hysterosalpingogram
4. intra-uterine insemination
5. in vitro fertilization

Ovulation normally occurs on day 14 in a 28-day cycle. It is controlled by hormones secreted from the anterior pituitary. Spermatogenesis is a temperature dependent process occurring in the seminiferous tubules, which leads to the production of mature sperm.

　　Infertility may arise due to problems in either partner and has a variety of causes. Anovulation, tubal disease and endometriosis are the common female causes. Infection, undescended testis and anti-sperm antibodies can all cause male infertility.

　　The chances of pregnancy occurring for a given couple having unprotected intercourse are 80% after 1 year. Investigations are therefore usually only started after this time. The simplest and least invasive tests should be performed first, such as confirmation of ovulation by measurement of day 21 serum progesterone and seminal fluid analysis.

妇科检查:子宫均匀性增大,表面光滑 质硬,有压痛,附件未扪及包块。

实验室检查:血红蛋白:110 g/L。

1. 该患者的诊断是什么?
2. 进一步需做何检查?
3. 如何治疗?

4.16　不孕症

关键词

1. 不孕症
2. 下丘脑-垂体-卵巢轴
3. 子宫输卵管造影
4. 人工授精
5. 体外受精

排卵一般发生在一个 28 天月经周期的第 14 天,是受垂体前叶分泌的激素调控的。精子发生是一个温度依赖性的过程,在曲细精管中产生成熟精子。

　　不孕症可由配偶任何一方出现问题引起,有多种病因。无排卵、输卵管疾病和子宫内膜异位症是常见女性因素。感染、隐睾和抗 精子抗体都能导致男性不育。

　　一对夫妇性生活正常,未采取避孕措施,1 年以后怀孕的概率为 80%。因此,通常 1 年后才开始临床检查。应该首先进行最简单和最少侵入性的检查,如第 21 天检测血清孕酮确认排卵以及男方精液分析。

Most forms of ovulatory failure can be corrected with clomiphene treatment. Assisted reproduction techniques, *e. g.* in vitro fertilization, are useful in the treatment of endometriosis, tubal disease and clomiphene-resistant ovulatory failure. Intracytoplasmic sperm injection (ICSI) is a useful treatment for severe male factor infertility.

4.16.1 General principles

4.16.1.1 Learning objectives

You should understand:

- ◆ How ovulation is controlled?
- ◆ How mature sperm is produced?

Infertility is defined as the inability to conceive after 1 year of unprotected intercourse. It affects 15% of all couples, but the incidence is increasing, largely because of a developing trend towards delayed childbearing. The average time fertile couples take to conceive is 6 months, with 80% conceiving within 1 year. Investigations into infertility are therefore not normally commenced until after 1 year of trying.

Female fertility is the highest in the age range 20-24 years and declines gradually after the age of 35 years. In men, aging has only a minor effect on fertility.

Infertility can be divided into:

- ◆ Primary infertility — no previous pregnancies of any kind
- ◆ Secondary infertility — previous pregnancy, but current difficulty in conceiving.

4.16.1.2 Normal sperm production and function

Spermatozoa are produced in the seminiferous tubules and undergo further maturation in the seminal vesicles. Production of mature spermatozoa takes around 70 days. Normal spermatogenesis requires an environment of 1 ℃ below normal body temperature, which is the reason the testicles hang outside the body in the scrotum. In cryptorchidism

大多数类型的排卵障碍可用氯米芬治疗恢复。辅助生殖技术,如体外受精,能有效治疗子宫内膜异位症,输卵管疾病和氯米芬抵抗的排卵障碍。卵胞质内单精子注射(ICSI)是一种对严重男性因素不育的有效治疗方法。

4.16.1 一般原理

4.16.1.1 学习目的

你应该理解:

- ◆ 排卵如何调控?
- ◆ 成熟精子如何生成?

不孕症定义为未避孕性交 1 年不能受孕。有 15% 的夫妇患病,但发病率逐年升高,主要原因为生育年龄有推后的发展趋势。一般夫妇平均 6 个月能受孕,一年内受孕率为 80%。因此,尝试怀孕 1 年后才正规开始进行不孕症检查。

女性在 20~24 岁之间生育能力最高,35 岁以后逐渐下降。男性的年龄对生育力的影响很小。

不孕症可分为:

- ◆ 原发不孕——从未有过妊娠。
- ◆ 继发不孕——以前有过妊娠,但现在难以受孕。

4.16.1.2 正常精子生成和功能

精子在曲细精管中产生,继而在精囊中成熟。成熟精子的生成需要约 70 天。正常精子生成需要环境温度低于正常体温 1℃,因此睾丸位于体外的阴囊中。隐睾患者的睾丸未下降,更高的温度损害了精子发生,可导

where the testis is undescended, the higher temperature impairs spermatogenesis, resulting in male infertility.

致男性不育。

Cervical mucus undergoes changes at the time of ovulation from being thick and tenacious to becoming thin and watery. This enables spermatozoa to penetrate readily through it. When the mucus is favorable, it will exhibit "spinnbarkeit", which means it can be stretched out into a long thread and will dry on a microscope slide into a characteristic ferning pattern.

宫颈黏液在排卵期发生变化,从浓稠变得稀薄,有利于精子从中穿透。此时的宫内黏液表现为黏液拉丝现象,即能伸展为一根长线,在玻片上干燥后显微镜下呈特征性羊齿样改变。

After swimming through the favorable cervical mucus, spermatozoa are transported to the ampullary portion of the fallopian tube by a combination of uterine contractions and the wafting action of the cilia which line the tube. Penetration and fertilization of the oocyte take place in the tubal ampulla.

在游过适宜的宫颈黏液后,精子依靠子宫收缩和输卵管表面纤毛摆动,被运输到输卵管壶腹部,在那里穿透卵子进行受精。

4.16.1.3　Normal ovulation

Ovulation occurs on a regular monthly basis, on around day 14 in a 28-day cycle. The ovaries are controlled by gonadotropin hormones secreted from the anterior pituitary gland, called luteinizing hormone (LH) and follicle-stimulating hormone (FSH). These are in turn controlled by the pulsatile secretion of gonadotrophin-releasing hormone (GnRH) from the hypothalamus. GnRH travels to the anterior pituitary via the hypothalamo-hypophyseal portal circulation, where it stimulates the secretion of FSH and LH.

4.16.1.3　正常排卵

正常排卵每个月规律地发生,通常在一个 28 天周期的第 14 天。卵巢受垂体前叶分泌的促性腺激素黄体生成素(LH)和卵泡刺激素(FSH)调控。这两种激素轮流受到下丘脑脉冲式分泌的促性腺激素释放激素(GnRH)调控。GnRH 通过下丘脑-垂体门脉循环到达垂体前叶,刺激 FSH 和 LH 的分泌。

These gonadotrophins are released into the blood stream and target the ovary. FSH acts on the granulosa cells, whilst LH acts on the theca, stroma, granulosa and luteal cells. The combined action of FSH and LH stimulates the development of ovarian follicles and the production of estrogen from the granulosa cells.

促性腺激素释放到血流中,靶器官是卵巢。FSH 作用于卵巢颗粒细胞,而 LH 作用于卵泡膜细胞、间质细胞、颗粒细胞和黄体细胞。FSH 和 LH 的共同作用刺激卵泡的生长和颗粒细胞雌激素的生成。

Estrogen initially exerts a negative feedback effect on gonadotrophin secretion, but as levels rise a

雌激素起初对促性腺激素的分泌产生负反馈作用,但当雌激

positive feedback develops，which culminates in a large surge of LH. This LH surge triggers maturation and ovulation of the dominant follicle. After ovulation，the follicle becomes luteinized to form the corpus luteum， which secretes progesterone. The released oocyte undergoes spontaneous demise within 48 hours in the absence of fertilization.

4.16.2　Causes of infertility

4.16.2.1　Learning objectives

You should understand：

♦ The mechanisms by which infertility may be caused. Common causes of infertility are：

- Male infertility：20%
- Defective ovulation：20%
- Tubal disease：25%
- Endometriosis：10%
- Unexplained infertility：20%
- Hostile cervical mucus：5%

It should be remembered that several causes may coexist.

4.16.2.2　Male infertility

Male infertility accounts for 20% of cases and can arise from a wide variety of causes. Most infertile men are entirely healthy in other respects except fertility，and it is unusual to find a serious underlying cause like a chromosomal disorder or an anatomical problem such as an undescended tests. Gonadotrophin insufficiency and testicular trauma are rare causes of male infertility.

Erectile failure may result from neurological problems or performance anxiety. Ejaculatory failure may be due to sympathetic denervation.

4.16.2.3　Defective ovulation

Absent or irregular ovulation is another common cause of infertility. Associated clinical manifestations of anovulation include oligomenorrhea，amenorrhea

素水平上升就形成正反馈的效应，到达最高峰时形成 LH 分泌峰，从而触发优势卵泡的成熟和排卵。排卵后卵泡黄素化形成黄体，可分泌孕酮。排出的卵细胞如未受精，会在 48 h 内自发死亡。

4.16.2　不孕症的病因

4.16.2.1　学习目的

应该理解：

♦ 不孕症的可能发病机制
不孕症的常见原因包括：

- 男性因素：20%
- 排卵障碍：20%
- 输卵管因素：25%
- 子宫内膜异位症：10%
- 原因不明：20%
- 条件不适的宫颈黏液：5%

应记住多种病因可以共同存在。

4.16.2.2　男性不育

男性因素占不育的 20%，可起于多种原因。大多数不育男性在其他方面是完全健康的，严重的病因如染色体异常或隐睾等解剖学因素 一般不常见。促性腺激素不足以及睾丸外伤是男性不育症的少见病因。

勃起障碍可由神经因素或焦虑导致。射精障碍可因去交感神经引起。

4.16.2.3　排卵障碍

无排卵或排卵不规律是不孕症的另一个常见原因。无排卵的相关临床表现包括月经稀发、闭

and the polycystic ovary syndrome.

Anovulation usually results from a reversible dysfunction of the hypothalamic-pituitary-ovarian (HPO) axis. This may be associated with an abnormal body mass index. A woman needs to have 26%-28% of her body weight as fat in order to have regular fertile ovulatory cycles. Body for percentage above or below this range may result in a reversible hypothalamic dysfunction. Estrogen and gonadotrophin levels often remain in the normal range, but because of a lack of coordination between ovary and pituitary, ovulation becomes sporadic. In severe weight loss there tends to be a greater degree of hypothalamic dysfunction with both gonadotrophin and estrogen levels being low. This is called hypogonadotrophic hypogonadism.

Other typical examples of HPO axis dysfunction include the polycystic ovary syndrome and hyperprolactinaemia. For the former, high LH levels interfere with normal follicular development. For the later, the raised prolactin levels interfere with the pulsatile secretion of gonadotrophins.

Anovulation rarely results from irreversible failure of the hypothalamus, pituitary or ovaries. Premature ovarian failure may occur secondary to anti-ovarian antibodies, or may occur when the ovaries become pre-maturely exhausted of ovarian follicles.

Tubal disease

Damage to the delicate cilial lining of the fallopian tubes interferes with transport of both oocyte and spermatozoa. Sexually transmitted pelvic infection is the usual cause of the damage, with chlamydia and gonorrhea being the common pathogens. In severe cases, the fimbrial ends of the tube adhere together and become sealed. Other causes of tubal damage include previous pelvic surgery and endometriosis, both of which may cause

经以及多囊卵巢综合征。

无排卵通常是由下丘脑-垂体-卵巢（HPO）轴的可逆性功能紊乱造成的。可能与体重指数异常有关。女性的体脂需要达到26%到28%才能维持规律的有生育力的排卵周期，高于或低于这个范围都可能造成可逆性下丘脑功能紊乱。雌激素和促性腺激素水平通常保持在正常范围，但由于卵巢和垂体功能不协调，排卵变得稀发。当体重急剧下降时，下丘脑功能紊乱更严重，同时促性腺激素和雌激素水平降低，被称为促性腺激素分泌不足的性腺功能减退症。

其他典型的HPO轴功能紊乱有多囊卵巢综合征，表现为高LH水平干扰正常卵泡发育，还有高泌乳素血症，表现为升高的泌乳素水平干扰促性腺激素的脉冲分泌。

无排卵很少由下丘脑、垂体或卵巢的不可逆功能障碍导致。卵巢早衰可能由抗卵巢抗体导致，也可能由于卵巢的卵泡提前耗竭。

输卵管因素

输卵管上皮纤毛损伤会影响卵子和精子的运输。性传播疾病导致的盆腔感染是常见的损伤因素，衣原体和淋球菌是主要病原体。在严重的病例中，输卵管伞的末端粘连闭合。其他导致输卵管损伤的原因包括既往盆腔手术史和子宫内膜异位症，两者都可以导致输卵管粘连和疤痕。

tubal adhesions and scarring.

Endometriosis

In severe cases, endometriosis causes mechanical distortion of the fallopian tubes and destruction of the ovaries. However, even minor degrees of endometriosis are associated with infertility although the exact mechanism is unknown.

Hostile cervical mucus

In this condition, the cervical mucus is unreceptive to spermatozoa, causing agglutination or immobilization. It may be associated with the presence of antisperm antibodies.

Unexplained infertility

In 20% of couples, no satisfactory explanation for infertility can be found. In this situation, all tests of fertility are normal, but the couple are still having difficulty in achieving a pregnancy.

Rare causes of infertility include fibroids distorting or impinging on the uterine cavity and thereby preventing implantation, and psychosexual problems resulting in decreased coital frequency.

4.16.3　Investigation of infertility

4.16.3.1　Learning objectives

You should:

♦ Be able to use infertility investigations selectively, according to the history and clinical findings.

4.16.3.2　General

A couple should be seen and investigated together as possible as they can, since either or both partners may have an underlying cause for the infertility. The history must be taken carefully. Although infertility is not a life-threatening or physically painful disease, the emotional distress and bereavement experience by childless couples can be great. Specific details should be sought regarding the duration of infertility, any previous pregnancies and

子宫内膜异位症

在严重的子宫内膜异位症中，输卵管可发生机械性扭曲变形，卵巢也可受损。尽管具体机制不明，即使轻度的子宫内膜异位症也与不孕症有关。

宫颈黏液异常

如宫颈黏液对精子产生排斥，可以导致精子凝集或固定不动。可能与抗精子抗体的存在有关。

原因不明的不孕症

约有 20% 的不孕症夫妇找不到明确的病因，他们所有有关不孕症的检查都正常，但是仍然存在受孕障碍。

少见的不孕症病因包括使子宫扭曲变形，可以阻碍着床的肌瘤以及导致性交频率降低的性心理因素。

4.16.3　不孕症的检查

4.16.3.1　学习目的

应该：

♦ 能够根据病史和临床表现选择合适的不孕症检查。

4.16.3.2　一般检查

一对夫妇应该尽可能同时就诊，因为任何一方或双方都可能存在不孕的病因。病史的采集应该谨慎。尽管不孕症不是一种性命攸关或生理上痛苦的疾病，但是精神上的痛苦和失去孩子的经历可以对人造成严重的影响。应该对不孕症的时间、既往的任何妊娠和相关的疾病进行仔细

relevant past illnesses.

The male should be examined for any hernia or varicocele. The location and size of the testes should be noted. The prostate gland should be palpated by rectal examination for any tenderness, which would be suggestive of prostatitis. Female pelvic examination should be done to confirm normal anatomy, exclude pregnancy, and detect the rare occurrence of a congenital anatomical malformation like vaginal atresia.

The nature of any investigations to be performed should be explained to the couple. Unless the history and examination findings point strongly to a particular cause, it is usual to commence tests with a seminal fluid analysis and confirmation of ovulation with a day 21 serum progesterone level. Rubella antibodies should be checked, and imunological examinations should be recommended if needed.

If the duration of infertility is short, the sperm count is normal and ovulation is confirmed, there may be no need to investigate further at this stage as the majority of couples will achieve a pregnancy within 2 years. Conversely, many couples will be concerned about their age and be keen to have further investigations as soon as possible. Specialist referral is then necessary for tests of tubal patency.

4.16.3.3　Seminal fluid analysis

Seminal fluid analysis provides information about the number of sperm and their motility. Two semen specimens should be collected, 6 weeks apart and after 3 days abstinence, by masturbation into a sterile container. Specimens should be kept at room temperature and handed in to the laboratory within 2 hours of production. A normal analysis shows a volume of between 2 and 6 ml, a sperm density of 20-250 million per ml, an abnormality rate of less than 30% and a motility of 60% at 1 hour. Oligospermia is defined as less than 20 million spermatozoa per ml,

询问。

男方应检查有无疝气和精索静脉曲张。注意睾丸的位置和大小。应行肛门指捡触诊前列腺，如有触痛，提示前列腺炎。女方应做盆腔检查，确认正常解剖结构，排除妊娠，可以发现少见的生殖道解剖异常，如阴道闭锁。

应向就诊夫妇解释所有检查的目的。除非病史和检查发现很特殊的原因，一般从精液分析和月经第 21 天检查血孕酮确认有无排卵开始。应检测风疹病毒抗体，如有指证还需做相关免疫检查。

如不孕症病程尚短，精子计数正常且确定有排卵，此时可能不需要更多检查，因为大多数夫妇可在 2 年内获得妊娠。反而，很多夫妇因为担心年龄问题而要求尽快进行更多的检查，这样就有必要专业推荐输卵管开放性检查。

4.16.3.3　精液分析

精液分析可以反映精子的数量和活力。应该进行 2 次取样，相隔 6 周并且在禁欲 3 天后用手淫法射精到一个无菌的容器中。样品应该室温保存并在 2 h 内送检。正常标准为精液量2～6 ml，精子密度(20～250)×10⁶/ml，异常率小于 30%，1 h 活力为 60%。少精子症定义为每毫升精液少于 20×10⁶ 精子。无精子症定义为完全看不到精子。精液中如出现

and azoospermia as complete absence of spermatozoa. Large numbers of white cells in the semen are suggestive of genital tract infection. The presence of antisperm antibodies in serum or semen is suggestive of immunological infertility.

More sophisticated tests of sperm function such as the swim-up test and computer-assisted seminal analysis are generally only performed in tertiary referral centers. There is no satisfactory test of the actual fertilizing ability of sperm, but the ability of human sperm to penetrate oocytes from the golden hamster gives some correlation with fertility, but it is rarely used in practice.

4.16.3.4　Other male investigations

If azoospermia or severe oligospermia is found, measurement of FSH levels and karyotyping will be required. If these are normal, vasal or epididymal obstruction is likely. In this situation, a testicular biopsy can be useful to confirm normal spermatogenesis, prior to consideration of exploratory surgery. Occasionally clinical signs of a chromosomal disorder like Klinefelter's syndrome may be seen. This can present with male infertility, small testes and gynecomastia.

4.16.3.5　Tests for ovulation

There are several indications of ovulation. A history of regular monthly periods is suggestive, as anovulation usually results in oligomenorrhea. A simple method which the woman can undertake herself at home is daily temperature recording. The oral temperature is taken every morning before rising and recorded on a special chart. A rise of 0.5 ℃ over the last 14 days of the cycle is suggestive of ovulation. However, these indicators are unreliable, and the good standard is measurement of a day 21 serum progesterone level. If ovulation has occurred this should be greater than 30 nmol/L. Timing of test is crucial as the corpus luteum produces

大量白细胞提示生殖道感染。血清或精液中出现抗精子抗体提示免疫性不育。

更复杂的精子功能检测,包括上游试验以及计算机辅助精液分析,一般仅在第三方检测机构开展。目前还没有准确的对精子实际受精能力评估的检测,但人类精子穿透金黄色仓鼠卵细胞的试验在一定程度上能反映精子受精能力,但实际工作中较少用。

4.16.3.4　其他男科检查

如发现无精子症或严重少精子症,应检查 FSH 水平和染色体核型。如上述检查正常,可能为血管或附睾梗阻。在这种情况下,在考虑探查性手术之前行睾丸活检对于确定生精功能是否正常很有用。偶尔可见到染色体异常疾病的临床表现,如克氏综合征,表现包括男性不育症、小睾丸和男性乳腺发育。

4.16.3.5　排卵检测

出现这些情况提示排卵。排卵通常有规律的月经史,而不排卵一般导致月经稀发。女性自己在家能采用的一种简单的测排卵的方法就是测定每日基础体温。每早起床前测量口腔体温,并记录在专门的表格上。在月经周期的第 14 天出现基础体温升高0.5 ℃提示有排卵。但是,这些指征并不可靠,检测排卵的金标准是月经周期第 21 天测定孕酮水平。如有排卵,孕酮值应达到30 nmol/L 以上。测孕酮的时间

progesterone during the luteal phase of the cycle with a peak 7 days before the next period. This would be on day 21 in a 28-day cycle, 7 days before the next period in a cycle of any other length.

If ovulation is not confirmed, the hypothalamic/pituitary/ovarian endocrine axis will require further investigation. FSH and LH are measured in the early follicular phase of the cycle, together with testosterone, prolactin and thyroid function. Low gonadotrophin levels are suggestive of a hypothalamic disorder, whilst grossly elevated levels suggest primary ovarian failure. Elevated prolactin levels would suggest a pituitary tumor. An LH : FSH ratio greater than 3 : 1 accompanied by a slightly raised testosterone level suggests polycystic ovary syndrome.

4.16.3.6　Tests for tubal patency

Tests of tubal patency are usually delayed until last as they are both more invasive and carry a small risk of pelvic infection. They should be performed during the first 10 days of the cycle to prevent disruption of an early pregnancy.

4.16.3.7　Hysterosalpingogram

A hysterosalpingogram entails injecting radiopaque dye through the cervix under radiographic control. The dye demonstrates the internal contours of the uterus and fallopian tubes and should be seen to spill freely from the fimbrial ends into the peritoneal cavity. Fimbrial occlusion of the tubes results in distension with dye but no spillage. Mullerian duct abnormalities such as bicornuate uterus and intra-uterine pathological changes like polyps can also be detected.

4.16.3.8　Laparoscopy

This allows a full visual inspection of the abdomen and pelvis via a telescope inserted through a

很关键,因为黄体在黄体期中下次月经来潮前 7 天达到高峰。在 28 天的月经周期中即第 21 天,其他周期中为下次月经来潮前 7 天。

如没有排卵,需进一步检查下丘脑/垂体/卵巢内分泌轴。在卵泡早期可检测 FSH、LH、睾酮、泌乳素和甲状腺功能。低促性腺激素水平提示下丘脑功能紊乱,而促性腺激素明显升高提示原发卵巢早衰。泌乳素水平升高可能提示垂体肿瘤。LH/FSH 的比例如大于 3,并伴有轻度升高的睾酮水平提示多囊卵巢综合征。

4.16.3.6　输卵管通畅性检查

输卵管通畅性检查一般推迟到最后进行,因为它是侵入性的,并有增加盆腔感染的轻度风险。应该在月经周期的前 10 天进行该项检查,以免阻碍可能的早期妊娠。

4.16.3.7　子宫输卵管造影

子宫输卵管造影是在放射影像的监控下通过宫颈注射造影剂成像。染料显示出子宫和输卵管的内部轮廓,正常情况下应见到造影剂从输卵管伞端自由进入腹腔。输卵管堵塞时造影剂滞留输卵管扩张,但没有造影剂的泄漏。苗勒氏管异常如双角子宫和子宫内的病变如息肉等也可以被检测出来。

4.16.3.8　腹腔镜手术

全身麻醉下通过一个小切口插入脐下全面地观察腹部和盆

small subumbilical incision under general anaesthetic. The peritoneal surfaces of the uterus, tubes and ovaries can be inspected for the presence of adhesions or endometriosis, and follicular development in the ovaries can be assessed. Previous acute salpingitis may result in fine peritubal adhesions and clubbing of the delicate fimbrial ends. A solution of methylene blue dye is then injected through the cervix. This normally fills and then spills from the fimbrial ends of the tubes without resistance. Hysteroscopy may be undertaken at the same time to visualize the uterine cavity, and an endometrial sample can be sent for histology and culture if required.

4.16.3.9　Tests for sperm/mucus compatibility

The ability of sperm to penetrate cervical mucus can be assessed using the post-coital test. This has to be done at the mid-cycle when the mucus is favorable. It involves taking a sample of cervical mucus from the endocervical canal 6-12 hours after sexual intercourse. This is placed on a slide and examined under the microscope, and large numbers of progressively motile sperm should be seen.

4.16.4　Treatment of Infertility

4.16.4.1　Learning objectives

You should understand:

◆ How and why different treatment options are used in infertility?

4.16.4.2　General

Simple advice regarding the optimum timing for intercourse is usually helpful. The couple should be reassured and advised that pregnancy may still occur naturally even if the duration of infertility has been many years. This is especially so if all investigations have been normal. When a problem has been identified, accurate information should be given about the possible treatment options. Some couples

腔。检查腹膜表面的子宫和卵巢,是否存在粘连或子宫内膜异位症,还可以评估卵巢的卵泡发育。既往有急性输卵管炎可导致腹腔的粘连以及输卵管伞端杵状变。通过宫颈注入亚甲基蓝染料,在正常情况下,可无阻力地通过输卵管伞端并弥散。此外,可同时进行宫腔镜检查,观察宫腔情况并进行子宫内膜取样,需要时可进行组织学分析培养。

4.16.3.9　精子/黏液相容性测试

通过性交后测试可以评估精子穿透宫颈黏液的能力,这必须是在月经中期黏液较多时进行。性交后 6～12 h 从宫颈黏液取样,然后放置在一个玻片上在显微镜下检查,应该看到大量前向运动的精子。

4.16.4　不孕症的治疗

4.16.4.1　学习目标

你应该理解:

◆ 在不孕症的治疗中如何和怎样选择不同的治疗方案?

4.16.4.2　一般治疗

选择最佳性交时机的简单建议通常是有益的。夫妇双方应该确信,就算多年不孕,仍然还是有自然受孕的可能,尤其是所有检查都提示正常时。当存在某个异常时,应将可选择的治疗方案的信息准确告知患者。有些夫妇将需要时间来调整和表达自己的情

will need time to adjust and express their feelings, and if emotional difficulties arise the assistance of an understanding professional counselor may be helpful.

The option of adoption should also be discussed at an early stage. However, few babies are now available for adoption due to the changing social attitude towards single parenthood.

4.16.4.3　Disorders of ovulation

Correction of an abnormal body mass index will often restore ovulation. Under-or overweight women should therefore be advised that their fertility will be substantially improved by weight normalization.

If infertility persists despite efforts at weight correction, ovulation can be induced with drugs. This is usually successful, but there are some possible drawbacks, including an increased risk of multiple pregnancy. Drugs used for induction of ovulation include:

- Clomiphene
- Gonadotrophins
- Gonadotrophin-releasing hormone
- Dopamine agonists

Hyperstimulation

Ovarian hyperstimulation is a serious complication of ovulation induction. Women with polycystic ovarian disease appear to be at particular risk. It is characterized by ovarian cyst formation, accompanied by the escape of fluid and protein from the vascular space into the peritoneal and pleural cavities. This results in painful abdominal distension. If pregnancy has occurred, secretion of endogenous hCG causes further stimulation. Hyperstimulation is minimized by careful ovarian monitoring during ovulation induction regimens. Treatment consists of fluid replacement and correction of electrolyte imbalance.

Treatment of tubal disease

The choice lies between tubal microsurgery and

绪,如果情绪出现困难,需要专业顾问咨询和帮助。

在早期阶段也应讨论选择收养。然而,由于全社会对单亲态度的改变,现在很少有能够被收养的婴儿。

4.16.4.3　排卵障碍

纠正异常的体质指数往往会恢复排卵。应告知体重过轻或超重的妇女,其生育能力会因体重纠正而得到改善。

如果体重纠正后仍持续不孕,可予药物诱导排卵。这通常是成功的,但也有一些可能的弊端,包括多胎妊娠的风险增加。促排卵药物包括:

- 克罗米芬
- 促性腺激素
- 促性腺激素释放激素
- 多巴胺受体激动剂

卵巢过度刺激综合征

卵巢过度刺激是促排卵的一个严重并发症。多囊卵巢的妇女尤其危险。它的特点是卵巢囊肿的形成,伴随细胞间液和蛋白质从血管腔溢出到腹膜和胸膜腔,这样的结局是痛苦的腹胀。如果发生妊娠,内源性 hCG 的分泌会进一步加重刺激。在促排卵方案中仔细监测卵巢可以减少过度刺激的发生。治疗包括补液和纠正电解质失衡。

输卵管疾病的治疗

可选择输卵管显微手术或体

in vitro fertilization (IVF). In general, the results of tubal microsurgery are poor, with subsequent pregnancy rates of only 20%. Gross tubal disease destroys the cilia, so tubal function will not return even if patency is restored. When the tubes are not severely damaged, microsurgery is a useful treatment.

Endometriosis

Surgery is indicated for endometriosis to restore normal anatomy when it is causing mechanical distortion of the fallopian tubes. If unsuccessful, IVF can be offered, providing the ovaries are accessible and capable of yielding eggs. Small asymptomatic deposits of endometriosis should not be treated, as this will not improve fertility but merely delays attempts at conception still further.

4.16.5　Stages in IVF treatment

Ovarian stimulation

Several eggs are needed to ensure the best chance of a successful pregnancy. Controlled ovulation induction is performed using gonadotrophin injections. These must be started early in the cycle before the development of a dominant follicle.

Egg collection

Egg collection is carried out just prior to ovulation. This is done by transvaginal ultrasound-guided needle aspiration.

Fertilization

The eggs are mixed with a prepared sample of semen, which the male partner has been asked to produce. Fertilization should take place within a few hours. If the sperm count is very low or when the sperm have difficulties to penetrate the egg, a technique called inracytoplasmic sperm injection (ICSI) may be used to inject a single sperm directly

外受精（试管婴儿）。一般情况下，输卵管显微手术效果较差，妊娠率只有 20%。输卵管纤毛破坏后，输卵管功能很难恢复，即使输卵管被疏通后。当输卵管没有严重受损时，显微外科治疗有效。

子宫内膜异位症

当子宫内膜异位症造成输卵管机械变形时，可采用外科手术治疗恢复正常的解剖结构。如果不成功，可采用体外受精，前提是卵巢能够触及并得到卵子。小的子宫内膜异位症病灶不引起症状，可不进行治疗，因为并不会改善生育能力，而只是有所拖延备孕。

4.16.5　体外受精的治疗阶段

促排卵

为了得到最好的成功率，需得到多个卵子。通过注射促性腺激素进行控制性排卵。这些必须在优势卵泡形成之前进行。

卵子的收集

排卵前进行卵子收集。通过经阴道超声引导穿刺进行。

受精

男方提供精液后，用卵子与准备好的精液混合。受精一般需在几小时内完成。当精子数量很少或难以穿透卵子时，采用卵胞质内单精子注射技术（ICSI），将单精子直接注入卵子内。

into the egg.

Embryo transfer

When an embryo has reached the four cell stage, it is placed inside the uterus by gentle injection through the cervix using a fine plastic tube. This needs no anaesthetic, but the woman is advised to rest for a few hours afterwards. Progesterone injections may be given following embryo transfer in order to help implantation. Serum hCG measurements over the next 2 weeks are used to monitor process. Rising levels are an early indicator of a successfully implanted pregnancy before ultrasound can detect fetal heart activity.

Success rates of IVF

The success rate varies between different centers, but around 20% of woman treated by IVF will have a child to take home.

4.16.6 Ethical problems in infertility

Learning objectives

You should understand:

- how and why there are profound ethical issues in infertility

High multiple pregnancy

Triplets and higher order multiple pregnancies increase perinatal mortality and morbidity, and enormous demands for special care baby units are also increased. Early selective fetal reduction is a technique used to deliberately abort a number of fetuses at an early stage in order to improve the survival chances of the remaining ones.

Donor insemination

Couples need to be aware of the possible impact of donor insemination on their relationship and to consider their future plans with regard to telling the child the truth. Under current law, the anonymity of the donor is maintained. In some countries, donor

胚胎移植

当胚胎已达到四细胞期时，用特制的塑料管装载胚胎，通过宫颈轻柔地放置在子宫内。这不需要麻醉，但建议病人移植后休息几小时。胚胎移植后注射孕激素有助于植入。2 周后检测血清 hCG，其水平的增加提示妊娠成功。是 B 超能够检测到胎心前的一个妊娠成功的指标。

体外受精成功率

不同的中心 IVF 成功率各异，大约 20% 的妇女能够得到活产新生儿。

4.16.6 不孕症中的伦理问题

学习目标

理解：

- 为何不孕症有深刻的伦理问题存在？

多胎妊娠

多胎妊娠时围产期死亡率和发病率增加，并使对特殊婴儿护理机构的需求增加。早期选择性减胎术是在孕早期将多个胎儿人为流产的技术，使存留的胎儿提高生存概率。

供精人工授精

夫妇需要了解使用供精对其夫妻关系的影响，并考虑他们未来如何告诉孩子。在现行法律中捐精者的信息是保密的。在一些国家，供精人工授精可用于需要

insemination has been used in single women who wishes to have a family but does not have a male partner.

Surrogate mothers

A surrogate mother carries a pregnancy on behalf of a commissioning couple, usually by artificial insemination with semen from the male partner or by placement of a fertilized embryo into the uterus. Following birth, the baby is given to the commissioning couple.

Preimplantation diagnosis

This is achieved by removing one cell from the embryo at the eight cell stage, prior to implantation during IVF treatment. The cell can then be used for antenatal diagnostic testing. As the embryonic cells at this stage are pluripotential, normal fetal development is unaffected.

Objective Structured Clinical Examniation（OSCE）questions

A 29-year-old woman and her husband had been trying for a baby for 18 months. She had just seen her general practitioner （GP）, and following this initial consultation, she had some questions to ask you：

（1）Why has she been advised to have her rubella status being checked?

（2）Why has she been advised to start taking 0.4 mg folic acid daily?

（3）Why have they been advised to have regular intercourse throughout the cycle but not bother with temperature charts?

（4）The doctor said that it is only necessary to measure one hormone on the 21st day because she has a regular 28-day cycle. What about the other hormones such as thyroid hormones and prolactin?

（5）If she falls pregnant, how much alcohol can she safely drink?

一个家庭但又无男性伴侣的单身女性。

代孕母亲

代孕母亲是受一对夫妇的委托而妊娠。通常是用夫妇中男性的精液进行人工授精，或在子宫中植入受精的胚胎。婴儿出生后，将归于委托的夫妇。

植入前诊断

在 IVF 治疗中，在移植前通过获取八细胞阶段胚胎的一个细胞进行。获取的细胞可进行产前诊断检测。由于胚胎细胞在这个阶段具有全能性，所以胎儿的正常发育不受影响。

病例分析

29 岁的妇女和她的丈夫试图怀孕已有 18 个月。她刚刚看到她的全科医生（GP），并在这次咨询后，她有一些问题要问你：

（1）为什么建议她做风疹状态检查？

（2）为什么建议她开始每天服用 0.4 mg 叶酸？

（3）为什么建议他们规律性交，而不是使用温度图表？

（4）医生说，她的月经周期为 28 天，只需要测第 21 天的一个激素。那么其他激素，如甲状腺激素、催乳素需要测定吗？

（5）如果她怀孕了，她可以喝多少酒呢？

☑ANSWERS

(1) Maternal rubella infection in the first 8-10 weeks of pregnancy results in severe fetal abnormalities in up to 90% of cases. The rubella status of the female partner should therefore be checked, and rubella vaccination should be offered if seronegative.

(2) Folic acid supplementation is advised both whilst trying to conceive and during the first 12 weeks of pregnancy, in order to prevent fetal neural tube defects.

(3) There is no evidence that the use of temperature charts improves outcome. Advice to time intercourse has been evaluated by patients as being the most emotionally stressful element of infertility management.

(4) In the presence of regular menstruation, ovulation can be confirmed with a day 21 serum progesterone level. There is no value in measuring thyroid function, prolactin or any other hormones in the absence of symptoms, if the progesterone confirms ovulation.

(5) Excessive alcohol consumption reduces female fertility. The safe limit for consumption in pregnancy is not known. The usual advice is not to drink more than one or two units of alcohol once or twice a week when trying to become pregnant.

答案

(1)孕期8～10周的风疹感染会导致90%的病例出现严重胎儿异常。应该检查女方风疹感染情况,如果是阴性,应接种风疹疫苗。

(2)建议孕前及怀孕前12周补充叶酸,以防止胎儿神经管缺陷。

(3)没有任何证据表明,体温表的使用能改善结果。在不孕症的治疗中,对患者指定时间同房最易增加患者的紧张情绪。

(4)当月经规律时,第21天的血清孕酮水平可确定排卵。如果孕酮检测确定有排卵,在无症状存在时,甲状腺激素、催乳素检查没有临床意义。

(5)过度饮酒降低女性生育。孕期饮酒的安全底线目前尚不清楚。通常的建议是在准备怀孕时,一周饮酒不超过1～2次,每次的量不超过1～2个单位。

Chapter 5　Family Planning

第 5 章　计划生育

5.1　Family Planning

5.1　计划生育

Key words

other methods

关键词

其他避孕方法

5.1.1　Condom

Condom is a male contraceptive method.

1. Method of use
Use before each intercourse.
2. Advantages and disadvantages
(1) Advantages：
① simple and inexpensive；highly effective in perfect use，no side-effects.
②safe，clean，protection against STDs.
(2) Disadvantages：
①can not use rubber product when allergy occures.

②May affect male interesting.

5.1.2　Spermicides

1. Types
It contains nonoxynol 9 and is provided in the forms of contraceptive gel，cream，films，suppositories and foam tablets.
2. Methods of use
Insert it into the posterior fornix of vagina 5 to 10 minutes before intercourse. In most cases，it is used with the condom.
3. Advantages and disadvantages
(1) Advantages：
①convenient，efficacious.

5.1.1　避孕套

避孕套也称阴茎套，为男用避孕方法。

1.使用方法
每次性交前使用。
2.优缺点
(1)优点：
①简便经济，如果正确应用，避孕高度有效，无副作用。
②安全卫生,能预防性传播疾病。
(2)缺点：
①对橡胶过敏者不能应用橡胶避孕套。
②可能影响快感。

5.1.2　外用避孕药(杀精子剂)

1.种类
成分为壬苯醇醚,剂型有避孕胶冻、乳膏、薄膜、栓剂和泡腾片。

2.使用方法
每次性交前 5~10 min 将杀精剂置入阴道后穹窿,大多数和避孕套配合使用。
3.优缺点
(1)优点：
①方便有效。

②clean and lubricating.

(2) Disadvantages：

①high failure rate when used alone.

②can not prevent STDs.

5.1.3　Natural family planning（NFP）(periodic abstinence)

1. Method of use

（1）Menstruation cycles must be regular. Ovulation generally occurs at the 14th day prior the onset of next menstruation.

（2）Calculate the fertile period by calendar method，combined temperature and calendar method，cervical mucus （ Billings ） method and symptothermal method. Adopt abstinence during this period.

2. Advantages and disadvantages

（1）Advantages：not affect normal sexual intercourse.

（2）Disadvantages：difficult in accurately predicting the time of ovulation；high failure rate.

5.1.4　Emergency contraception

Emergency contraception is a therapy used to prevent unwanted pregnancy after unprotected intercourse or rape within 72-120 hours. It can't be used as a routine contraceptive method.

1. Method of use

（1）Copper IUD：inserted within 120 hours after unprotected intercourse. It may not be removed soon if woman wants IUD contraception.

（2）Mifepristone：10 or 25 mg single dose PO within 120 hours after unprotected intercourse.

（3）Levonorgestrel：first dose of 0.75 mg PO within 72 hours after unprotected intercourse，and repeated 0.75 mg after 12 hours interval.

（4）OC：first 4 tablets OC within 72 hours，and repeat the same dose after 12 hours.

2. Advantages and disadvantages

（1）Advantages：It can be used as the compensation of

②有清洁、润滑作用。

（2）缺点：

①单独使用失败率高。

②对预防性传播疾病无效。

5.1.3　自然受孕法(周期性禁欲)

1.使用方法

（1）月经周期必须规律；排卵通常发生在下次月经开始之前的第14天。

（2）用日历法、日历结合体温法、宫颈黏液法或症状体温法计算能孕期。在能孕期内禁欲。

2.优缺点

（1）优点：不影响正常性生活。

（2）缺点：不易准确预估排卵期；失败率高。

5.1.4　紧急避孕

在无保护性生活后72～120 h内采取的避孕补救措施。适用于避孕失败或受性暴力侵害时。不能作为常规避孕方法使用。

1.使用方法

（1）带铜宫内节育器：在无保护性性交后5天内放置。如希望长期避孕可不取出。

（2）米非司酮口服：无保护性性交后5天内，米非司酮10 mg或25 mg顿服一次。

（3）左诀诺孕酮口服：无保护性性交72 h内左诀诺孕酮片0.75 mg，12 h后重复一次。

（4）口服复方短效避孕药4片，12 h重复4片。

2.优缺点

（1）优点：可作为避孕的补救

contraceptive failure and prevents 80%-85% of pregnancy.

Disadvantages：It can not ensure 100% contraception rate.

5.1.5　Termination of early pregnancy

5.1.5.1　Surgical abortion by vacuum aspiration

1. Indications

（1）Women who ask for termination of pregnancy within 10 weeks gestation and no contraindications.

（2）Pregnancy is not suitable because of some diseases or hereditary diseases.

2. Contraindications

（1）Acute stage of all diseases.

（2）Genital tract infections.

（3）Women can't stand for the operation due to poor health.

（4）Temperature ＞37.5 ℃ twice within 24 h.

3. Patients should be admitted for surgical abortion

（1）Hypertension with BP≥150/100 mmHg.

（2）Hb≤80 g/L.

（3）Pregnancy with uterine fibroma.

（4）Gestational period more than 10 weeks.

（5）Hyperemesis gravidarum.

（6）Congenital heart disease or rheumatic heart disease.

（7）Acute hepatitis.

（8）Dure to malformation of pelvis, spine, or limbs, patients can't be placed in the lithotomy position.

（9）Uterus perforation or vault crack.

（10）Induced abortion 3 times within 1 year, pregnancy after vaginal delivery within 3 months, or pregnancy within half a year after cesarean section.

措施,防止 80％～85％的妊娠。

（2）缺点：有效性未能达到 100％。

5.1.5　早期妊娠终止

5.1.5.1　人工流产负压吸引术

1. 适应证

（1）妊娠在 10 周以内要求终止妊娠而无禁忌证者。

（2）因某种疾病或遗传性疾病不宜继续妊娠者。

2. 禁忌证

（1）各种疾病的急性阶段。

（2）生殖道感染。

（3）周身情况不良不能承受手术。

（4）术前 24 h 两次体温在 37.5 ℃以上。

3. 下列情况应酌情住院手术

（1）高血压,血压≥150/100 mmHg。

（2）血红蛋白≤80 g/L。

（3）子宫肌瘤合并妊娠。

（4）妊娠 10 周以上。

（5）妊娠呕吐。

（6）先天性心脏病、风湿性心脏病。

（7）急性肝炎。

（8）盆腔或脊柱、肢体畸形不能采取膀胱截石位者。

（9）子宫穿孔或阴道穹窿部裂伤。

（10）一年内 3 次人工流产、阴道产后 3 个月内、剖腹产术后半年内妊娠。

5.1.5.2　Surgical abortion by dilatation and extraction（D & E）

1. Indications

（1）Women who ask for induced abortion with pregnancy 10-13 weeks due to disease or other causes.

（2）Abortion failure by other methods.

2. Contraindications

Same as above mentioned.

5.1.5.3　Medical abortion

1. Indications

（1）Health women who ask for medical abortion with pregnancy ≤7 weeks.

（2）Pregnancy with risk factors of curettage.

（3）Fearful and nervous to surgical abortion.

2. Contraindications

（1）Contraindications of mifepristone：endocrinological disease such as adrenal gland，diabetes and thyroid gland diseases，liver or kidney disorders，coagulopathy，history of thromboembolism，and tumors associate with steroid hormone.

（2）Contraindications of prostaglandin：cardiovascular disease，glaucoma，disorders of gastrointestinal tract，asthma，and epilepsy.

（3）Hypersensitive to mifepriston or prostaglandins，hyperemesis gravidarum.

（4）Hb≤100 g/L.

（5）Pregnancy with IUD-in-situ.

（6）Ectopic pregnancy or molar pregnancy.

（7）Smoking cigarette≥10/d or alcohol abuse.

（8）Infection of genital tract.

3. Methods of use

Mifepristone 150 mg combined with misoprostol 600 μg orally. Complete abortion rate is about 92% to 95%.

5.1.5.2　人工流产钳刮术
　　　　　（扩刮吸引）

1. 适应证

（1）凡妊娠 10～13 周，要求终止妊娠或因疾病等特殊情况不宜继续妊娠者。

（2）其他方法流产失败者。

2. 禁忌证

同上。

5.1.5.3　药物流产术

1. 适应证

（1）确诊为正常宫内妊娠≤7周，自愿要求药物终止妊娠的健康妇女。

（2）刮宫高危者妊娠。

（3）对手术流产有顾虑或恐惧心理者。

2. 禁忌证

（1）米非司酮禁忌证（如肾上腺、糖尿病、甲状腺等内心泌疾病），肝肾功能异常，凝血障碍史，血管栓塞病史，与皮质激素有关的肿瘤。

（2）前列腺素禁忌证、心血管系统疾病、青光眼、胃肠功能紊乱、哮喘、癫痫。

（3）对米非司酮或前列腺素过敏，妊娠呕吐。

（4）血红蛋白 100 g/L 及以下者。

（5）带器妊娠。

（6）宫外孕或葡萄胎。

（7）吸烟超过 10 支/天或酗酒。

（8）生殖道感染。

3. 用药方法

米非司酮 150 mg 配伍米索前列醇 600 μg 口服。完全流产率约 92%～95%。

（1）Mifepristone given in several doses：first dose mifepristone 50 mg is given fasting in the morning，second dose 25 mg is given 12 h apart，repeat same regimen on the second day（total mifepristone 150 mg）. In the morning of the third day，misoprostol 600 μg is given，and patient is kept under observation in hospital for 6 h.

（2）Mifepristone 150 mg given fasting single dose，and misoprostol 600 μg in the morning of the third day with patient observed in hospital for 6 h.

4. Advantages and disadvantages

（1）Advantages：convenient，painless.

（2）Disadvantages：Successful rate is not 100％. Longer bleeding period than surgical abortion.

5.1.6　Termination of midtrimester pregnancy

5.1.6.1　Indications

Pregnancy of 14-24 weeks；ask for termination because of family planning，some diseases or special reasons；no contraindications.

5.1.6.2　Contraindications

（1）Scar of uterus，hypoplasia of cervix or uterus.

（2）Acute and chronic liver，kidney diseases and liver or renal dysfunction.

（3）Acute stage of all diseases.

（4）Coagulopathy.

（5）Acute genital tract infection. Infection at the puncture site of abdominal wall is contraindicated for Rivanol injection.

（6）Recurrent bleeding during pregnancy and placenta previa confirmed by B-ultrasound are prohibited for waterbag induced abortion.

（7）Temperature ＞37.5 ℃ twice per day prior to surgery.

5.1.6.3　Methods for midterm induced abortion

（1）Rivanol intra-amniotic injection.

（2）Water bag intra-uterine cavity.

（1）米非司酮分服：早晨空腹服米非司酮 50 mg，隔 12 h 再服 25 mg，服用 2 天，共 150 mg，第 3 天晨一次服用米索前列醇 600 μg，留院观察 6 h。

（2）米非司酮顿服：第一天空腹顿服米非司酮 150 mg，第 3 天晨加用米非前列醇 600 μg，留院观察 6 h。

4. 优缺点

（1）优点：方便、无痛苦。

（2）缺点：流产成功率不是 100％。比手术流产出血时间长。

5.1.6　中期妊娠中止

5.1.6.1　适应证

妊娠 14～24 周，因计划生育、各种疾病或特殊原因需要终止妊娠而无禁忌证者。

5.1.6.2　禁忌证

（1）子宫疤痕、子宫或宫颈发育不良。

（2）急慢性肝、肾疾病及肝肾功能不全。

（3）各种疾病的急性期。

（4）凝血障碍。

（5）急性生殖道感染，腹部穿刺部位皮肤感染禁忌行利凡诺尔注射。

（6）妊娠期间反复出血，B 超确定为胎盘前置者，不应该进行水囊引产。

（7）术前 24 h 内两次体温在 37.5 ℃ 以上。

5.1.6.3　引产方法

（1）利凡诺尔羊膜腔内注射引产。

（2）宫腔水囊放置引产术。

参考文献

［1］ Alan H. DeCherney, Lauren Nathan , T. Murphy Goodwin, Neri Laufer, Ashley S. Roman. Current diagnosis & treatment obstetrics & gynecology (10th edition). New York：McGraw-Hill companies，2006.

［2］ Eugene C. Toy，Benton Baker III，Patti Jayne Ross，John Jennings. Case files obstetrics and gynecology. 3rd ed (Lange Case Files) [Kindle Edition]. New York：McGraw-Hill companies，2009.

［3］ John E. Clinical Protocol in Obstetrics and Gynecology (Third Edition). Informa Texas Healthcare，2008.

［4］ Practical obstetrics and gynaecology handbook for the general Practitioner. Singapore：Word Sientific Pub Co Inc，2006.

［5］ 丰有吉,陈晓军(译). 妇产科精要.北京:人民卫生出版社，2009.

［6］ 乐杰. 妇产科学(第七版).北京:人民卫生出版社，2011.

［7］ American College of Obstetricians and Gynecologists. Management of endometrial cancer. ACOG Practice Bulletin 65. Washington：American College of Obstetricians and Gynecologists，2005.

［8］ Hacker NF. Uterine corpus cancer. In：Hacker NF，Moore JG，Gambone JC，etc.. Essentials of obstetrics and gynecology. 4th ed. Philadelphia：Saunders，2004：478-4854.

［9］ Herbst AL. Neoplastic diseases of the uterus. In：Stenchever MA，Droegemueller W，Herbst AL，Mishell DR，et al. (eds). Comprehensive gynecology. 4th ed. St. Louis：Mosby-Year Book，2001：919-954.

［10］ D'Hooghe TM，Hill III JA. Endometriosis. In：Berek JS. (ed.) Berek & Novak's gynecology. 14th ed. Philadelphia：Lippincott Willianms & Wilkins，2007：1137-1184.

［11］ Robert L. Feig，Nicole C. Johnson，Latha G. Stead，Matthew Stead. First aid for obstetrics & gynecology clerkship etc. 北京:人民军医出版社，2007.

［12］ http：//www. cytopathology. org/guidelines/cervical-cytologyiii. php

［13］ American College of Obstetricians and Gynecologists http：//www. acog. org/ N-profit organization of women's health care physicians advocating highest standards of practice，continuing member education and public awareness of women's health care issues.

［14］ http：//red. 9thunder. com/html/showcontent. asp? ClassID＝172&ArticleID＝400

［15］ 中国妇产科网 http：//www. china-obgyn. net/

［16］ http：//contemporaryobgyn. modernmedicine. com/

[17] http://www.obgyn.net/medical.asp

[18] http://www.nccn.org/index.asp

[19] http://www.figo.org/

[20] http://www.medscape.com/

[21] American College of Obstetricians and Gynecologists. Uterine artery embolization. ACOG Committee opinion 293. Washington, DC: American College of Obstetricians and Gynecologists, 2004.

[22] Droegmueller W. Benign gynecologic lesions. In: Stenchever MA, Droegemueller W, Herbst AL, et al. Comprehensive gynecology. 4th ed. St. Louis: Mosby-Year Book, 2001: 479-530.

[23] Moore GJ, Nelson AL. Congenital anomalies and begign conditions of the uterine corpus and cervix. In: Haceer NF, Moore JG. Essentials of obstetrics and gynecology. 4th ed. Philadelphia: Saunders, 2004: 268-276.

内 容 提 要

　　本书分基础、生理产科、病理产科及胎儿医学、妇科及计划生育共五章 41 节,每一节均包含关键词汇、知识要点、实践应用案例、思考题、答案及案例分析、循证思维知识拓展六个部分。

　　本书重点突出,理论联系实际,以案例为导向,加深读者对概念的理解,锻炼妇产科临床思维,增强学习的兴趣和效果。

图书在版编目(CIP)数据

　　妇产科实践指南:英汉对照 / 凌奕,金松主编. —杭州:
浙江大学出版社,2013.9(2015.1 重印)
　　ISBN 978-7-308-11933-7

　　Ⅰ.①妇… Ⅱ.①凌… ②金… Ⅲ.①妇产科学—指南
—英、汉 Ⅳ.①R71-62

　　中国版本图书馆 CIP 数据核字(2013)第 175564 号

英汉对照妇产科实践指南

凌　奕　金　松　主编

丛书策划	阮海潮(ruanhc@zju.edu.cn)
责任编辑	阮海潮
封面设计	续设计
出版发行	浙江大学出版社
	(杭州市天目山路 148 号　邮政编码 310007)
	(网址:http://www.zjupress.com)
排　版	杭州中大图文设计有限公司
印　刷	杭州日报报业集团盛元印务有限公司
开　本	787mm×1092mm　1/16
印　张	22.5
字　数	680 千
版印次	2013 年 9 月第 1 版　2015 年 1 月第 2 次印刷
书　号	ISBN 978-7-308-11933-7
定　价	45.00 元